DIAGNOSING LEARNING DISORDERS

Diagnosing Learning Disorders

SECOND EDITION

A Neuropsychological Framework

Bruce F. Pennington

THE GUILFORD PRESS
New York   London

© 2009 The Guilford Press
A Division of Guilford Publications, Inc.
72 Spring Street, New York, NY 10012
www.guilford.com

Printed in the United States of America

This book is printed on acid-free paper.

Last digit is print number: 9   8   7   6   5   4   3   2   1

Library of Congress Cataloging-in-Publication Data

Pennington, Bruce Franklin, 1946-
    Diagnosing learning disorders : a neuropsychological framework /
Bruce F. Pennington. — 2nd ed.
        p. ; cm.
    Includes bibliographical references and index.
    ISBN 978-1-59385-714-1 (hardcover : alk. paper)
    1. Learning disabilities—Diagnosis.   2. Autism in children—Diagnosis.
3. Attention-deficit hyperactivity disorder—Diagnosis.   I. Title.
    [DNLM: 1. Learning Disorders—diagnosis.   2. Attention Deficit Disorder
with Hyperactivity—diagnosis.   3. Autistic Disorder—diagnosis.   4. Language
Development Disorders—diagnosis.   5. Neuropsychology. WS 110 P414d 2008]
    RJ496.L4P46 2008
    618.92′85889075—dc22

                                                        2008032101

*For children everywhere
and those who try to help them*

About the Author

Bruce F. Pennington, PhD, is a developmental neuropsychologist who has earned an international reputation for his research on dyslexia, attention-deficit/hyperactivity disorder (ADHD), and autism. He has published 163 articles in refereed journals and was selected to appear on ISIHighlyCited.com because of his exceptional citation count in the field of Psychology/Psychiatry. He is particularly interested in using genetic and neuropsychological methods to understand comorbidity among disorders, such as the comorbidity between dyslexia and ADHD.

Dr. Pennington is a John Evans Professor of Psychology at the University of Denver, where he heads the Developmental Cognitive Neuroscience Program. His honors include Research Scientist, MERIT, and Fogarty awards from the National Institutes of Health; the Samuel T. Orton Award from the International Dyslexia Association; and the Emanuel Miller Memorial Lecture from the British Association for Child and Adolescent Mental Health. He is also a Fellow of the American Association for the Advancement of Science.

Dr. Pennington has also been the primary research mentor for 35 doctoral and postdoctoral students, many of whom are now pursuing their own research on developmental disabilities. The Guilford Press published his other book, *The Development of Psychopathology: Nature and Nurture*, in 2002. Both that book and this one emphasize a close relation between research and practice. In addition to being a researcher and research mentor, Dr. Pennington is also a child clinical neuropsychologist, and has been active in clinical practice and training throughout his career.

Preface

Since the first edition of this book was published, 18 years have passed, and the field of learning disorders has gone from being a fledgling science to becoming a key part of developmental cognitive neuroscience. Now it makes sense to speak of a science of learning disorders, whereas when I began my career over 30 years ago, there was debate about whether several of these learning disorders (e.g., dyslexia and attention-deficit/hyperactivity disorder [ADHD]) even existed. There has been considerable scientific progress both in understanding most of the disorders covered in the original volume (dyslexia and other language disorders, ADHD, and autism spectrum disorder [ASD]) and in understanding additional disorders covered in this expanded edition (intellectual disability [ID], mathematics disorder [MD], and developmental coordination disorder [DCD]). So the time was overripe for a new edition of this book, which was rapidly becoming out of date.

Therefore, one goal for the new book has been to update both the research and clinical sections with new advances. Modern genetic and neuroimaging methods have led to many discoveries about the neurobiology of these disorders, including in some cases the discovery of candidate genes and their role in early brain development. Our cognitive models of these disorders have also become much more sophisticated. The new book differs radically from the old one in embracing a multiple-cognitive-deficit model of learning disorders, in contrast to the modular, single-deficit model described in the first edition. Also, empirically based practice has had a major impact on how we diagnose and treat these disorders. So this second edition is a new book for a new century, and one of its major goals is to make the new science of learning disorders accessible to both practitioners and researchers.

After the first edition was published, I was quite gratified to hear from clinicians, professors, and students that they found it useful. It was used as a text in numerous graduate classes and was translated into Portuguese in 1997 (*Diagnostico de Disturbios de Aprendizagem*, São Paulo: Editeria Pionervia). So another goal for the revision was to make it even more useful for these various audiences. To this end, I have updated the clinical sections of the chapters on major disorders with new case descriptions that use modern test instruments and that focus on well-validated cognitive constructs. I have also added research and clinical summary tables to these chapters, so that readers can easily learn about the basic features of these disorders.

The book is organized into three main sections: "Basic Concepts," "Reviews of Disorders," and "Implications for Practice and Policy." Part I, "Basic Concepts," covers ideas and issues that are fundamental to understanding what learning disorders are, how they develop, and how we diagnose them. It also includes a chapter on less well-validated disorders that do not have the same scientific support as the disorders covered in Part II of the book. In Part II, "Reviews of Disorders," the presentation of each of the main disorders follows a common format. First, there is a research review with sections on history, definition, epidemiology and comorbidities, etiology, neural correlates, and neuropsychology. Next, there is a clinical review, which includes sections on presenting symptoms, developmental history, behavioral observations, and results of testing. Chapters 6–10 also include two case presentations apiece, followed by a section on treatment.

There is not as much clinical detail for three of the disorders covered in Part II, DCD (Chapter 11), MD (Chapter 12) and Nonverbal Learning Disability (NVLD; Chapter 13). That is because there is less basic and applied research on each of them, and we have had much less clinical experience with them. But there is clearly enough research to qualify each as a valid learning disorder that clinicians and researchers should know about. Let us hope that the work already done on the other learning disorders presented will facilitate future research on MD, DCD, and NVLD.

A final goal for this new book was to extend the science of learning disorders into public health and educational policy. Part III of the book, "Implications for Practice and Policy," is an effort to achieve this goal. It also includes a fairly comprehensive review of controversial therapies for learning disorders, so that practitioners, educators, and parents can more easily avoid therapies without proven effectiveness.

The long-term scientific objective of future research on learning disorders is to achieve a complete, integrated neuroscientific understanding of the development of each of these disorders and their relations, including their etiology, neurobiology, neuropsychology, diagnosis, and treatment. What is presented in this volume documents how much progress has been made since 1991 toward fulfilling that ambitious objective.

Acknowledgments

Our laboratory's research contributed considerably to the science presented in this book, and so I want to acknowledge the funding that made this research possible. Our lab has been supported by several grants from the National Institutes of Health (Nos. HD04927, HD027802, HD35468, HD17449, and HD04024).

I have been very fortunate to have outstanding collaborators. In the dyslexia research, these collaborators include Richard Boada, Shelley Smith, Richard Olson, John C. DeFries, Claudia Cardoso-Martins, Rebecca Treiman, Larry Shriberg, Barbara Lewis, and Sudha Iyengar. Dorothy Bishop and Maggie Snowling have provided invaluable consultation on our speech sound disorder (SSD) project. In the ADHD research, my main collaborator has been Erik Willcutt. In the work on ASD, I have worked with Sally Rogers, Sally Ozonoff, and Susan Hepburn. Finally, in the work on ID, I have collaborated with Linda Crnic, Carolyn Mervis, and David Patterson.

My wonderful graduate students and postdoctoral fellows, present and past, have made very important contributions to this work; some of them have become long-term collaborators, like Sally Ozonoff, Erik Willcutt, and Richard Boada. Two current graduate students, Lauren McGrath and Robin Peterson, have helped specifically with this revision by coauthoring research reviews, by preparing case descriptions and other material in the clinical sections, and by very carefully editing the whole volume. They are listed as coauthors of several chapters, and they were absolutely critical in helping this revision get done in a form that is much clearer and more complete than the original.

The University of Denver has provided a very supportive setting for my work over the last 18 years. I wrote the first edition shortly after joining the faculty here, and most of our research that is reported in the present book was conducted here.

Suzanne Miller, my administrative assistant, again provided invaluable assistance in preparing the manuscript. She has now seen me through three books that span a large portion of my career. Although I composed part of this book on a PC, in moments of great inspiration I regress to writing by hand on yellow tablets. Suzanne has become an expert at deciphering my handwriting and following the often intricate maze of revisions. I would also like to thank Sally Ozonoff, Deborah Waber, and Sally Shaywitz for their helpful comments on an earlier version of the manuscript of this book.

Finally, I would like to thank my editors at The Guilford Press, Rochelle Serwator and Seymour Weingarten. Seymour opined about 7 years ago that this revision would be "easy." He and Rochelle have waited patiently for me to complete that easy task.

BRUCE F. PENNINGTON

Contents

PART I
BASIC CONCEPTS

CHAPTER 1

How Learning Disorders Develop

This book is about "learning disorders," which is a broader term than the more familiar "learning disabilities." As used here, the term "learning disorder" means any neurodevelopmental disorder that interferes with the learning of academic and/or social skills. So traditionally defined learning disabilities, such as dyslexia or reading disability (RD) and mathematics disorder (MD), constitute a subset of learning disorders. The category also includes developmental disabilities, such as autism spectrum disorder (ASD), intellectual disability (ID, formerly called "mental retardation"), developmental coordination disorder (DCD), speech sound disorder (SSD), language impairment (LI), and attention-deficit/hyperactivity disorder (ADHD). All these disorders are congenital, genetically influenced variations in brain development. This book is not about brain disorders acquired in childhood (e.g., traumatic brain injury), although acquired brain disorders can produce some of the same kinds of learning problems found in the learning disorders considered here.

Understanding learning disorders and most psychiatric disorders requires a developmental perspective, because these disorders have their origins in genetic and environmental risk factors that generally act early in development and change the developmental trajectory in particular domains of functioning. As children with a particular learning disorder encounter different developmental tasks, different symptoms emerge, so there is only heterotypic continuity in the symptoms of a disorder across ages.

For instance, a preschool child at family risk for dyslexia may have speech problems, as well as some delays in vocabulary development and expressive syntax. By kindergarten, this child is likely to be having trouble learning letter names and color names. In first grade, phoneme awareness will nearly always be difficult, as will learning to decode new printed words and reliably recognizing familiar ones. In the later elementary grades, prob-lems in reading fluency and comprehension will be more evident, in addition to problems memorizing math facts. Somewhat later, there are likely to be difficulties with math "word" problems, as well as with foreign languages.

Another important feature of the developmental model employed in this book is that it encompasses multiple levels of analysis, recognizes bidirectional causal influences across levels, and is probabilistic rather than deterministic. There are four levels of analysis in this model: etiology, brain development, neuropsychology, and behavior (Figure 1.1).

These levels of analysis are explained in more detail elsewhere (see Pen-nington, 2002), but I describe them briefly here. Etiology is concerned with the distal causes of disorders—the particular genetic and environmental risk and protective factors that cause one child to have a disorder and another child not to have the disorder (see Box 1.1 at the end of this chapter). These distal causes act on brain development, often *in utero*, changing the wiring and/or the neurotransmitter systems of the brain. These structural and neu-rochemical changes in the brain (see Box 1.2 at the end of this chapter) alter its functions in ways we can detect with neuropsychological tests, and these alterations in neuropsychological functions affect behaviors observable by teachers, parents, and peers. These changes in behavior are the symptoms that define various learning disorders.

But because brain development is an open process that continues throughout the lifespan, the environment, including the social environment, affects brain development. So a child without genetic risk factors for dys-lexia may end up with RD because the environment does not provide ade-quate spoken language and preliteracy input. And a child with genetic risk

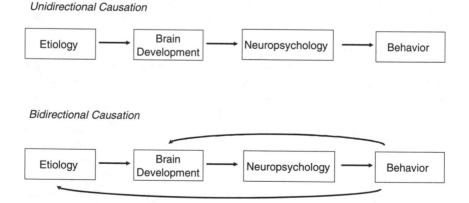

FIGURE 1.1. Models of causation.

factors for a particular learning disorder may benefit from compensating environmental protective factors and end up with only a subclinical form of the disorder. This is why the model is probabilistic rather than deterministic, and why the causal influences are bidirectional. This also means that achieving a complete scientific understanding of why one child has a disorder and another does not is a very ambitious goal, since it requires disentangling complex developmental pathways. Nonetheless, considerable progress toward this ambitious goal has been made in the roughly two decades since the first edition of this book was published, and progress is accelerating because of technical advances in both genetics and neuroscience. Whereas a true science of learning disorders seemed almost unimaginable when I began my career in 1977, it is now emerging rapidly.

So one goal of this book is to make the emerging science of learning disorders accessible to practitioners who help children with learning disorders. The other goal is to show concretely how science informs practice by thoroughly presenting actual examples of diagnosis and treatment planning, and by reviewing less well-validated disorders and controversial therapies.

I now turn to an example of an important way in which science has changed our thinking about learning disorders. Unlike the first edition of this book (Pennington, 1991), this edition is based on a multiple-deficit model of the etiology and neuropsychology of learning disorders (Pennington, 2006). The earlier version espoused a modular single-deficit model of the neuropsychological causes of learning disorders (see also Morton & Frith, 1995, and Morton, 2004). Since this is the simplest and most parsimonious model, it made sense for the field to test it first. Now enough evidence has accumulated to force us to abandon this simple model, although there is still considerable controversy within cognitive psychology about whether there are innate "cognitive modules," especially for language (see Ramus, 2006). The view taken in this book is that cognitive modules (i.e., brain regions specialized for processing certain kinds of input, such as language or faces) are not innate, but instead are the products of a developmental process that shows considerable plasticity. Moreover, the function of these developed modules is not encapsulated, but instead depends on their connections and interactions with other brain structures. Consequently, it is too simplistic to completely localize such a complex cognitive operation as recognizing faces or spoken words in just one part of the brain.

Our research group's own work on the reasons why disorders co-occur (i.e., "comorbidity") has led us to abandon the single-deficit model (Pennington, Willcutt, & Rhee, 2005). The single-deficit model posits that a single cognitive deficit is sufficient to explain the symptoms of a given disorder, and that different disorders have different single deficits. We and others have found that the frequent phenomenon of comorbidity is often explained by partially shared etiological and cognitive risk factors. So, as will be reviewed later, RD and ADHD have a partial genetic overlap, as do RD and SSD. This overlap at the etiological level is consistent with the widely accepted multifactorial model of the etiology of behaviorally defined disorders—that is, virtually all psychiatric disorders and nonsyndromal developmental disorders. (Syndromal developmental disorders, such as the three genetic syndromes discussed in connection with ID in Chapter 10, are defined by etiology, not by behavior.) In the multifactorial model, multiple genetic and environmental risk factors combine to produce a given disorder. In order to produce disorders with a high prevalence, some of these etiological risk factors must be fairly common (e.g., the DAT1 "risk" allele for ADHD is often found in more than 50% of population samples). Because these risk factors are common, they are more likely to be part of the etiology of multiple disorders. In fact, the sharing of etiological risk factors across disorders has been confirmed empirically.

We came to realize that the multifactorial model of etiology did not fit well theoretically with the single-cognitive-deficit model of learning disorders, which was also challenged by the empirical finding of multiple cognitive deficits in all the learning disorders considered in this book. If a cognitive deficit is shared by two distinct disorders, it cannot be sufficient to produce either one, but it may act as a cofactor with other cognitive deficits not shared by the two comorbid disorders. So we have proposed and are now testing a multiple-cognitive-deficit model of learning disorders (Figure 1.2).

Similar to the complex disease model in medicine (Sing & Reilly, 1993) and the quantitative genetic model in behavioral genetics (e.g., Plomin, DeFries, McClearn, & Rutter, 1997), the current model proposes that (1) the etiology of complex behavioral disorders is multifactorial and involves the interaction of multiple risk and protective factors, which can be either genetic or environmental; (2) these risk and protective factors alter the development of the neural systems that mediate cognitive functions necessary for normal development, thus producing the behavioral symptoms that define these disorders; (3) no single etiological factor is sufficient for a disorder, and few may be necessary; (4) consequently, comorbidity among complex behavioral disorders is to be expected because of shared etiological and cognitive risk factors; and (5) the liability distribution for a given disease is often continuous and quantitative rather than discrete and categorical, so that the threshold for having the disorder is somewhat arbitrary. Applying the model to two comorbidities considered in this book (RD + ADHD and RD + SSD), we can see that each individual disorder will have its own profile of risk factors (both etiological and cognitive), but that some of these risk factors will be shared by another disorder, resulting in comorbidity.

Figure 1.2 illustrates the complex disease model as applied to complex behavioral disorders. As in Figure 1.1, there are four levels of analysis in

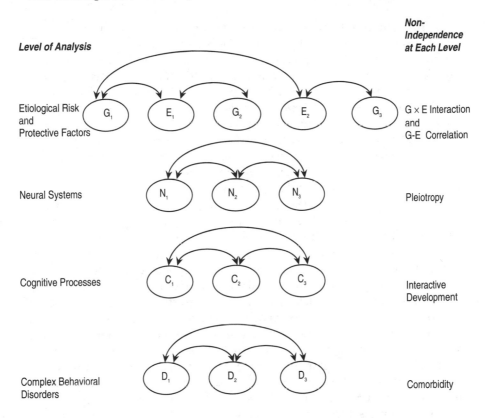

FIGURE 1.2. Multiple-deficit model. G, genetic risk or protective factor; E, environmental risk or protective factor; N, neural system; C, cognitive process; D, disorder.

this diagram: etiological, neural, cognitive, and symptom (where clusters of symptoms define complex behavioral disorders). For any such complex behavioral disorder, it is expected that there will be many more etiological risk and protective factors than the five shown in Figure 1.2. Bidirectional connections at each level indicate that constructs are not independent. For instance, at the etiological level, there are likely to be gene × environment (G × E) interactions and gene–environment (G-E) correlations. At the neural level, a single genetic or environmental risk factor will often affect more than one neural system ("pleiotropy"). Even if the risk factor initially only affects one neural system, this alteration is likely to have downstream effects on the development of other neural systems. At the cognitive level, constructs are correlated because their developmental pathways overlap and because cognition is interactive. Overlap at the cognitive level leads to comorbidity at the symptom level. So, whereas the single-deficit model conceptualizes the relation between disorders in terms of double dissociations, the multiple-deficit model conceptualizes this relation in terms of partial overlap. At the symptom level, there is comorbidity (i.e., greater than chance co-occurrence) of complex behavioral disorders. Omitted from the diagram are the causal connections *between* levels of analyses, some of which would include feedback loops from behavior to brain or even to etiology, as in Figure 1.1. The existence and strength of these various causal connections must be determined empirically. The weights on the connections between levels of analysis will tell us to what extent different etiological and cognitive factors contribute to comorbidity at the symptom level.

This model makes it clear that achieving a complete understanding of the development of such disorders as SSD, RD, or ASD will be very difficult because of the multiple pathways involved. But this kind of model is needed, because it is becoming increasingly clear that there are shared processes at the etiological, neural, and cognitive levels across such disorders.

In this book's chapters on disorders, I consider their comorbidities and discuss how the multiple-deficit model applies to them. For instance, in the case of dyslexia or RD, we used to think that a deficit in phoneme awareness was the single cognitive deficit that caused RD in most children. But when we learned that children with SSD can have a similar deficit in phoneme awareness and not develop RD, we began to question whether this single deficit is sufficient to produce RD. Moreover, children with RD, compared to children with SSD but not RD (SSD only), have deficits in processing speed; this suggests that intact processing speed is a protective factor for children with SSD, despite their having a deficit in phoneme awareness. And we have also learned that deficits in processing speed are shared by RD and ADHD (Shanahan et al., 2006), helping to explain their comorbidity.

In Chapters 6–13, this model is applied to specific learning disorders. Each chapter begins with a research review of what is known about a disorder's etiology, brain mechanisms, neuropsychology, and comorbidities. This is followed by a discussion of how our scientific understanding of each disorder informs its diagnosis and treatment. So the overall goal is to integrate science and practice in the field of learning disorders.

In the next chapter, I explain in more detail the neuropsychological constructs that are important for understanding learning disorders. To provide readers with background knowledge about two other levels of analysis in Figures 1.1 and 1.2, Boxes 1.1 and 1.2 cover key concepts in genetics, neuroanatomy, and neuroimaging.

BOX 1.1. Genetic Tests and Terms

TESTS

Familiality?—Does a condition occur more frequently in relatives of people with the condition than in the general population? The usual measure of familiality is lambda (λ), which is the rate in biological siblings of probands per rate in population. Typical lambda values for a behaviorally defined disorder are 3–10, meaning that the disorder is 3–10 times more frequent in siblings than in the general population. Familiality can be caused by genes, environments, or some combination of the two.

Heritability?—Is the familiality of a condition partly caused by genes? Answering this question requires comparing relatives who differ in degree of genetic relations (e.g., monozygotic, or MZ, twins with dizygotic, or DZ, twins). If MZ twins are significantly more similar for the trait in question, then familiality is partly genetic. A twin design also estimates the shared environment effect, the other component of familiality. Heritability and environmentality are measured as proportions of the total phenotypic variance, and so their value can range from 0 to 1.0. Most behaviorally defined disorders have moderate heritabilities (roughly .30–.80), and smaller values for shared environmentalities. So, for these disorders, genes explain more of their familiality than do shared environments. Other possible components of phenotypic variance may be due to environmental effects that siblings do not share, gene–environment (G-E) correlations, gene $\times$ environment (G $\times$ E) interactions, and error.

Gene locations?—If a disorder is familial and heritable, which are the actual genes involved? There are two main methods for locating genes: linkage and association. Linkage tests whether known genetic markers tend to be inherited along with a given disorder. Because only genes that are close together on the same chromosome are inherited together, finding a marker linked to a disorder tells us the approximate location of a risk gene for that disorder (its genetic "neighborhood"). Association tests whether a particular variant (allele) of a gene or marker occurs more frequently in those with the disorder than in those without it, and only detects effects in a much smaller region of the genome than linkage.

Candidate genes?—Once there is replicated linkage or association for a disorder, the next step is to identify the responsible gene(s) and the causative mutations in them. This step requires fine mapping of the linkage region or the much smaller association region to identify genes that are expressed in the brain, and systematically screening those genes for mutations associated with the disorder. Candidate genes can also be tested in animal models.

(continued)

BOX 1.1. *(continued)*

TERMS

Mendelian locus—A gene variant that is sufficient to cause a disorder. Examples include the mutations of single genes that cause phenylketonuria, sickle cell anemia, and Huntington disease.

Quantitative trait locus (QTL)—A gene variant that is neither necessary nor sufficient to cause a disorder, but affects a continuous phenotype whose extreme end may be a disorder, such as obesity, hypertension, RD, or ADHD.

BOX 1.2. Neuroanatomy and Neuroimaging

NEUROANATOMY TERMS

Cerebrum—The entire brain except for the cerebellum and brainstem. It is divided into two hemispheres. The outer layer of the cerebrum is the neocortex ("new bark"). Inside the cerebrum are white matter, ventricles, and subcortical structures. The white matter consists of axons covered in a fatty sheath (myelin) that connect various brain regions. The ventricles are fluid-filled cavities that expand when there is brain atrophy. Subcortical structures include the limbic system, the basal ganglia, and the thalamus.

Cerebellum—A roughly plum-sized structure located underneath the occipital lobe of the neocortex and at the top of the brainstem. It is important for both motor coordination and higher cognitive processes.

Lobes of the Neocortex

Occipital—Located at the back of the brain, these lobes receive and process visual input.

Parietal—Located in front of the occipital lobes and above the temporal lobes, these lobes are involved in processing spatial, proprioceptive, and tactile information important for planning body movements. The left parietal lobe also contains structures (e.g., the angular gyrus) that are important for language and mathematics.

Temporal—Located partly underneath the temples of the head, and below the parietal and frontal lobes, these lobes are important for auditory processing (bilaterally), language processing (usually on the left), and visual object recognition, including faces and printed words (fusiform face and word areas).

Frontal—Located at the front of the brain, these lobes are important for planning and executing actions over different time scales. The frontal lobes receive inputs from all the rest of the brain, allowing decisions about actions to integrate perception, memory, cognition, and emotion.

Subcortical Structures

Limbic system—Includes structures involved in both emotion (e.g., the amygdala) and long-term memory (e.g., the hippocampus).

Basal ganglia—Part of the extrapyramidal motor system; they include the caudate nucleus, putamen, and globus pallidus. Part of the basal ganglia (i.e. caudate nucleus and putamen) is also known as the striatum. The basal ganglia have reciprocal connections with the frontal lobes (corticostriatal loops) and are involved in implicit learning based on reinforcements.

Thalamus—A large grey matter nucleus in the center of the cerebrum that relays sensory input to the neocortex.

(continued)

BOX 1.2. *(continued)*

TYPES OF NEUROIMAGING

Structural—Used to measure the size, shape, and integrity of brain structures. There are two main structural neuroimaging methods, both of which use magnetic resonance imaging (MRI). One is morphometry, which produces a detailed, 3-D picture of grey matter, white matter, and ventricles that form the boundaries of the brain structures listed above. The other is diffusion tensor imaging (DTI), which yields a 3-D picture of white matter tracts connecting regions of neocortex.

Functional—Used to measure both global and local brain activity. The main methods are event-related potential (ERPs), functional MRI (fMRI), and positron emission tomography (PET). ERPs are based on scalp measures of electrical activity in the brain (electroencephalography, or EEG). ERPs have excellent temporal resolution but poor spatial resolution. Both fMRI and PET measure local blood flow changes associated with brain activity. They have good spatial resolution but poor temporal resolution.

CHAPTER 2

Neuropsychological Constructs

Just as Chapter 1 has described a model for how learning and behavioral disorders develop, this chapter describes a model of neuropsychological development, focusing on neuropsychological domains that are relevant for understanding learning disorders. Because work on diagnosing cognitive differences in children began with a fairly atheoretical psychometric approach, and because a cognitive science approach to such differences is much newer, the model presented here is a hybrid model including both psychometric and cognitive constructs. However, the long-term goal is to ground all these constructs in cognitive theory.

Before I turn to specific constructs, it is important to sketch a developmental model that guides the thinking presented here. This model is based on the key principles of "constructivism" and "interactive specialization" (Elman et al., 1996; Johnson, 2005; Oliver, Johnson, Karmiloff-Smith, & Pennington, 2000); it may be contrasted with "modular" or "maturational" models, in which specialized cortical processors (for phonemes, faces, etc.) are either innate or emerge according to a strict maturational timetable. Whereas modular or maturational models propose a strict one-way direction of causality from brain to behavior, a constructivist or interactive model conceives of the relation between brain and behavior as bidirectional. Accordingly, while brain structures certainly constrain learning and development, learning also changes the brain. The mature brain does have somewhat localized, specialized "modules" for different tasks (such as perceiving faces and phonemes), but a constructivist model holds that such specializations emerge from a developmental process and are not innate. So cognitive functions become more localized with development on both large and small time scales. During initial language acquisition, the whole brain is involved, but over a course of years structural language processing becomes localized

13

to the left hemisphere in most people. On a small time scale, learning a new task (e.g., playing the computer game Tetris) initially activates more brain areas, including the prefrontal cortex, than are activated when one is skilled at the task.

The model embraced here also depends on a connectionist view of how the brain learns and processes information (O'Reilly & Munakata, 2000). Connectionist models simulate learning and processing with layers of neuron-like elements that have adjustable connections between elements. Each learning trial adjusts the connections according to a learning rule. O'Reilly and Munakata (2000) have identified three different kinds of processing performed by the real neural networks in the human brain, and have simulated each kind of processing with computational neural networks. These three kinds are (1) the slow learning of overlapping distributed representations of the environment, performed by the posterior cortex; (2) active maintenance by the prefrontal cortex of limited amounts of information over short time intervals, to enable problem solving; and (3) rapid acquisition of unique conjunctions of novel information by the hippocampus and related structures. Each of these kinds of processing is related to constructs in our neuropsychological model. The first kind, slow learning of distributed representations, is the basis of accumulated knowledge about the world, which is related to semantic memory and crystallized intelligence. The second kind, active memory, is related to working memory, executive functions, and fluid intelligence. The third kind, rapid acquisition of novel information, is related to episodic memory, which turns out to be less important for understanding learning disorders. Let us next consider constructs from the psychometric tradition.

A key contribution of the psychometric approach is the recognition that virtually all cognitive processes are positively correlated with each other (Spearman's "positive manifold"), so a model of neuropsychological constructs must represent this important fact. On the other hand, to understand a particular cognitive process (such as memory, reading, or language comprehension), we must break it into cognitive components and test which components are most important for understanding individual differences in that domain, including learning disorders. These two considerations dictate that the model of neuropsychological constructs should be hierarchical, with constructs becoming more global as we move up the hierarchy and more discrete as we move down. Different learning disorders are likely to require different levels of this hierarchy for their explanation. For instance, understanding ID may require only more global levels of the hierarchy, whereas understanding a subtype of RD may require a much more fine-grained level. Nonetheless, as explained in Chapter 1, it is unlikely that we will be able to reduce any developmental learning disorder to a single cognitive component. Any disorder will present us with a range of cognitive deficits, some more global and some more specific.

Another important consideration is that development in any cognitive domain involves both "bottom-up" and "top-down" influences. As an example of a bottom-up influence, limits in a low-level skill (e.g., phoneme perception) could drive individual differences in a higher-level domain (e.g., vocabulary acquisition). In contrast, a top-down developmental influence would be one in which individual differences in the higher-level cognitive domain lead to individual differences in the lower-level skill. Because of the fundamental interactivity of cognitive processing and development, it is unlikely that we will be able to reduce individual differences to initial differences in either bottom-up processes or top-down processes. Let us next review relevant constructs for our model, starting with psychometric constructs and then presenting cognitive neuroscience constructs.

PSYCHOMETRIC CONSTRUCTS

The psychometric constructs come from hierarchical models of intelligence, such as Carroll's (1993) three-stratum model. Figure 2.1 illustrates the hierarchical model of intelligence applied to the Wechsler Intelligence Scale for Children—Fourth Edition (WISC-IV; Wechsler, 2003). At the top of the hierarchy is general psychometric intelligence—the thing that is reflected in the Full Scale IQ on the WISC-IV. The next level of the hierarchy has four broad constructs: fluid intelligence, crystallized intelligence, working memory, and processing speed. The lowest level of the hierarchy consists of more specific constructs, which are represented in Figure 2.1 as specific WISC-IV subtests, with the subtests standing for constructs like spatial reasoning (Block Design), vocabulary knowledge (Vocabulary), or phonological short-term memory (Digit Span). However, in Carroll's (1993) model, the lowest-level constructs are more than just individual tasks. Instead, they are narrow latent traits that capture what is common across multiple measures of that particular construct.

In the standardization of the WISC-IV, this hierarchical four-factor structure was well supported by both exploratory and confirmatory factor analyses (Wechsler, 2003). I first focus on the broad constructs of fluid and crystallized intelligence, and then consider working memory and processing speed.

The psychometric theory of fluid and crystallized intelligence was proposed and tested by Spearman's student Cattell (1943, 1963), and elaborated by Cattell's student Horn (Cattell & Horn, 1978; Horn & Noll, 1997). The distinction between the concepts of fluid and crystallized intelligence has been made by numerous psychologists both before and after Cattell's work, using many different but conceptually similar labels for these constructs (Table 2.1). Some of these psychologists were attempting to understand the cognitive deficits associated with acquired brain damage or aging. So

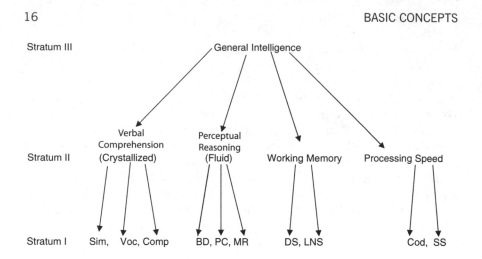

FIGURE 2.1. Carroll's (1993) hierarchical model of intelligence, illustrated by the WISC-IV. Sim, Similarities; Voc, Vocabulary; Comp, Comprehension; BD, Block Design; PC, Picture Completion; MR, Matrix Reasoning; DS, Digit Span; LNS, Letter–Number Sequencing; Cod, Coding; SS, Symbol Search.

these constructs have a long history in psychology and have been extensively validated by psychometric, developmental, and neuropsychological studies. These two constructs also correspond to two widespread intuitive notions of what it means for someone to be smart—namely, either being good at solving new problems or knowing a lot. So, simply put, fluid intelligence involves novel problem-solving ability, and crystallized intelligence involves accumulated (mostly verbal) knowledge. Because fluid intelligence is much more vulnerable to brain damage or aging than is crystallized intelligence, these two kinds of intelligence also each have a distinct developmental course. Fluid intelligence reaches a lifetime peak in late adolescence and slowly declines thereafter (e.g., Wechsler Adult Intelligence Scale—Third Edition [WAIS-III] norms for Matrix Reasoning show that the highest average raw score is attained by 16- to 17-year-olds), whereas crystallized intelligence keeps increasing until at least middle age (e.g., WAIS-III norms for Vocabulary show that the highest average score is attained by 45- to 54-year-olds) (Wechsler, 1997). A paradigmatic fluid intelligence task is the WISC-IV Matrix Reasoning task, and a paradigmatic crystallized intelligence task is the Vocabulary test.

The WISC-IV has two factors that correspond closely to these two constructs. The Verbal Comprehension Index corresponds to crystallized intelligence and is measured by three subtests that tap accumulated verbal knowledge (Similarities, Vocabulary, and Comprehension). The Perceptual Reasoning Index corresponds to fluid intelligence and is measured by three

TABLE 2.1. Two Kinds of Intelligence

Fluid	Crystallized	Source
Flexibility and elasticity	Routine or accustomed work	Proctor (1873)
Adaptability and rapid adjustment	Accumulated experience	Foster & Taylor (1920)
Capacity to develop new patterns of response	Functioning of already developed patterns of response	Hebb (1942)
Productive	Reproductive	Wertheimer (1945)
Capacity to acquire a new way of thinking	Ability to recall acquired information	Raven (1948)
Problem solving	Accumulated knowledge	Hebb (1949)
Ability to acquire information	Previously learned or stored information	Birren (1952)
Don't hold	Hold	Wechsler (1955)
Abstract intelligence	Accumulated experience	Jones (1959)
Mental agility	Ordered knowledge	Welford (1962)
Immediate problem-solving ability	Previously accumulated experience	Fitzhugh, Fitzhugh, & Reitan (1967)
Nonroutine	Routine	Sternberg (1985)
Current processing efficiency	Accumulated products of prior processing	Salthouse (1988)

subtests that tap novel problem-solving ability (Block Design, Picture Concepts, and Matrix Reasoning).

Now let us consider working memory and processing speed. Working memory involves the transient storage and processing of information, so it is essentially the same thing as active memory in the O'Reilly and Munakata (2000) model. The construct of working memory is closely related to the construct of short-term memory. Of the four cognitive constructs considered here, working memory is the most "respectable" from the point of view of cognitive theory. Much current research in cognitive neuroscience is focused on understanding working memory. Indeed, the inclusion of a Working Memory Index in the WISC-IV represents a positive trend toward the gradual integration of the psychometric and cognitive approaches. The construct of working memory will come up again in the discussion of cognitive neuroscience constructs.

We might say, in contrast to working memory, that the construct of processing speed is the least "respectable" from the point of view of cognitive theory. But it is a very robust psychometric factor, and it is useful in understanding cognitive disorders, including learning disorders. The reason it is less respectable is that it does not map onto established cognitive constructs. Nonetheless, reduced processing speed is a pervasive finding across both developmental and acquired cognitive disorders, as well as in aging (Salthouse, 1991). Moreover, there are marked developmental changes in processing speed that help explain cognitive development (Kail, 1991). This pervasive role of processing speed in both individual and developmental differences in cognitive skill may arise because processing speed actually requires the integrated activity of the whole brain. Although some processing speed measures, such as choice reaction time, are deceptively simple, performing consistently well on them requires the concerted activity of brain networks involved in perception, attention, motivation, and action selection (as well as inhibition). Furthermore, processing speed may affect the efficiency of cognitive components, like working memory, necessary for complex problem solving.

For instance, Fry and Hale (1996) used path analyses to test relations among age, processing speed, working memory, and fluid intelligence. They found that working memory mediated 41% of the total relation between age and fluid intelligence, and that processing speed mediated 71% of the relation between age and working memory. In other words, their results support a developmental cascade in which age-related increases in processing speed lead to age-related increases in working memory, which in turn lead to age-related increases in fluid intelligence. Although this was a cross-sectional, correlational study, which cannot establish the direction of causality, these authors were able to reject an alternative, top-down model in which fluid intelligence mediates the developmental relation between age and speed. So this study and other related work give us a view of how one key aspect of intelligence, fluid reasoning, may develop. A later section of this chapter considers models of how crystallized intelligence develops.

In sum, four basic psychometric constructs are important for understanding developmental and individual cognitive differences, including the learning disorders covered in this book. For instance, as we will see later, reduced processing speed is an important correlate of two of the learning disorders discussed in Part II, RD and ADHD, and helps to explain their co-occurrence.

COGNITIVE NEUROSCIENCE CONSTRUCTS

Whereas psychometric constructs grew out of applied research aimed at predicting individual differences in educational and occupational settings, cognitive neuroscience constructs come from basic research aimed at developing a universal theory of human cognition and understanding how it is mediated by the human brain. So developing and testing competing theories of cognitive processes is at the heart of this enterprise. Like the psychometric approach, the cognitive neuroscience approach has both broad and narrow constructs that may be arranged hierarchically. But the critical difference is that the subordinate constructs are based on an analysis of the cognitive components necessary to perform a given task—whether it be pronouncing a printed word, solving the Tower of Hanoi puzzle, or encoding a new memory. Increasingly, as discussed earlier, this theoretical analysis is implemented as a functioning computational model. In other words, a satisfactory cognitive theory would enumerate the underlying processing mechanisms used by real humans in sufficient detail that human performance could be simulated by a machine. From a cognitive theorist's point of view, all the lowest-level, Stratum I constructs in the psychometric model (Figure 2.1) require further analysis into cognitive components, and the relations across strata require a theoretical explanation in terms of shared cognitive processes. So, for a cognitive theorist, it is not enough to say that measures of numerical analogies and Piagetian reasoning both load on a fluid factor. What is required is an empirically tested cognitive explanation of why they do so, framed in terms of shared cognitive processes.

Some of the broad constructs in cognitive neuroscience are such things as perception, language, memory, executive functions, and social cognition, but each of these domains is divided into subtypes (e.g., short-term memory, long-term memory, and implicit memory), each of which is then subjected to a componential analysis. So, for a cognitive scientist, it is not very meaningful to talk about individual differences in language or memory. Nonetheless, cognitive analysis is proving very useful for understanding the broad individual differences described by psychometricians.

The three broad cognitive constructs that are most relevant for understanding the learning disorders covered in this book are language (which is important for understanding SSD, LI, and RD, as well as ASD and ID), executive functions (which are important for understanding ADHD, ASD, and ID) and social cognition (which is important for understanding ASD). Therefore, I next provide a cognitive analysis of two of these broad domains, language and executive functions. The components of social cognition are discussed in connection with ASD in Chapter 8.

Language

We may divide language into two broad categories (Figure 2.2): structural and functional. To learn a given language, a child must learn about its particular structure: its sound system (phonology), its grammar (syntax), and its vocabulary (lexical semantics). But mastery of structural language is not sufficient for a child to be able to use a language effectively as a tool for communication. In addition, a child must learn about the socially appropriate

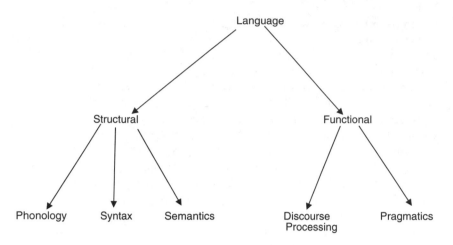

FIGURE 2.2. A cognitive analysis of language.

use of language (pragmatics), which includes social rules for conversation, such as taking turns, maintaining relevance, and monitoring the comprehension of the listener; it also includes the use of paralinguistic cues to convey meaning, such as intonation (or prosody) and gestures. And, to go beyond the single-sentence level of communication, children must learn to produce and comprehend both narratives and explanations (discourse processing).

The main language problems in SSD, LI, and RD are with aspects of structural language. LI is typically defined by deficits in syntax and lexical semantics. SSD is almost by definition a disorder of phonological development. And most individuals with developmental dyslexia, the main form of RD, also have deficits in phonological development. ID inevitably impairs at least some aspects of language development, although which aspects are most affected vary across particular ID syndromes, as described in Chapter 10.

Since discourse processing builds on structural language, it is not too surprising that individuals with these disorders have discourse problems as well, but this is not inevitably true. Primary problems with pragmatic language are more associated with problems in social cognition, such as those found in ASD.

The cognitive constructs of structural language and semantic memory have a close correspondence to the psychometric construct of crystallized intelligence. Poorer performance than that of otherwise similar controls on crystallized intelligence measures, such as the WISC-IV Verbal Comprehension Index score, is a well-replicated finding in SSD, LI, and RD, although the degree of deficit varies by disorder and across individuals. Almost by definition, a child with LI cannot have an average or better Verbal Comprehension score, whereas some children with SSD or RD do score well above average because their structural language problem is restricted to aspects of phonology.

One may ask how structural language develops and what underlies individual differences in crystallized intelligence. Because structural language has several components, as described above, the answer to this question varies somewhat by component. Nonetheless, work on typical and atypical language development is providing some initial answers to these questions. One developmental model to answer this question (in the domain of vocabulary development) has been proposed and tested by Gathercole and Baddeley (1990b). In their model, a key cognitive mechanism underlying learning new vocabulary words is phonological short-term memory, which is often measured by a nonword repetition task. When children learn a new word for a concept they already possess, they must hold the new name in short-term memory while they map it onto the appropriate concept, and then store the name–concept combination in long-term memory. In preschool children, individual differences in phonological short-term memory predict later differences in vocabulary, but not the reverse, providing empirical support for this developmental model (Avons, Wragg, Cupples, & Lovegrove, 1998; Bowey, 2001; Gathercole & Baddeley, 1989; Gathercole, Willis, Emslie, & Baddeley, 1992). There is also theoretical and empirical support for a developmental relation between phonological short-term memory and syntax (Adams & Gathercole, 1995; Daneman & Case, 1981; Laws & Gunn, 2004).

Executive Functions

"Executive functions" is an umbrella term for a set of cognitive processes that are important in the control of cognitive processes and action selection, especially in novel contexts, or in familiar contexts that strongly evoke prepotent but maladaptive responses. Executive functions are necessary for cognitive flexibility and for controlled or effortful processing. Neuropsychologically, executive functions are mediated by the prefrontal cortex and closely connected structures, such as the basal ganglia and the anterior cingulate gyrus. A key construct for understanding executive functions is the construct of working memory or active memory (O'Reilly & Munakata, 2000), mentioned earlier in the discussion of the WISC-IV. Working memory is a limited-capacity memory system that must be constantly reconfigured (updated) as one solves a problem, and that must be protected from interference by associated but irrelevant information (inhibition). Working memory allows one to generate alternative possibilities and evaluate them, and so it allows one to shift cognitive set if necessary. Therefore, a list of executive functions includes updating, inhibiting, generating, and set shifting.

Some of these functions can be illustrated by the games of bridge and chess. To succeed at these games, one must (1) generate alternative lines of play and look ahead several moves to see where they lead; (2) inhibit prepotent but maladaptive moves; and (3) constantly update the contents of working memory to reflect the current state of the game, which in turn leads to shifting cognitive set. Practiced bridge and chess players rely on heuristics to reduce the processing demands of play. These heuristics are generally useful tactics, such as occupying the center squares of the board in chess or drawing trumps in bridge. But these heuristics are not appropriate in every situation. So to perform at a high level of skill, a player must be able to inhibit an overlearned heuristic, shift cognitive set, and generate novel solutions for the problem at hand. Hence expert performance in these games at least occasionally requires executive functions and the fluid intelligence they support.

Miyake et al. (2000) performed a confirmatory factor analysis of popular executive function tasks in the literature, including the Wisconsin Card Sorting Test (WCST), the Tower of Hanoi, and operation span. They found three distinct but moderately correlated latent traits that corresponded conceptually to three of the executive functions discussed here: shifting (e.g., the WCST), inhibiting (e.g., the Tower of Hanoi), and updating (e.g., operation span). In other studies (Fagerheim et al., 1999; Friedman et al., 2006), they tested the relations between these three traits and fluid and crystallized intelligence. They found that updating was strongly related to both intelligence constructs, whereas shifting and inhibiting were not related to either construct. An earlier cognitive analysis of fluid intelligence (Carpenter, Just, & Shell, 1990) also found that working memory capacity was a key contributor to individual differences in fluid intelligence. So although it may be tempting to equate psychometric intelligence with executive functions or frontal lobe functions, the relation appears more complex, because not all executive functions are equally related to intelligence. Nonetheless, our broader everyday construct of intelligence would include all three functions discussed here—shifting, inhibiting, and updating.

This concludes the review of neuropsychological constructs relevant for understanding learning disorders. The chapters that follow will examine the roles these constructs play in different learning disorders and the ways they contribute to differential diagnosis. Although the psychometric and cognitive neuroscience approaches to these constructs are converging, more work is needed to achieve a full integration.

CHAPTER 3

Issues in Syndrome Validation

An alternative title for this chapter might be "The Rocky Road from Symptoms to Syndromes." The point of this alternative title is that not all symptom clusters noticed by clinicians qualify as valid syndromes. Symptoms are atypical behaviors. Obviously, the variety of symptoms found in children is vast. By randomly combining subsets of these symptoms, we could create a very large number of potential syndromes. So we have to address the question of why some clusters of symptoms qualify as valid syndromes and others do not. Basically, the answer is that valid syndromes consist of groups of symptoms that reliably co-occur, are associated with functional impairment, are theoretically meaningful, and are not redundant with an already validated disorder. What "theoretically meaningful" means will become clearer below. The point here is that a putative syndrome must undergo a variety of scientific tests before it is considered valid. Even then, future research may demonstrate that it should be lumped with another disorder or split into subtypes. So our current list of valid psychiatric syndromes or learning disorders is provisional and will evolve as our scientific understanding increases.

Understanding how syndromes are validated is important for practitioners, because it will help them be more critical about the less well-validated disorders they will encounter in the field of learning disorders. Chapter 4 reviews two less well-validated learning disorders and explains why they do not satisfy the scientific tests required to validate a syndrome.

The learning disorders presented in this book represent a nosology (i.e., a taxonomy) for classifying learning problems in childhood. In this chapter, the issues involved in validating both a nosological scheme and individual syndromes within a nosology are considered. The concepts of "nosology" and "syndrome" imply that the domain of behavior can be divided in meaningful ways—that it is not just a smooth continuum. Therefore, we must ask what validates one division versus others. These issues have been well discussed by Fletcher (1985) and Rapin (Rapin, 1987; Rapin & Allen, 1982), and I draw on their discussions.

The two basic goals of a nosology are to identify clusters of symptoms that (1) reliably co-occur and (2) are distinct at the level of etiology, pathogenesis, or response to treatment. A reliable cluster that is also distinct at one or more of these levels may be a valid syndrome, although extensive research is required to test its validity. These two goals of reliable co-occurrence and distinct mechanisms concern internal and external validity, respectively.

INTERNAL AND EXTERNAL VALIDITY

"Internal validity" might also be termed "internal consistency." Fletcher (1985) lists five criteria for internal validity: (1) coverage, or number of patients classified; (2) homogeneity of the subtypes; (3) reliability of the classification procedures; (4) replicability across techniques; and (5) replication in other samples. Clearly, a sample- or test-specific subtype would necessarily lack consistency.

"External validity" essentially concerns the explanatory significance of a subtype or its syndrome validity. To qualify as a valid disorder, any behaviorally defined syndrome must be associated with functional impairment— that is, problems in social relations and/or educational or occupational functioning. A syndrome or subtype may be reliable in terms of the variables used to define it, and may be associated with functional impairment, yet may lack a distinctive relation to any external variables of interest. In that case, it would lack *discriminant* external validity and should not be distinguished from other syndromes or subtypes with a similar external validity profile. As discussed in Chapter 4, central auditory processing disorder (CAPD) lacks discriminant external validity.

Fletcher (1985) lists three possible criteria for discriminant external validity: (1) differential response to treatment; (2) clinical meaningfulness; and (3) differential relation to processing measures independent of those used to define the subtype, such as neuropsychological measures. To this list, I would add (4) differential etiology; (5) differential pathogenesis; and (6) differential prognosis or developmental course (see Table 3.1 and Figure 3.1).

Fletcher (1985) emphasizes that the search for external validity is essentially a hypothesis-generating and hypothesis-testing affair; that is, it is a search for construct validity (Cronbach & Meehl, 1955). A good subtype or syndrome is a fruitful hypothesis about how to "parse" the domains of

TABLE 3.1. Criteria for a Valid Nosology

Internal	External
Coverage of cases	Etiology
Homogeneity of subtypes	Pathogenesis
Reliability	Neuropsychology
Replicability	Developmental course
	Response to treatment
	Clinical meaningfulness

both disordered and nondisordered behavior, as well as how to "parse" the various levels of the underlying causes of behavior. If a syndrome is valid, it will satisfy tests of both convergent and discriminant validity across levels of analysis: etiology, brain mechanisms, neuropsychology, and symptoms. Satisfying these tests makes it theoretically meaningful.

The ultimate goal of syndrome analysis is discovering a meaningful causal chain across these different levels of analysis, although recognizing that some of these causal paths are bidirectional. We would like to know which etiologies specifically cause the syndrome in question, what aspects of brain development they perturb, what deficits in neuropsychological processes this leads to, how these underlying neuropsychological deficits lead to the symptoms of the disorder, how the symptoms and underlying deficits

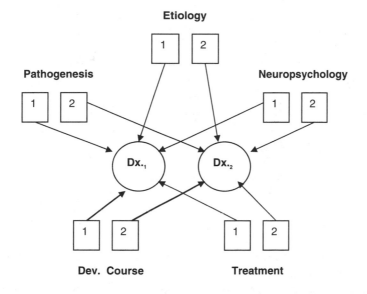

FIGURE 3.1. Ideal discriminant validity for diagnoses.

change with development, and how all of this information helps explain the response to treatment. Thus a valid syndrome (or subtype of a syndrome) is a theoretical construct below the level of observable behaviors or symptoms, which provides a meaningful explanation of why certain symptoms co-occur in different patterns across development, as well as a meaningful explanation of why some treatments are efficacious and others are not.

The concepts of convergent and discriminant validity are closely related to the concept of external validity. An ideal nosology would have a complete and unique set of external, converging validators for each of its different syndromes, thereby guaranteeing discriminant validity. This ideal situation is depicted in Figure 3.1, but as we have seen in Chapter 1, this ideal situation does *not* apply to learning disorders or most behaviorally defined disorders. Instead, there is partial overlap of external validators for many pairs of disorders, so that what is unique to a given disorder is the overall pattern and not each specific validator.

The scientific descriptions of the learning disorder syndromes discussed in this book review the evidence for external validity in the areas of etiology, brain mechanisms (pathogenesis), neuropsychology, and developmental course. Evidence for differential response to treatment is included in the clinical section of each chapter. There is at least some evidence for differential etiology, brain mechanisms, neuropsychology, and response to treatment across these disorders. In general, we know the least about the brain mechanism level of analysis in these behaviorally defined disorders, but in some cases we know a fair amount about the genetic factors involved in their etiologies. As we will see, there are known genetic and environmental risk factors for nearly all these disorders, and sometimes evidence for etiological subtypes. It is less certain that subtypes exist that are defined by differences in brain mechanisms or underlying neuropsychological deficits, but the issue of possible neuropsychological subtypes is considered for each learning disorder. Therefore, instead of a one-to-one correspondence between etiological and neuropsychological subtypes, the correspondence may be many-to-one. Different etiologies may produce similar symptoms by acting on the same underlying brain mechanisms.

A many-to-one situation may turn out to be quite common in the case of complex behavioral disorders generally, and may not be restricted to the developmental learning disorders we are considering here. Recent discoveries about the genetics of bipolar illness, schizophrenia, and Alzheimer disease suggest both major gene effects and genetic heterogeneity in etiology, but it is less clear that the genetic subtypes of these disorders are associated with clearly distinguishable phenotypic subtypes in a one-to-one fashion. It is also important to note that this kind of etiological heterogeneity, by itself, does not invalidate the construct of a behavioral syndrome. If the different etiologies affect the same or similar brain mechanisms and produce the same underlying neuropsychological deficit, then it seems reasonable to retain the concept of the behavioral syndrome and not divide it into subtypes. As discussed by Shaywitz and Shaywitz (1988), there are valid medical syndromes, such as hypertension and hydrocephalus, that are definitely heterogeneous in their etiologies. A similar point is made by Folstein and Rutter (1988) in reviewing the genetics of autism; although autism is undoubtedly heterogeneous in its etiology, it may not be heterogeneous in its pathophysiology.

The next chapter illustrates the process of syndrome validation by examining putative syndromes that have not passed the tests described here. In contrast, Chapters 6–13 present current better-validated disorders. I hope that contrasting these better-validated disorders with less well-validated ones will make the process of syndrome validation clearer.

CHAPTER 4

Less Well-Validated Learning Disorders

This chapter provides an example of how we can close the gap between science and practice in the field of learning disorders. Implications for practice are discussed more fully in Part III of this book, which describes evidence-based practice (EBP) and reviews controversial therapies.

Chapter 3 has discussed how a putative disorder is tested for validity, and Part II of this book reviews how those tests have been applied to various disorders. To review this process briefly, a behaviorally defined disorder begins with a cluster of symptoms that reliably co-occur and are associated with impairment. But to become a valid syndrome, a putative disorder must exhibit external validity. Nonetheless, future research may lump disorders together, split a disorder, or even eliminate a disorder. Diagnostic constructs are not set in stone. Instead, they are hypotheses that are constantly being tested and refined by science.

We turn now to learning disorder categories that are frequently encountered in clinical practice, but are much less well validated by research. The two such disorders considered here are central auditory processing disorder (CAPD) and sensory modulation disorder (SMD). Neither of these disorders is in the *Diagnostic and Statistical Manual of Mental Disorders*, fourth edition, text revision (DSM-IV-TR) or *International Classification of Diseases*, 10th revision (ICD-10). The three main issues regarding the validity of these two disorders are (1) their theoretical plausibility; (2) an insufficient empirical knowledge base; and (3) questions about whether they are distinct from other, better-validated disorders.

We do not know whether CAPD is distinct from either the speech, language, and literacy disorders (RD, SSD, and LI) or from ADHD, and whether SMD is distinct from ADHD, anxiety, or ASD. So, even though the clusters of symptoms that define CAPD and SMD may be reliable and associated with clinical impairment, they lack discriminant external validity.

Advocates for one of these disorders might argue that historical precedence (which is similar to "senior water rights" in the western United States) is not a good reason for deciding validity, and they would be entirely correct! Even if CAPD or SMD were totally redundant with a better-validated disorder (i.e., it provided no increase in coverage), if it provided a better theoretical and empirical account of the disorder or a better treatment, then the old category should be replaced by the new one. So that is why it is incumbent on proponents of these diagnoses and the field generally to gather more data on their validity. In the meantime, both practitioners and parents need to be cautious and skeptical about the claims sometimes made by proponents of these disorders. In what follows, I review the research on the validity of these two learning disorders.

CENTRAL AUDITORY PROCESSING DISORDER

History and Definition

CAPD was proposed by audiologists in the 1970s (e.g., Willeford, 1977) and it is defined as a cortical-level deficit in processing auditory stimuli. The definition also includes two important exclusionary criteria—namely, that CAPD is not due either to a peripheral hearing problem or to higher-order language, cognitive, or attentional problems. In other words, CAPD must be central, not peripheral, but it also must be modality-specific. So the localization of CAPD in the brain must be in primary or secondary auditory cortex. The theoretical claim is that these auditory brain areas fail to extract acoustic features that are necessary for higher multimodal language and cognitive processing.

As discussed in Chapters 6 and 7, this kind of bottom-up auditory hypothesis has been very controversial in research on RD, SSD, and LI, and empirical support for it is weak in those areas. So the challenge faced by proponents of CAPD is to meet the empirical tests that proponents of the auditory hypothesis for these other disorders have failed to meet.

The National Institute of Deafness and Other Communication Disorders (2004) lists the symptoms that are associated with CAPD. These include "trouble paying attention to and remembering information presented orally," "problems carrying out multistep directions," "poor listening skills," needing "more time to process information," "low academic performance," "behavior problems," "language difficulty," and "difficulty with reading, comprehension, spelling, and vocabulary." If we use this list of symptoms to define CAPD, it is not a distinct disorder, because this list overlaps completely with the symptoms found in ADHD, LI, and RD.

A different definition of CAPD has been provided by the American Speech–Language–Hearing Association (ASHA) which produced a technical report on CAPD in 2005. This report concludes that the scientific evidence supports CAPD as a diagnostic entity and audiologists as the professionals who should diagnose it. Instead of being symptom-based, as are all the diagnoses in Chapters 6–13 of this book (and all the diagnoses in DSM-IV-TR), the ASHA (2005) definition of CAPD is based on audiological tests. Basically, the definition poses the two exclusionary criteria discussed earlier (not peripheral and not multimodal), and then says that the difficulty in CAPD is demonstrated by poor performance in one or more of the following auditory skills: "sound localization and lateralization; auditory discrimination; auditory pattern recognition; temporal aspects of audition, including temporal integration, temporal discrimination (e.g., temporal gap detection), temporal ordering, and temporal masking; auditory performance with competing acoustic signals (including dichotic listening); and auditory performance with degraded signals."

Review of Validity

What is problematic about the ASHA (2005) definition, besides not being symptom-based, is that this list of auditory skills is essentially a list of skills tapped by a typical CAPD battery administered by an audiologist. So CAPD is reduced to doing poorly on one or more of the tests that audiologists give! Moreover, if the skills listed are discrete auditory constructs, then there are potentially 11 subtypes of CAPD—one for each construct.

In addition, many of these tests given by audiologists use linguistic stimuli. For instance, auditory discrimination means auditory discrimination of spoken words, dichotic listening uses speech stimuli, and so on. But if the stimuli are linguistic, it is very difficult to rule out the possibility that poor performance is due to a higher-order language problem, which is excluded by the definition of CAPD. So it is not clear how higher-order attention or cognitive problems are to be ruled out by an audiologist making the diagnosis of CAPD, even though the presence of such a disorder excludes this diagnosis. In other words, the ASHA definition of CAPD is incomplete and therefore not operational, because it does not include a procedure for excluding key confounding conditions. Finally, there are important psychometric problems with this test battery approach to diagnostic definition. How often will healthy individuals do poorly on one of these measures by chance alone? How are these 11 measures correlated with each other? Do they have incremental validity in predicting real-world performance beyond related language and cognitive measures? The questions go on and on, because the appropriate validity research has not been done.

The criticisms made here are not new. There is a fairly extensive literature criticizing the validity of CAPD (Cacace & McFarland, 1998; Kamhi

& Beasley, 1985; Vellutino & Scanlon, 1989). And there is a corresponding lack of evidence supporting the reliability and construct validity of CAPD tests. For instance, Cacace and McFarland (1998) cite data indicating that the median test–retest reliability of such CAPD tasks as filtered words, auditory figure–ground, and competing words is .41. Moreover, these tasks correlate at about .38 with the Peabody Picture Vocabulary Test—Revised, a measure of receptive vocabulary; this means that virtually all the reliable variance on these measures overlaps with a measure of supramodal language skill.

In sum, several concerns about CAPD call its validity into question. These include its definition, the psychometric properties of the tests used to diagnose it, its distinctness from other disorders, and the lack of sufficient empirical research to test its validity.

SENSORY MODULATION DISORDER

History and Definition

SMD is also called "sensory integration dysfunction" and "sensory processing disorder." For a recent review, see Schaaf and Miller (2005). SMD was first described in the writings of Jean Ayres (1972, 1979), an occupational therapist who worked with adults and children with brain damage. At that time, rehabilitation of such patients was focused on their most obvious sensory and motor problems. Ayres realized that their most disabling problems were more subtle ones involving deficits in processing and integrating information (Mangeot et al., 2001), and that understanding how the brain accomplished information processing and integration was important for diagnosing and treating these patients' problems. Although most clinical neuropsychologists would have come to a similar conclusion, they would have focused on problems in behavior regulation and cognition—attention, memory, language, and executive functions—and would have been concerned with how to rehabilitate these deficits.

In contrast, Ayres (1979) focused on apparent altered vestibular functioning in these patients and on the integration of information across sensory modalities to guide adaptive behavior. Ayres was correct about the importance of cross-modal integration in the brain. Since most of the neocortex consists of polymodal association areas as opposed to unimodal areas, most of the neocortex is involved in cross-modal intergrations. Modern cognitive neuroscience has learned that these polymodal association areas accomplish the integration of information across sensory modalities by constructing amodal cognitive and affective representations of the environment, always with reference to planning and selecting actions. But Ayres's concept of sensory integration had much more limited scope than the concept has in modern cognitive neuroscience.

Ayres was particularly struck by the extreme reactions her patients exhibited to sensory stimuli, including gravity, and she traced the cause of these hypo- and hypersensitivities to sensory integration dysfunction. So while Ayres was right to realize the importance of less obvious deficits in her patients, her neuropsychological model had "tunnel vision." It was overly focused on extreme reactions to sensory stimuli, and it assumed rather than tested the cause of these extreme reactions. So one important criticism of SMD as a disorder is that it lacks theoretical plausibility, given our current understanding of how the brain functions.

The symptoms of SMD (Mangeot et al., 2001) are described as sensation-seeking and sensation-avoiding behaviors; these are hypothesized to be reactions to sensory stimuli in different domains, such as tactile (touching too much vs. avoidance of touch), vestibular (overactive and risky motor behaviors vs. avoidance of playgrounds and car rides), and proprioceptive (seeking vs. avoiding deep pressure). Healthy sensory modulation is defined as "the capacity to regulate and organize the degree, intensity, and nature of responses to sensory input in a graded and adaptive manner so that an optimal range of performance and adaptation to challenges can be maintained" (Mangeot et al., 2001, p. 399). So this definition of SMD is based on behavioral symptoms selected with a hypothesized sensory integration problem as their explanation. This symptom definition has been partly validated by a study of electrodermal responses (EDRs) to sensory challenges (McIntosh, Miller, Shyu, & Hagerman, 1999). In this study, the group with SMD had larger EDRs to these challenges and took longer to habituate than controls. So parents' reports of extreme sensory reactions were related to actual EDRs to sensory challenges. Nonetheless, there are various problems with the validity of SMD.

Review of Validity

Although Ayres's analysis of the problems exhibited by her patients with brain damage did not include the cognitive problems they were very likely to have had, she was nonetheless quite ready to hypothesize that sensory integration dysfunction *caused* cognitive problems, just as proponents of CAPD assume that auditory problems cause cognitive problems. For instance, she stated: "About five to 10 percent of the children in this country today have enough trouble with sensory integration to cause them to be slow learners or to have behavior problems" (Ayres, 1979, p. 8). She went on in this passage to trace academic problems (in understanding instructions and reading, writing, and arithmetic) and social problems (in turn taking and control of aggressive impulses) to sensory integration dysfunction in children who nonetheless had average or above-average intelligence. In other words, she claimed that sensory integration dysfunction causes both learning disabilities and behavior disorders. This claim persists in contemporary work on SMD. But the symptoms of SMD described by Mangeot et al. (2001) and the EDR results (McIntosh et al., 1999) are open to alternative explanations. Some of these symptoms overlap with symptoms of ADHD, anxiety, or ASD. For instance, several studies have found a high rate of comorbidity of ADHD with SMD (Mangeot et al., 2001; Yochman, Parush, & Ornoy, 2004). Other studies have found that SMD symptoms correlate with symptoms of anxiety and depression (Pfeiffer, Kinnealey, Reed, & Herzberg, 2005). This result is not surprising, since the definition of sensory modulation itself is not that different from the definition of emotion regulation. Children with emotion regulation problems are known to have exaggerated startle responses and may well have exaggerated EDRs to sensory challenges. So, once again, we face the question of whether the causative problem is actually in sensory integration or in some higher-order cognitive process. And, once again, there is not enough research on the validity of SMD to answer this question.

As discussed in Chapter 15, Ayres (1972, 1979) developed a therapy to deal with the hypothesized deficit in sensory integration. Basically, this therapy consists of enhanced sensory input, partly based on research on the effects of "enriched" environments on laboratory rats, which at that time had recently demonstrated enhanced brain development in such environments. Whereas typical children spontaneously seek out environmental stimulation to foster their brain development, Ayres postulated that children with sensory integration dysfunction avoid the very kinds of sensory stimuli they need to overcome their dysfunction. So her therapy provides enriched vestibular, proprioceptive, tactile, and other sensory input to facilitate the development of normal sensory integration. Once this is achieved, it is hypothesized that the higher-level problems caused by sensory integration dysfunction, such as problems in reading, language, attention, and behavior, will also be alleviated. In sum, Ayres's (1972, 1979) concept of sensory integration proposed a grand vision of the cause and treatment for most of the learning disorders described in this book! So this is a second problem with theoretical plausibility, which is that the explanatory scope of sensory integration dysfunction or SMD is far too broad. As Part II of this book makes clear, these various learning disorders have distinct etiologies, brain mechanisms, and treatments. It is extremely implausible that they could all be reduced to one cause. And as we will see in Chapter 15, the claim that a single treatment can cure multiple disorders is a "red-flag" indicator that the treatment is likely to be unscientific.

In sum, there are several important questions about whether SMD is a valid disorder: It lacks theoretical plausibility; it may not be distinct from other better validated disorders; and there is very little research on its external validity. Since the therapy based on sensory integration theory is also not validated, practitioners should be very skeptical about this diagnosis.

SUMMARY

Neither CAPD nor SMD currently meets scientific criteria for validity. Consequently, they do not belong in evidence-based practice (EBP), just as unvalidated treatments do not. There are ethical concerns about unvalidated diagnoses in practice. A child with a learning disorder who receives an unvalidated diagnosis may be delayed or prevented from receiving an accurate diagnosis and appropriate treatment.

CHAPTER 5

Differential Diagnosis

The previous chapters have provided a scientific perspective on what diagnoses are and how their validity is tested. This chapter discusses the diagnostic process and the value and limitations of diagnosis. Teachers, parents, and even clinicians are inherently suspicious of behavioral diagnoses for children. Many have seen examples of the diagnostic process gone awry: a child mislabeled, a diagnosis improperly conveyed, or a child receiving inappropriate or even harmful treatments. Furthermore, some children change so much in such a short amount of time that it may not be appropriate to label them at all. These are important reservations, and in what follows I try to deal with some of them (see also Appendix A for a list of user-friendly resources that can be recommended to parents or teachers).

The process of making a diagnosis has important similarities to the process of testing a hypothesis in scientific research. A good hypothesis or theory accounts for many observable data in diverse domains and sometimes makes predictions in unexpected domains. As discussed earlier, a diagnostic category is a theory or construct; convergent validity for this theory is provided by data from different levels of analysis. Most importantly, a good hypothesis or diagnosis should be more than just a descriptive relabeling of the data and should contain explicit criteria for ruling it in or out. Obviously, one of the main differences between hypothesis testing in research and in the diagnostic process is that research usually focuses on a group, usually carefully chosen to test the hypothesis at hand, whereas diagnosis focuses on an individual patient, not chosen but referred. So the clinician always deals with an N of 1, and cannot exclude confounding factors a priori. In this way, the hypothesis testing of the diagnostician is inevitably less powerful and precise than that of the researcher.

However, the diagnostician has some important compensating advantages. One is that he or she has many more data about the one subject than a researcher typically has about his or her group of subjects. This additional data can be used to test for both convergent and discriminant validity of a particular diagnostic hypothesis. If a child has dyslexia, then certain things ought to be true and not true across heterogeneous domains of data, including presenting symptoms, the early developmental history, the school history, the behavior during testing (including kinds of errors), and the test results. A particular diagnosis is supported by a converging pattern of results across these different domains of data and by a diverging pattern of results for competing diagnoses. As will be described, our diagnostic model makes this process of testing for convergent and discriminant validity explicit. A second advantage the diagnostician presumably has is that the diagnostic hypotheses being tested in an individual patient have already been tested on groups of patients in research studies. His or her main task should be to see whether a given patient fits an established, well-articulated pattern, not to develop these patterns.

Before presenting this diagnostic model, I should say something more about the "medical model" approach to diagnosis advocated here. For some mental health practitioners, this kind of approach is aversive, because it does not capture the individuality of the patients' problems. Robin Morris (1984) has said, "Every child is like all other children, like some other children, and like no other children." In other words, some characteristics are species-typical; some are typical of groups within the species; and some are unique to individuals. For diagnosticians and therapists, it is important to have a good grasp of which characteristics fall into which category. Some patients have symptoms that they feel are unique to them, but that are in fact virtually species-typical. Other symptoms are fairly specific to a particular diagnosis, and still others are unique to a given patient. Although a good clinician must be aware of and make use of a patient's unique attributes, scientific progress in understanding and treating mental disorders depends on there being "middle-level" variation—differentiating characteristics of groups within our species. If not, mental health work is reduced either to just treating the life problems everyone faces or to recreating the field for each unique individual. On the one hand, we say that there are no mental disorders because everyone is "in the same boat." On the other hand, we say that there are no mental disorders because everyone is different. A science of mental health is not tenable at either extreme. Although much confusion and many limitations exist in the current state of knowledge about mental disorders in children, this state of affairs hardly means that a science of developmental psychopathology is impossible.

Another important point to remember is that the patient has the diagnosis, rather than vice versa (e.g., Achenbach, 1982). In other words, most diagnoses don't provide an explanation for every aspect of a patient's being. A related point is that nosologies classify disorders, not people. It is easy to fall into the shorthand of talking about "dyslexics," "autistics," or "schizo-phrenics," but these labels can be just as stereotyping and potentially stigma-tizing as other labels based on ethnicity, religion, or certain medical illnesses. So mental health practitioners and advocates prefer "people-friendly" language. A person with autism is not reducible to an "autistic."

There are several other reasons why diagnoses are important. Diagnoses permit efficient identification and treatment, and research on a given diagnosis can lead to early identification/prevention. As discussed earlier, studies of diagnostic groups can contribute to basic research on human development. Finally, diagnosis itself can be therapeutic for parents and patients, because an accurate diagnosis provides an explanation for troubling symptoms and a focus for the efforts the parents and child patient are already making to alleviate the symptoms.

Another criticism of the medical model is that it presupposes a single biological model for the cause of all behavioral disorders. However, Mechl (1973) pointed out that within medicine itself there is no single causal model. This point is even more true today. Recent medical research on disorders like heart disease espouses a multifactoral causal model and acknowledges the contribution of genetic, psychological, and cultural factors in etiology. So the medical model that has been castigated by social scientists may increasingly be a "straw man." Moreover, our search for the causes of behavioral and learning disorders should be just as broad as the search for causes of "medical" disorders, and not hampered by a priori assumptions about what kinds of causes will prove important.

A MODEL OF DIFFERENTIAL DIAGNOSIS

The process of differential diagnosis requires generating a list of possible diagnoses (hypotheses) based on the presenting complaints and the developmental history, and then testing these hypotheses with new data (parent and teacher reports, family history, behavioral observations of the child during the evaluation, and neuropsychological testing). This is the process we have followed for many years in our Developmental Neuropsychology Clinic at the University of Denver. So this process essentially applies the scientific method to understanding an individual's problem. Just as in science, supporting or rejecting a hypothesis requires converging evidence from multiple methods and levels of analysis.

Clearly, then, diagnosis requires more than just applying DSM-IV-TR or other diagnostic criteria in a "cookbook" fashion. A parent's or teacher's ratings of symptoms may exceed the threshold for a given diagnosis, but those symptoms may have an alternative explanation. Or the parent's or teacher's ratings may not reach the diagnostic threshold, but the balance of evidence may support a given diagnosis nonetheless. So differential diagnosis requires clinical judgment—the weighing of all the evidence to achieve an integrated formulation. Both clinical experience *and* research aid diagnostic skill. The more knowledge we have about a diagnostic construct, the richer the network of knowledge that surrounds it, allowing more tests of whether that diagnosis is present.

So it is very important that clinical experience be supplemented by research, because the generalizations garnered from clinical experience have not been systematically tested and may be biased or mistaken. Many clinical "chestnuts" have later been proven to be untrue, such as the association of dyslexia with left-handedness (Bishop, 1990; Pennington, Smith, Kimberling, Green, & Haith, 1987) or the existence of Gerstmann syndrome (defined as the co-occurrence of finger agnosia, right–left confusion, agraphia, and acalculia).

The apparent association of left-handedness with dyslexia is an example of referral bias. The association is found in referred samples but not in general population samples, and the most plausible explanation is that referred samples are more likely to have multiple problems. Left-handedness (and reading problems) can be caused by early brain insults, and children with such problems will be found more often in a referred sample.

Benton (1961, 1977, 1992) demonstrated that although the four symptoms that define Gerstmann syndrome all occur after parietal lesions, there is not a greater than chance association of all four symptoms among patients with parietal lesions. In other words, clinicians selectively remembered the cases that fit the Gerstmann profile, but discounted all the cases with only one, two, or three symptoms.

So diagnosticians are susceptible to human information-processing biases (Dawes, 1994), such as the "availability heuristic" (Groopman, 2007). The availability heuristic is the likelihood that diagnosticians will think more often of diagnoses they encounter frequently. As the saying goes, "If you only have a hammer, everything looks like a nail." Research and a skeptical attitude are necessary to guard against such biases.

Therefore, good diagnosticians must be good scientists in several ways. They must evaluate their hypotheses about a given case systematically; they must confront their own cherished beliefs drawn from clinical experience with the same skeptical scrutiny that they would apply to peer reviews of others' hypotheses; they must be up to date on research bearing on the diagnosis; and they must be open to unexpected patterns in the clinical data. A patient who fits diagnostic criteria for a given disorder may nonetheless have characteristics that contradict some key aspect of the current theoretical model of the diagnosis. For example, one might encounter a child with dyslexia but without a phoneme awareness problem, or a child with ADHD without an executive inhibition problem. Such patients are important stimuli for new research and new theories. So the relation between science and practice should be a two-way street, with each informing the other.

My colleagues and I view the process of diagnostic decision making as being similar to the constraint satisfaction problem in cognitive psychology, rather than being similar to an exercise in formal logic. That is, diagnoses are "fuzzy sets," membership in which depends on many soft constraints and a few hard constraints. Not every patient with autism has motor stereotypies or gaze aversion, even though these are frequent symptoms of autism. Thus these symptoms provide evidence for that diagnosis, but their absence does not violate a hard constraint. On the other hand, a child with an IQ of 100 cannot receive a diagnosis of ID, since IQ level is a hard constraint for that diagnosis. Diagnostic decision making involves weighing the goodness of fit of different competing diagnoses against the soft and hard constraints provided by the data, and deciding which one (or few) fits best. A good fit is determined in part by the convergent and discriminant validity checks discussed above.

Another important component of the diagnostic process is the recognition that it is a process, and that diagnostic decisions are not possible until there are enough data. Diagnosis is like the process of perception in slow motion. Thus one must consciously experience the frustrating and sometimes painful intermediate stages of uncertainty. It is important for diagnosticians to be aware of their own sense of uncertainty, and not to flee from it into a premature diagnostic decision. Anxiety and confusion about a case are important signals that more data are probably needed.

I now present in abbreviated form the patterns of converging and diverging data that are used in the differential diagnosis of learning disorders (Tables 5.1 and 5.2). The first table presents patterns of history data associated with each learning disorder. The second table presents patterns of test results associated with each learning disorder. The patterns for each disorder are for that disorder in isolation: RD without LI, SSD, or ADHD; SSD without LI or RD; and so on. Comorbid cases combine the characteristics of the particular individual diagnoses that are comorbid. The chapters that follow present the research supporting these patterns, so these tables are intended to be just simplified summaries.

One can see from these tables that each disorder has its own pattern of findings, but the patterns are not totally distinct. For instance, deficits in phonological memory and processing speed are shared by several disorders. This overlap is consistent with the multiple-deficit model presented earlier.

The chapters in Part II illustrate the application of these diagnostic principles via case studies of the following disorders: dyslexia or RD, SSD, LI, ASD, ADHD, and ID. Each of these chapters provides two case studies that are prototypical of the types of clients we see in our Developmental Neuropsychology Clinic at the University of Denver. No case study repre-

TABLE 5.1. Patterns of History Supporting Different Diagnoses

	Family History	Developmental history	School history
RD	Yes	Problems with speech, letter names, color names	Problems with reading, spelling, dictation
LI	Yes	Late talker, low vocabulary, syntax errors	Poor language comprehension
SSD	Yes	Unclear speech	Can be OK
ADHD	Yes	Active, accident-prone	Problems with seatwork and homework
ID	Yes–no	Motor, speech, and adaptive behavior delays	Problems with all subjects
ASD	Yes	Social and language delays	Problems with peer relations

TABLE 5.2. Patterns of Test Results That Support Different Diagnoses

	RD	LI	SSD	ADHD	ID	ASD
Crystallized intelligence	+	–	+	+	–	–
Fluid intelligence	+	+/–	+	+	–	–
Processing Speed	–	–	+	–	–	–
Reading						
Word recognition	–	–	+	+	+/–	+/–
Phonological coding	–	–	+	+	+/–	+/–
Fluency	–	–	+	+	+/–	+/–
Comprehension	+/–	–	+	+/–	–	–
Oral language						
Semantics	+	–	+	+	–	–
Syntax	+	–	+	+	–	–
Phonological awareness	–	–	–	+	+/–	+/–
Verbal working memory	–	–	–	+/–	–	+
Executive functions						
Inhibition	+	+/–	+	–	–	+
Generating	+	+/–	+	–	–	–
Set shifting	+	+/–	+	+/–	–	–
Sustained attention	+	+/–	+	–	–	–
Visual–spatial skills	+	+	+	+	–	+
Social and communication skills	+	+/–	+	+/–	–	–

Note. +, intact; –, impaired.

sents an individual client; instead, each is a composite reflecting the typical presentation of clients with a certain disorder. Because I wanted to stay as close as possible to our experience in clinical settings, these cases are not "pure" or simplified. Rather, they illustrate the difficulties of differential diagnosis, particularly when there is comorbidity or considerable variability within a diagnostic category.

Each of the case studies includes a history, test results, and an integrated discussion. The test results correspond closely to the cognitive constructs listed in Table 5.2. Although at our clinic we employ a flexible testing battery that is responsive to the presentation of each client and each referral question, in practice the testing battery often looks similar across clients, because we have found certain tests very useful for particular cognitive and academic domains. I provide further information about the tests included in the clinical case studies in Appendix C. Nevertheless, there are many available tests that could accomplish similar goals. As long as a test has adequate reliability and validity, we consider the particular test employed to be less important than the cognitive construct that is being measured. Therefore, I organize the test results by construct, in order to highlight points of convergence and divergence that would be expected for the profile of a particular disorder as depicted in Table 5.2. In the discussion of each case, I integrate the information from the history and the test results, consider different hypotheses, and provide a rationale for the diagnosis or diagnoses selected.

PART II
REVIEWS OF DISORDERS

CHAPTER 6

Dyslexia

WITH ROBIN L. PETERSON AND LAUREN M. MCGRATH

Three main types of abnormal language development are discussed in this chapter and Chapter 7: (1) developmental dyslexia or reading disability (RD), in which the defining problems are in written rather than spoken language; (2) speech sound disorder (SSD), in which the defining problem lies in the development of speech production; and (3) language impairment (LI), in which the defining problem is in the expression and/or comprehension of spoken language. There are proposed subtypes of each of these three broad types, but the external validity of these subtypes is still an open issue, as we will see. At the same time, these three disorders are comorbid and share etiological risk factors, so we may be able to collapse across the broad types to some extent. For instance, many children with SSD also have LI and later develop RD. Do such children have three distinct disorders, or are all three disorders different manifestations of the same neuropsychological deficits and underlying etiology? Although we do not yet have complete answers to these questions, relevant evidence is reviewed in these two chapters.

Robin L. Peterson, earned her BA in 1998 from Harvard University and worked as an elementary school teacher before entering the Child Clinical and Developmental Cognitive Neuroscience Programs at the University of Denver, where she is currently a fifth-year graduate student. Her research focuses on speech, language, and literacy disorders.

Lauren M. McGrath, earned her BS in 2001 from Brandeis University and worked as a research assistant for Helen Tager-Flusberg, doing autism research before entering the Child Clinical Psychology and Developmental Cognitive Neuroscience Programs at the University of Denver. She is currently completing a predoctoral clinical internship in the department of psychiatry at the University of Illinois at Chicago. Her research focuses on gene × environment interactions in speech and reading disorders.

HISTORY

Dyslexia or RD was first described over 100 years ago by Pringle-Morton (1896) and Kerr (1897), but real advances in our understanding of its cognitive phenotype have only come in the last 25 years. These advances have made it much clearer that dyslexia is a type of language disorder, and that one of its underlying neuropsychological deficits is faulty development of phonological representations. Earlier theories of dyslexia postulated a basic deficit in visual processing. These theories focused on the reversal errors made by individuals with dyslexia, such as writing "b" for "d" or "was" for "saw." Orton (1925, 1937) termed this deficit "strephosymbolia," which means "twisted symbols," and hypothesized that this visual problem arose because of a failure of hemispheric dominance. According to Orton's hypothesis, mirror images of a visual stimulus in the typically nondominant right hemisphere were not inhibited, thus leading to reversal errors. Vellutino (1979) demonstrated that such reversal errors in dyslexia were restricted to processing print in one's own language, and were thus really linguistic rather than visual in nature. However, it is still possible that other sorts of visual processing problems may be correlated with dyslexia.

DEFINITION AND EPIDEMIOLOGY

Children with RD have difficulties with accurate and/or fluent word recognition. The current definition of RD has two parts: (1) a diagnostic threshold; and (2) a list of exclusionary conditions, which usually include a peripheral sensory impairment (e.g., deafness), acquired neurological insults, environmental deprivation, and other more severe developmental disorders (e.g., intellectual disability [ID] and autism spectrum disorder [ASD]). Setting a diagnostic threshold for RD on what is essentially a continuum is inevitably somewhat arbitrary. A further issue is whether the diagnostic threshold should be relative to age or IQ expectations for the particular ability involved.

Traditional definitions of RD have required that the reading deficits be significantly below the child's IQ level. This means that many children with reading problems will not fit the definition, even though their reading is significantly below age expectations, and even though these problems are interfering with everyday functioning. Besides excluding some children from services, IQ discrepancy definitions face a fundamental logical problem. Measures of IQ, even nonverbal IQ, are moderately correlated with measures of both reading and language, but we do not fully understand the causal basis of this correlation. IQ could influence reading and language development, or reading and language development could influence IQ, or all three could be related to a third variable. As an example of a potential third variable, certain cognitive skills that are important for reading and language development, such as verbal short-term memory, are also part of what is measured by an IQ test. IQ discrepancy definitions assume that the causal basis of this correlation is that IQ influences reading and language development. According to this logic, children with lower IQs will inevitably have poor reading and language skills, and for a *different* reason (i.e., their low IQs) than children with higher IQs. But it is very likely that the other two possibilities are also involved in these correlations between reading and IQ. Reading and language skills are very likely to affect IQ scores, even nonverbal IQ scores, and these measures also share cognitive components. Therefore, children with age discrepancies but not IQ discrepancies may be the children with the most severe cases of RD, and they are likely to have the *same* underlying cognitive deficits as children who meet the IQ discrepancy definition. It seems ironic that a definition of a disorder should systematically exclude those with the most severe form of the disorder!

There is an emerging research literature on the external validity of the distinction between age and IQ discrepancy definitions of RD (see review in Fletcher, Foorman, Shaywitz, & Shaywitz, 1999). It is now broadly accepted that there is no evidence for the external validity for this distinction in terms of either the underlying deficits (i.e., in phonological processing) or the kinds of treatments that are helpful. So retaining this distinction seems hard to justify if the same treatments are efficacious for children with and without IQ discrepancies. At a practical level, children should be identified and treated for RD if they meet either definition. An IQ discrepancy approach is most useful for identifying children with above-average IQ scores and relatively weaker reading ability. Case Study 2 below provides an illustration of such an IQ-discrepant case. Although most of this child's reading scores fall in the average range, they are substantially weaker than would be predicted from her strong verbal IQ.

Both age and IQ discrepancy definitions face the problem that any particular threshold is arbitrary. However, both clinicians and researchers must regularly decide whether or not a particular individual meets criteria for RD. A reasonable age-based criterion for dyslexia requires an age-based standardized score of 80 or lower, which represents a 1.3 standard deviation (SD) cutoff, and identifies approximately 9% of the population. By this definition, an average of 2.5 children will meet criteria for dyslexia in an elementary school classroom with 28 students.

IQ-based cutoffs are based on an individual's expected reading score, which in turn depends on the strength of the relationship between IQ and reading. Since the correlation is not perfect, predicted reading scores regress toward the population mean. Many standardized tests of reading correlate with IQ measures at approximately 0.6. Thus, while an IQ of 100 gives a predicted reading score of 100, an IQ of 130 gives a predicted reading score of 118, and an IQ of 70 gives a predicted reading score of 82. The chosen discrepancy can then be subtracted from the predicted reading score to determine whether or not a child meets an IQ discrepancy definition. If a discrepancy of at least 20 standardized score points (again, 1.3 SD) is required, then a child with an IQ of 100 would still qualify for dyslexia based on a reading score of 80 or lower, while a child with an IQ of 130 would need a reading score of 98 or lower, and a child with an IQ of 70 would require a reading score no better than 62.

Comorbidities

Population-based studies have found a slight male predominance for RD (approximately 1.5:1) (Flannery, Liederman, Daly, & Schultz, 2000; Shaywitz, Shaywitz, Fletcher, & Escobar, 1990; Smith, Gilger, & Pennington, 2001). However, the male–female difference is even higher in referred samples, ranging from about 3:1 to 6:1 (Smith et al., 2001). The difference in gender ratios between epidemiological and referred samples indicates that girls with RD are less likely to be referred for services. The reason for this differential rate of referral appears to be higher rates of comorbid externalizing disorders (attention-deficit/hyperactivity disorder [ADHD], oppositional defiant disorder, and conduct disorder) in boys with RD, whereas girls with RD are more likely to have comorbid internalizing disorders, such as dysthymia. We (Willcutt & Pennington, 2000) found in our population-based sample that the overall male–female ratio was 1.3:1, similar to that in other epidemiological samples. However, among subjects with RD and a comorbid externalizing disorder, the male predominance was twice as great (2.6:1), and in the range found in referred samples. So it appears that girls with RD are less likely to be referred for services because they have lower rates of comorbid externalizing disorders.

Clearly, besides the comorbidities with SSD and LI mentioned earlier, RD is also comorbid with externalizing and internalizing disorders. We (Willcutt & Pennington, 2000) found that the presence of ADHD accounted for the other externalizing comorbidities of RD (i.e., conduct disorder and oppositional defiant disorder). Boetsch (1996) found in a longitudinal study of children at family risk for RD that an increased rate of ADHD was already evident in the at-risk children before kindergarten, whereas dysthymia only emerged after the beginning of reading instruction. So it appears that internalizing symptoms in RD are secondary to the stress and frustration of reading problems, but that ADHD is not a secondary comorbidity. Other research in our lab has shown that RD and ADHD share both cognitive and genetic risk factors (Pennington et al., 2005).

ETIOLOGY[1]

Dyslexia is an interesting example of the intersection between an evolved behavior (language) and a cultural invention (literacy). Although there cannot be genes for relatively recent cultural inventions (e.g., chess, banking, and football), there can be genetic influences on evolved cognitive and behavioral traits necessary for proficiency in such cultural inventions. Because there is now extensive evidence of genetic influences in individual differences on most domains of cognition and behavior, it is not surprising that there are genetic influences on reading and spelling skills.

In the last two decades, our understanding of the etiology of dyslexia has increased considerably, due to advances in both behavioral and molecular genetics. For 50 years after it was first described by Kerr (1897) and Pringle-Morgan (1896), evidence for recurrence in families was repeatedly documented in case reports, leading Hallgren (1950) to undertake a more formal genetic epidemiological study of a large sample of families. Besides conducting the first test of the mode of transmission, his comprehensive monograph also documented several characteristics of dyslexia that have recently been rediscovered: (1) As noted above, the male–female ratio is nearly equal (Shaywitz et al., 1990; Wadsworth, DeFries, Stevenson, Gilger, & Pennington, 1992); and (2) there is not a significant association between dyslexia and left-handedness (Pennington, Smith, Kimberling, Green, & Haith, 1987). Hallgren also documented that dyslexia co-occurs with other language disorders.

Familiality

Although Hallgren and his predecessors provided considerable evidence that dyslexia is familial, all of this evidence came from referred samples. Modern family studies using epidemiological samples have confirmed the familiality of RD (Gilger, Pennington, & DeFries, 1991). Roughly between 30% and 50% of the children of a parent with RD will develop RD—a relative risk roughly four to eight times that found in controls (Gilger et al., 1991; Pennington & Lefly, 2001). It has taken modern twin studies to demonstrate that this familiality is substantially genetic, and modern linkage studies to actually begin locating the genes involved. Unlike the situation in Hallgren's time, we now have very strong, converging evidence that dyslexia is both familial and heritable (see DeFries & Gillis, 1993, for a review). We can also reject the hypotheses of classic X-linked or simple recessive autosomal transmission, at least in the vast majority of cases.

Hallgren (1950) found evidence for autosomal dominant transmission of dyslexia, as we did (Pennington et al., 1991). In the latter study,

---

[1] For a description of genetic technical terms, see Box 1.1 in Chapter 1.

we performed segregation analysis on four large family samples, and found sex-influenced major locus (additive or dominant) transmission in three of the four samples. However, we now know that there are multiple genetic loci linked to dyslexia, and that the environment influences how heritable dyslexia is (a gene × environment [G × E] interaction that will be discussed later). Consequently, dyslexia, like virtually all complex behavioral disorders, is currently conceptualized as having a multifactorial etiology in which there are multiple genetic and environmental risk factors involved.

Candidate Genes

The cognitive dissection of dyslexia described below proceeded hand in hand with decades of work demonstrating that dyslexia and its cognitive components are familial and heritable (Pennington & Olson, 2005), and are linked to several quantitative trait loci (QTLs) across the genome (Fisher & DeFries, 2002). Seven replicated QTLs have been identified on chromosomes 1p36–p34 (DYX8), 2p16–p15 (DYX3), 3p12–q13 (DYX5), 6p22 (DYX2), 15q21 (DYX1), 18p11 (DYX6), and Xq27.3 (DYX9) (Table 6.1).

Two additional genetic loci for dyslexia are included on the most recent Human Gene Nomenclature Committee list (*www.gene.ucl.ac.uk/nomenclature*). These are on 6q13–q16 (DYX4; Petryshen et al., 2001), and 11p15 (DYX7; Hsiung, Kaplan, Petryshen, Lu, & Field, 2004). So there are currently nine genetic risk loci, but two of these need additional replication to be convincing.

This linkage work has now been followed by the initial identification of four candidate genes in three of these linkage regions: 3p12–q13 (ROBO1), 6p22 (DCDC2 and KIAA0319), and 15q21 (DYX1C1, initially labeled as EKN1). These candidate gene studies are reviewed elsewhere (Fisher & Francks, 2006; McGrath et al., 2006). The identification of candidate genes is a rapidly progressing area of research in dyslexia, so additional candidate genes are likely.

The first candidate gene to be identified was DYX1C1, so it has been the target of the most replication attempts, six so far (Bellini et al., 2005; Cope et al., 2005b; Marino et al., 2005; Meng et al., 2005a; Scerri et al., 2004; Taipale et al., 2003; Wigg et al., 2004). Five of these failed to find any association between DYX1C1 variants and dyslexia phenotypes, but the study by Wigg et al. (2004) found an association in the opposite direction, such that the more common, nonrisk alleles of the haplotypes proposed by Taipale et al. (2003) were associated with the dyslexia phenotype. They also found a significant association with an additional single-nucleotide polymorphism that was not tested by Taipale et al. (2003). So more work is needed to confirm or reject this candidate gene.

TABLE 6.1. Linkage and Association Studies for Replicated Linkage Peaks

Linkage regions	Supportive results	Negative results
1p36–p34 (DYX8)	Rabin et al. (1993) Grigorenko et al. (2001) Tzenova et al. (2004)	
2p16–p15 (DYX3)	Fagerheim et al. (1999) Fisher et al. (2002) Francks et al. (2002) Petryshen et al. (2002) Kaminen et al. (2003) Peyrard-Janvid et al. (2004)	Chapman et al. (2004)
3p12–q13 (DYX5)	Nopola-Hemmi et al. (2001) Fisher et al. (2002)	
6p22.2 (DYX2)	Smith et al. (1991) Cardon et al. (1994, 1995) Grigorenko et al. (1997) Fisher et al. (1999) Gayán et al. (1999) Grigorenko et al. (2000) Fisher et al. (2002) Kaplan et al. (2002) Turic et al. (2003) Marlow et al. (2003) Grigorenko et al. (2003)	Field & Kaplan (1998) Nöthen et al. (1999) Petryshen et al. (2000) Chapman et al. (2004)
15q15–q21 (DYX1)	Smith et al. (1983) Smith et al. (1991) Fulker et al. (1991) Grigorenko et al. (1997) Nöthen et al. (1999) Nopola-Hemmi et al. (2000) Morris et al. (2000) Chapman et al. (2004)	Rabin et al. (1993) Bisgaard et al. (1987)
18p11.2 (DYX6)	Fisher et al. (2002) Marlow et al. (2003)	Chapman et al. (2004) Schumacher et al. (2006)
Xq27.3 (DYX9)	Fisher et al. (2002) de Kovel et al. (2004)	

Note From McGrath, Smith, and Pennington (2006). Copyright 2006 by Elsevier Limited. Reprinted by permission. See original article for references.

The other three candidate genes, ROBO1 (Hannula-Jouppi et al., 2005), DCDC2 (Francks et al., 2004; Meng et al., 2005b), and KIAA0319 (Francks et al., 2004), were identified more recently and thus have been tested less for replication. Nevertheless, both DCDC2 (Schumacher et al., 2006) and KIAA0319 (Cope et al., 2005a; Harold et al., 2006) have been replicated.

One of the most exciting aspects of the work on the four recent candidate genes is that the role of each in brain development has been studied in animal models. Joseph LoTurco (using RNA interference technology) found that shutting down the expression of DCDC2 (Meng et al., 2005b), KIAA0319 (Paracchini et al., 2006), and DXY1C1 (Rosen et al., 2007; Threlkeld et al., 2007; Wang et al., 2006) interferes with neuronal migration. These findings are consistent with the pioneering work of Galaburda, Sherman, Rosen, Aboitiz, and Geschwind (1985), who discovered ectopias (neurons that did not migrate properly during brain development) in the brains of deceased individuals with dyslexia. The remaining candidate gene for dyslexia, ROBO1, is known to be involved in brain development, specifically in axon path finding. Andrews et al. (2006) genetically modified mice so that they were lacking ROBO1 completely (a ROBO1 knockout). Although the knockout mice died at birth, they demonstrated prenatal axonal tract defects and neuronal migration defects in the forebrain.

These results from animal models indicate that alterations in DCDC2, KIAA0319, ROBO1, and DYX1C1 could disrupt human brain development in a way that is consistent with what little is known about the neuropathology of dyslexia. But really proving causation will require several more steps: (1) The functional and/or regulatory mutations in these particular genes have to be identified; (2) it has to be demonstrated that these particular mutations disrupt brain development in animal models; and, most difficult of all, (3) it has to be shown that humans with dyslexia and these mutations have similar disruptions in brain development. In sum, the identification of candidate genes for dyslexia has taken us all the way from cognitive dissection to developmental neurobiology, so that we are now able to test specific hypotheses about how brain development is disrupted in this prevalent disorder. This work is now developing rapidly, so new insights about brain development in dyslexia are likely.

BRAIN MECHANISMS[2]

As stressed throughout this chapter, reading builds on earlier-developing language skills, and RD is a kind of language disorder. Therefore, the neural networks serving reading in the brain are very likely to include networks

---

[2] For a description of neuroanatomical technical terms, see Box 1.2 in Chapter 1.

that serve spoken language, plus some extra components to deal with the fact that printed language is processed visually by a sighted person. It would be much less parsimonious for the brain to develop an entirely separate system for reading printed text. The second theoretical constraint on the neural basis of reading is that it cannot be innate, but instead must be a product of learning, because reading is culturally transmitted. So learning to read must change the structure of the brain, at least at the level of synapses, and also must change brain function.

So we should seek the neural correlates of normal and abnormal reading in (1) language areas of the brain; (2) visual areas necessary for processing printed words; and (3) pathways connecting all these areas, whose connections will change as the skill of reading is learned. As we will see, what has been found in structural and functional neuroimaging studies of typical reading and RD generally fits these broad theoretical expectations, but also provides some surprises.

Structural Studies

Galaburda and colleagues (Galaburda, Menard, & Rosen, 1994; Galaburda et al., 1985; Humphreys, Kaufmann, & Galaburda, 1990; Livingstone, Rosen, Drislane, & Galaburda, 1991) conducted an influential set of autopsy studies of a small number of brains of people with RD. They found symmetry differences in the planum temporale (the posterior portion of the superior temporal gyrus, which overlaps in the left hemisphere with Wernicke's area), histological anomalies (e.g., ectopias) consistent with failure of neuronal migration, and structural differences in the magnocellular portion of the thalamus. Structural magnetic resonance imaging (MRI) studies have failed to replicate the planum temporale findings (Best & Demb, 1999; Eckert et al., 2003; Haaga, Dyck, & Ernst, 1991; Heiervang et al., 2000; Hugdahl et al., 2003; Robichon, Levrier, Farnarier, & Habib, 2000; Rumsey et al., 1997a; Schultz et al., 1994), but the evidence for abnormal neuronal migration is consistent with the function of the candidate genes for RD reviewed earlier.

Structural MRI studies of RD have also found replicated differences in perisylvian language areas. These include various portions of the temporal lobes, including the insula (Badian, 1997; Brambati et al., 2004; Brown et al., 2001; Eliez et al., 2000; Hynd, Semrud-Clikeman, Lorys, Novey, & Eliopulos, 1990; Pennington et al., 1999; Vinckenbosch, Robichon, & Eliez, 2005); the inferior frontal gyrus (IFG; Brown et al., 2001; Eckert et al., 2003); and two language-related parietal lobe structures, the supramarginal gyrus (Eckert et al., 2005) and parietal operculum (Robichon et al., 2000). These findings support our theoretical expectation that language areas will differ in RD.

But there have been surprises as well, most notably reductions in cerebellar volumes (Eckert et al., 2003; Leonard et al., 2001; Rae et al., 2002).

Several research groups have also found reductions in total cerebral volume in RD, even after controlling for IQ (Casanova, Araque, Giedd, & Rumsey, 2004; Eckert et al., 2003; Phinney, Pennington, Olson, Filley, & Filipek, 2007), although such reductions have not been found by some investigators (e.g., Vinckenbosch et al., 2005). The theoretical significance of the cerebellar and total cerebral volume findings are not as clear as the findings in perisylvian language areas.

Researchers have only recently begun to examine how white matter connections among brain regions vary as a function of reading skill. These studies utilized diffusion tensor imaging (DTI), which measures white matter pathways. Both Klingberg et al. (2000) and Deutsch et al. (2005) found bilateral white matter disturbances in temporoparietal regions in groups with RD. It remains possible that these white matter differences are a result of reading less rather than a cause of RD—a possibility that applies to many of the structural findings reviewed here (but not to the ectopias found by Galaburda and colleagues, since neuronal migration occurs prenatally).

In sum, structural results for RD fit two of our broad theoretical expectations—that language areas will be involved, and that connections between areas (in white matter) may play a role—but they do not address the third one. That is, structural studies have not clearly identified a part of the visual cortex that differs in RD. As we will see next, functional neuroimaging studies have identified such a structure.

Functional Findings

Numerous investigators have attempted to elucidate the neural bases of RD further by examining brain function during reading and language tasks, using positron emission tomography (PET) and functional MRI (fMRI). This literature has been marked by many of the same methodological concerns as the anatomical literature (e.g., different definitions of both RD and of various brain regions). Interpretation of functional results is further limited in studies that use a case–control design but do not equate performance across the two groups (see Price & McCrory, 2005). In these cases, it is not clear whether the neural differences are a cause or a result of impaired performance.

Functional neuroimaging studies of reading and language tasks have identified aberrant activation patterns in participants with RD across a distributed set of left-hemisphere sites, including many of the same regions implicated by the anatomical literature. The most common findings have been reduced activation of left occipitotemporal (Badian, 1997; Brunswick, McCrory, Price, Frith, & Frith, 1999; Paulesu et al., 2001; Rumsey et al., 1997b; Shaywitz et al., 2003) and temporoparietal (Shaywitz et al., 2002, 2003; Temple et al., 2001) regions. Findings in the region of the left IFG have been mixed, with several studies reporting increased activation in RD

(Brunswick et al., 1999; Shaywitz et al., 1998; Temple et al., 2001), while others have reported decreased activation (Aylward et al., 2003; Corina et al., 2001; Georgiewa et al., 1999). Both task and participant characteristics have probably contributed to the difference in findings. Increased IFG activity in RD has most often emerged in the context of reading aloud (Price & McCrory, 2005). In silent reading or other language tasks, decreased activity in this region is more likely among the most impaired readers (Shaywitz et al., 2003). A common interpretation of the full pattern of results is that decreased occipitotemporal activity corresponds to deficits in word recognition processes; decreased temporoparietal activity corresponds to phonological processing difficulties; and increased IFG activity relates to compensatory processes. Notably, very few studies have equated performance across groups of participants with RD and controls. This limitation particularly complicates the interpretation of temporoparietal findings, which (to date) have emerged only in the context of group performance differences (Price & McCrory, 2005).

Some authors have argued that the left occipitotemporal region includes a "visual word form area" (McCandliss, Cohen, & Dehaene, 2003) that is specifically responsible for orthographic processing of words. This interpretation would be consistent with the close proximity of this region to other occipitotemporal structures that mediate expertise in recognition of visual objects, such as faces (i.e., the fusiform face area). These occipitotemporal structures are part of the ventral stream of visual processing, sometimes called the "what" pathway because the ventral stream mediates visual object identification (in contrast to the dorsal "where" pathway). Supporting this visual object expertise view is the fact that functional activity during reading in this visual word form area only emerges later in reading development in typical readers (and after remediation in readers with RD).

However, we can ask whether it is only *visual* word forms that activate this area, or whether its expertise is exclusive to reading. Some neuroimaging studies of reading have found that this area is more activated by pseudowords than by unpronounceable letter strings (see McCandliss et al., 2003), so the processing in this region cannot be exclusively lexical and instead generalizes to pronounceable letter strings. Other evidence suggests that this area phonologically recodes the "visual" word form (Sandak et al., 2004).

A PET study (see McCrory, Mechelli, Frith, & Price, 2005) tested whether aberrant activation of this region in RD is specific to word reading. The authors compared adults with RD and controls on both a picture-naming task and a word-reading task. Behavioral performance was comparable across the two groups. The participants with RD exhibited reduced left occipitotemporal activation for both tasks; furthermore, there was no group × task interaction. The authors concluded that the left occipitotemporal area is important in the integration of visual and phonological information, and that this process is impaired in RD. Given the relative recency of written language, it is unsurprising that the neural basis for reading in general, and impaired reading in particular, would relate to more general cognitive processes.

Consistent with the anatomical literature, some studies of RD have also reported activation differences in the cerebellum. For example, Brunswick et al. (1999) found that, compared to controls, adults with RD underactivated the cerebellum bilaterally during reading tasks. Another study by the same research group (McCrory, Frith, Brunswick, & Price, 2000) reported that participants with RD exhibited reduced activity in the left cerebellum during a word repetition task. These findings make sense in light of the growing appreciation for the cerebellum's importance in a wide variety of cognitive processes, including language (e.g., Schmahmann & Caplan, 2006). However, the precise role of the cerebellum in RD, including the specific regions that are implicated, is not yet well understood.

Exciting new research is using fMRI to investigate the neural correlates of improved performance following treatment for RD (Aylward et al., 2003; Richards et al., 2006; Shaywitz et al., 2004; Temple et al., 2003). In general, these studies have reported that successful behavioral treatment correlates with a normalization of brain activation patterns, such that participants with RD begin to resemble controls more closely.

The Shaywitz et al. (2004) study particularly merits discussion because it had the largest sample size and longest follow-up time, and in-scanner performance was comparable across groups. The study compared three groups of 6- to 9-year-old children: participants with RD receiving an intensive, year-long experimental treatment; participants with RD receiving standard community intervention; and controls. The experimental treatment was significantly more effective than the community treatment in promoting reading fluency. Brain activation was measured during a letter identification task. Following treatment, the experimental group but not the community group demonstrated increased activation in a number of left-hemisphere sites, including the IFG and the posterior middle temporal gyrus. Importantly, the control group showed similar activation changes to the experimental group, and previous work demonstrated that left IFG activation correlates positively with age in reading-related tasks (Shaywitz et al., 2002). Thus these results suggest that in the absence of successful treatment, the community group did not exhibit normal age-related changes in brain activity.

Summary

In summary, RD is associated with differences across multiple brain regions. The most consistent evidence points to aberrant structure and function of left-hemisphere networks important to reading and language, some of which are involved in oral language apart from reading, and some of which learn to map visual words onto the language system (i.e., the visual word form area). Furthermore, correlational and treatment studies indicate that these brain differences have meaningful behavioral consequences. However, these regions do not appear to tell the whole story in RD. The cerebellum is one structure likely to be fruitful for future research, since it has been implicated by histological, structural, and functional studies, but its role in RD is not yet well understood. One proposal is that it is related to automaticity in reading (Nicolson & Fawcett, 1990). Another important direction for future work will be to continue to investigate the connections among the brain regions involved in RD. The recent application of DTI to RD research (e.g., Deutsch et al., 2005; Klingberg et al., 2000) holds promise for addressing this question. Because reading is a culturally transmitted skill, and reading proficiency requires extensive training and practice, we must expect that learning to read changes the brain; therefore, an important challenge for neuroimaging studies of RD will be to distinguish differences in brain structure and function that cause later RD from those that result from RD because of reduced practice and expertise in reading.

NEUROPSYCHOLOGY

Cognitive Findings

As shown in Table 5.2, RD has a fairly consistent cognitive phenotype, and cognitive testing is a necessary part of the diagnosis of RD. As will be reviewed below, most children with RD have a core phonological deficit, but this single deficit is not sufficient to account for all cases of RD. As will be discussed later, other deficits, in language and processing speed, are needed in a multiple-deficit model of RD.

Among complex behavioral disorders, dyslexia is unusual because it is so well defined at the cognitive level of analysis. We understand both the typical and atypical development of reading much better than we understand the typical and atypical development of other domains (e.g., emotion regulation) that are relevant for psychopathologies (Pennington, 2002). The cognitive analysis of dyslexia has provided us both with a fairly precise diagnostic phenotype and with cognitive components of that diagnostic phenotype. These cognitive components have proved useful as endophenotypes in genetic and neuroimaging studies of dyslexia and typical reading (discussed earlier).

Since the goal of reading is reading comprehension, we begin our cognitive analysis with the components of reading comprehension (Figure 6.1). This figure shows that reading comprehension can be first broken down into cognitive components and then into developmental precursors of these cognitive components. One key component is fluent printed word recognition, which is highly predictive of reading comprehension, especially in the early years of reading instruction (Curtis, 1980). The other key component is listening comprehension—that is, *oral* language comprehension. Hoover and Gough (1990) proposed a simple model of skill in reading comprehension in which there are only these two components of reading comprehension: fluent printed word recognition and listening comprehension. Figure 6.1 adds a third component, discourse-specific comprehension skills, to this simple model because understanding a text (or lecture) requires greater use of other comprehension skills (e.g., inferencing, monitoring comprehension, and building a mental representation of the meaning of the text) than does conversational speech or reading single sentences.

Because fluent printed word recognition is necessary (but not sufficient) for reading comprehension, the field of dyslexia research long ago made a key simplifying assumption. That is, it defined dyslexia as problems in printed word recognition rather than as problems in reading comprehension. Consequently, reading comprehension problems without a word recognition problem are not counted as dyslexia. Instead, individuals with such problems are called "poor comprehenders." and the cognitive causes of their reading comprehension problems are considered to be distinct from those that interfere with word recognition (Nation, 2005).

As we will see later, although this simplifying assumption is valid, individuals with dyslexia as a group have oral as well as written language problems. For instance, more recent research (e.g., Keenan, Betjemann, Wadsworth, DeFries, & Olson, 2006) has found that dyslexic individuals as a group also have problems with *oral* language comprehension, not just reading comprehension. Nevertheless, because this assumption greatly simpli-

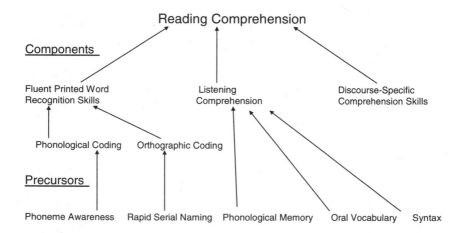

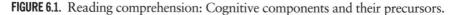

FIGURE 6.1. Reading comprehension: Cognitive components and their precursors.

fied the cognitive analysis of dyslexia, it eventually led to the major genetic breakthroughs described earlier. The analogy in psychiatry would be that instead of taking on the entire syndrome of schizophrenia or major depression, cognitive neuroscientists should tackle one key feature, understand its development thoroughly at a cognitive level, and then use that feature and its cognitive components in genetic studies. Then, as the features are understood, they can be recombined into appropriate syndromes based on a common genetic etiology.

So the diagnostic phenotype in dyslexia is an idiopathic deficit in the speed and accuracy of printed word recognition. "Deficit" is usually defined relative to age norms, although IQ discrepancy definitions are also used, and "idiopathic" means that the reading deficit cannot be explained by an uncorrected hearing or visual problem, inadequate reading instruction, an acquired neurological insult, or ID.

Printed word recognition can be broken into two component written language skills: phonological and orthographic coding (see Figure 6.1). "Phonological coding" refers to the ability to use knowledge of rule-like letter–sound correspondences to pronounce words that have never been seen before (usually measured by pseudoword reading), and "orthographic coding" refers to the use of word-specific patterns to aid in word recognition and pronunciation (see Harm & Seidenberg, 2004, for a neural network model of reading that implements both phonological and orthographic coding). Words that do not follow typical letter–sound correspondences (e.g., "have" or "yacht") must rely, at least in part, on orthographic coding to be recognized, as do homophones (e.g., "rows" vs. "rose"). So phonological coding and orthographic coding are essentially two endophenotypes of dyslexia. It has been established that dyslexia is characterized by deficits in both types of coding, and that such deficits are coheritable with dyslexia (Gayan & Olson, 2001) and linked to dyslexia genetic loci (Table 6.1).

But the cognitive analysis of dyslexia doesn't end with phonological and orthographic coding. Because reading development depends on earlier development of spoken language, dyslexia researchers have investigated the oral language precursors of reading skill and disability. These precursors include phonological awareness and rapid serial naming, but also broader language skill (Figure 6.1). Phonological awareness is measured by tasks that require a child to manipulate the sound structure of spoken words (e.g., "What is 'cat' without the /k/?"). Tasks that require the manipulation of individual phonemes (phoneme awareness), as opposed to syllables, are most highly linked to reading skill. Rapid serial naming is assessed by presenting the child a card with rows of color patches or familiar objects and asking him or her to name each item in each row as rapidly as possible. Broader language skill is measured by tests of vocabulary and syntax. On average, predyslexic children have deficits on all these precursors to reading skill (Pennington & Lefly, 2001; Scarborough, 1990), and these deficits are likewise coheritable with dyslexia (Gayan & Olson, 2001) and linked to dyslexia genetic loci (see Table 6.1; Fisher & DeFries, 2002). So these precursors qualify as endophenotypes for dyslexia, although they are not exclusively related to dyslexia, since children with SSD also have problems with phoneme awareness, as is discussed later, and children with ADHD have problems with rapid serial naming and other processing speed measures.

Despite agreement about the importance of phoneme awareness deficits in RD, there is disagreement about whether or not these difficulties are themselves caused by lower-level processing deficits. Phoneme awareness is a complex metalinguistic skill that clearly involves multiple components. One argument is that phoneme awareness deficits arise from impaired phonological representations (Fowler, 1991; Swan & Goswami, 1997a, 1997b). Another argument postulates that the central deficit is not specific to language, but occurs at a lower level of auditory processing (Tallal, 1980). This hypothesis will be discussed later.

Our view is that the most parsimonious explanation for current data is that deficits in phonological representations lead to both phoneme awareness and phonological coding difficulties in RD. An important caveat is that the relationship between phoneme awareness and reading is bidirectional, so that over time, poor reading also causes poor phoneme awareness (Morais, Cary, Alegria, & Bertelson, 1979; Perfetti, Beck, Bell, & Hughes, 1987; Wagner, Torgesen, & Rashotte, 1994). Although some lower-level sensory problems are correlated with RD, there is not much evidence for a causal relationship. We now briefly review the evidence for the phonological representations hypothesis.

The phonological representations hypothesis is appealing because it helps explain why RD is associated not only with deficits in phoneme awareness, but also with impairments on a wide variety of phonological tasks, including phonological memory (Byrne & Shea, 1979; Shankweiler, Liberman, Mark, Fowler, & Fischer, 1979), confrontational naming (Fowler & Swainson, 2004; Swan & Goswami, 1997b), and rapid naming (Bowers & Wolf, 1993; Denckla & Rudel, 1976)—though there is debate as to whether rapid naming tasks are best conceptualized as phonological (see Vellutino, Fletcher, Snowling, & Scanlong, 2004, for a discussion). It is important to note that these are all *oral* language tasks, buttressing the argument that RD is a language disorder. Researchers have proposed a number of ways in which phonological representations might be impaired. For example, the representations of individual phonemes may be somehow distorted (Harm & Seidenberg, 1999). An alternative proposal, the segmentation hypothesis (Bird & Bishop, 1992; Fowler, 1991; Metsala, 1997b), is concerned with the grain size of phonological representations. During language acquisition, typically developing children build increasingly fine-grained phonological representations, from the whole-word level to the level of the syllable and, eventually, the phoneme (Metsala, 1997a; Metsala & Walley, 1998; Walley, 1993). The segmentation hypothesis holds that RD results from a delay in this process. Because alphabetic languages require establishing mappings between phonemes and letters, phonological representations specified at the level of the demisyllable or the syllable would greatly complicate the task of learning to read.

A recent study in our laboratory (Boada & Pennington, 2006) compared 11- to 13-year-old children with RD to both age-matched and reading-level controls on tasks designed to be sensitive to the grain size of phonological representations. For example, a syllable similarity task provided a measure of whether children were more likely to confuse nonsense words that were similar in syllabic structure or that shared an initial phoneme. There is normal developmental change in this task; compared to adults, children, whose phonological representations are presumably less well segmented, are more likely to confuse words that share syllabic structure (Treiman & Breaux, 1982). Another task investigated whether participants' identification of a spoken word was aided by a very short prime that primarily carried initial phoneme information, versus a longer prime that carried more information about the whole first syllable. Finally, a gating task investigated whether groups differed in how much of a spoken word was needed to achieve word identification. Across all three tasks, the performance of participants with RD was consistent with the segmentation hypothesis. For example, in the priming task, participants with RD benefited from the longer prime as much as controls, but did not benefit from the shorter prime. These performance differences were evident in comparisons to both age-matched and reading-level controls; this suggested that they did not result solely from reduced exposure to print. Furthermore, results did not vary as a function of whether the participants with RD had a history of SSD or LI, so segmentation deficits are not just a result of comorbid speech or language problems.

Of course, language is a highly interconnected system (Bishop, 1997). Many children with phonological impairments might be expected to show difficulties with other aspects of language, such as semantics (word meanings) or syntax (grammar). In fact, on IQ tests, children with RD tend to underperform relative to their typically developing counterparts not only on phonological tasks, such as digit span, but on all verbal subtests (D'Angiulli & Siegel, 2003). Some of this performance deficit is likely to have resulted from RD, since children with reading difficulties have impoverished opportunities to learn from print (e.g., Stanovich, 1986—but see Scarborough & Parker, 2003); however, some may well reflect subtle, wide-ranging language difficulties. Nonverbal reasoning skills are relatively, but not absolutely, spared in RD. Children with RD tend to obtain lower nonverbal IQ scores than typically developing children, though the effect size is typically smaller than for verbal IQ (D'Angiulli & Siegel, 2003; Snowling, Gallagher, & Frith, 2003). This finding is unsurprising, given that in the population as a whole, verbal and nonverbal IQ scores are highly correlated (Sattler & Dumont, 2004).

In summary, RD is associated with performance deficits on a wide variety of phonological tasks, including tasks that do not require metalinguistic awareness. Evidence suggests that many of the deficits result from poorly segmented phonological representations. More severe cases of RD may additionally be complicated by distortions within the representations. Future longitudinal studies should attempt to establish that poorly segmented phonological representations cause the phonological coding deficits that are central to RD. Although RD-related impairments are most striking on phonological tasks, linguistic difficulties also extend to verbal conceptual measures.

However, despite the widespread support for the phonological model of RD, recent evidence raises the question of whether a phonological deficit is sufficient to cause RD. As discussed elsewhere (Pennington, 2006) and in Chapter 7, children with SSD have phonological deficits like those found in RD, but usually do not develop RD unless they have comorbid LI. It appears that their normal performance on rapid serial naming tasks (Raitano, Pennington, Tunick, Boada, & Shriberg, 2004) is a protective factor. Rapid serial naming, and processing speed more broadly, are impaired in both RD and ADHD (Shanahan et al., 2006), so processing speed appears to be a cognitive risk factor shared by RD and ADHD. We recently used structural equation modeling to test this hypothesis (Shanahan et al., 2007). We found that processing speed was a unique predictor of both RD and ADHD symptoms and reduced the correlation between them to a nonsignificant value. Phoneme awareness and language skill were unique predictors of RD symptoms, and inhibition was a unique predictor of ADHD symptoms. These results support a multiple-deficit model of both RD and ADHD. The total variance explained in RD symptoms by phoneme awareness, language skill, and PS was over 80%. So our best current understanding of the neuropsychology of RD is that at least three cognitive risk factors are involved.

Sensory–Motor Findings

An influential single-deficit theory of RD and LI (Tallal, 1980) holds that phonological impairments in RD arise from lower-level deficits in auditory processing that are not specific to language. This theory developed out of earlier work demonstrating auditory processing deficits in LI (Tallal & Percy, 1973a, 1975). Indeed, as a group, individuals with RD have demonstrated impaired performance on a variety of nonspeech auditory tasks (Farmer & Klein, 1995; Tallal, Miller, Jenkins, & Merzenich, 1997). Methodological concerns have been raised about this literature (Vellutino et al., 2004). Perhaps more importantly, the argument for causality is damaged by a case-by-case inspection of data, which has consistently revealed that many participants with RD do not have auditory deficits, while some control participants do (see Ramus, 2003, for a review). For example, Ramus et al. (2003) compared 16 participants with RD to 16 controls on an extensive battery of phonological, auditory, and other sensory–motor tasks. Although there was a mean group difference on the nonspeech auditory tasks, a minority of individual RD cases (approximately 6, or 38%) showed evidence of a deficit. This result contrasted with the phonological tasks, on which 100% of the participants with RD (and only 6% of the controls) were impaired.

The auditory processing hypothesis assumes that a low-level sensory deficit causes a higher-level linguistic deficit. However, it is also possible that linguistic deficits have top-down effects on audition. Longitudinal studies have generally failed to establish a connection between earlier auditory deficits and later reading problems (Heath & Hogben, 2004; Share, Jorm, Maclean, & Matthews, 2002). Similarly, Boets, Wouters, van Wieringen, and Ghesquiere (2006) compared preschoolers at high and low familial risk for later RD on a variety of low-level auditory tasks and did not find group differences. Instead, consistent with earlier studies (Pennington & Lefly, 2001; Scarborough, 1998), the high- and low-risk groups were distinguished by measures of phonological skill and letter knowledge.

Anatomical results from animal models are also more consistent with a top-down than with a bottom-up relationship between cognitive and sensory processing in RD (see Ramus, 2004, for a discussion). Galaburda and colleagues (Rosen, Press, Sherman, & Galaburda, 1992) have developed a rat model of RD that depends on induction of the kinds of cortical anomalies found in RD brains on postmortem examination (see discussion above). Although the rats obviously cannot demonstrate reading difficulties, they have shown evidence of learning deficits (Rosen, Waters, Galaburda, & Denenberg, 1995). Some of the rats with cortical damage later developed anomalies in the medial geniculate nucleus of the thalamus, which in turn impaired auditory processing (Herman, Galaburda, Fitch, Carter, & Rosen, 1997; Peiffer, Rosen, & Fitch, 2002). Of course, much more research would be needed to establish whether a similar phenomenon exists in humans. However, this work serves as a good reminder that while a bottom-up explanation often seems more intuitive, top-down processes are equally plausible.

There is a long history of theories positing a causal visual deficit in dyslexia (Hinshelwood, 1907; Orton, 1925, 1937; Pringle-Morgan, 1896). The most straightforward of these theories have long been discredited (Vellutino, 1979, 1987). However, participants with RD have shown reliable group deficits on certain low-level visual processing tasks, including motion perception and detection of low spatial frequencies (Badcock & Lovegrove, 1981; Eden et al., 1996; Martin & Lovegrove, 1984). Because such tasks specifically engage the magnocellular pathway of the visual system, these findings have led to a magnocellular theory of RD (Stein & Walsh, 1997). Further support for the theory comes from the autopsy findings discussed earlier, since thalamic abnormalities in RD brains were found in magnocellular layers of the lateral geniculate nucleus. As a causal hypothesis, this theory has faced some of the same challenges as the auditory theory.

Studies have generally found that many individual participants with RD do not have visual deficits, while some control participants do (Ramus, 2003; Vellutino et al., 2004). Furthermore, this theory lacks surface validity to explain the word recognition deficit in RD. The magnocellular system is responsible for large-scale visual tasks, such as detection of motion and rapid changes in the visual field. In contrast, the parvocellular system is responsible for fine, high-frequency discriminations (Gazzaniga, Ivry, & Magnun, 2002). Although it is conceivable that a magnocellular deficit could negatively affect the reading of connected text, it is not clear how such a deficit could influence single-word reading under central fixation (Hulme, 1988). And yet a deficit in reading single words is the defining symptom in RD!

Studies have also reported tactile deficits (Laasonen, Service, & Virsu, 2001; Stoodley, Talcott, Carter, Witton, & Stein, 2000) and motor skill deficits (Fawcett, Nicolson, & Dean, 1996; Nicolson & Fawcett, 1990; Ramus, 2003) in some participants with RD. The magnocellular theory has been proposed as an overarching explanation for these diverse findings, since there are magnocellular pathways within every sensory modality, and because the cerebellum receives massive magnocellular input (Stein, 2001). As discussed above, such a theory cannot account for all cases of RD, and probably not even for the majority of cases. Thus one interpretation is that RD sometimes co-occurs with more general sensory–motor difficulties that are not the cause of the central phonological coding deficit (Hulslander et al., 2004; Ramus, 2003).

Given some of the brain findings discussed earlier (i.e., reduced cerebral volume, widespread neural differences), it is not surprising that RD might be associated with a variety of symptoms. Extrapolating from the rat model, Ramus (2004) has advanced a specific brain-based hypothesis for why a sensory–motor syndrome should sometimes, but not always, accompany RD. In rats, cortical disruption only sometimes leads to thalamic abnormalities, with the likelihood being moderated by the presence of fetal testosterone (Rosen, Herman, & Galaburda, 1999). Ramus has suggested that RD results from phonological impairments caused by cortical damage, and that under certain hormonal conditions, the cortical damage also leads to thalamic damage, which in turn causes the sensory–motor syndrome. This is an intriguing hypothesis that merits future research.

As noted earlier, individuals with dyslexia as a group have problems with oral language comprehension. This result might be expected, given that they have been shown to have problems with broader language skill as preschoolers (Scarborough, 1990). Since various components of oral and written language interact in development (e.g., phonological skill facilitates the acquisition of new words and thus helps build lexical networks, but lexical development also promotes phonological development), these various components are correlated. So, almost inevitably, individuals selected because they are deficient in one component of language development (e.g., printed word recognition) will have deficits in other components of language development. This consideration means that various speech and language disorders will almost inevitably be comorbid, and raises the problem of determining which cognitive and etiological risk factors cause the particular comorbidity in question.

So even when we begin with a developmental disorder with a very narrow diagnostic phenotype (such as dyslexia), the disorder will almost inevitably have broader correlated cognitive features and comorbidities, because development is interactive. This appears to be a generic problem in neurodevelopmental disorders—a category that includes virtually all psychiatric diagnoses. This means that expecting that a specific causal pathway runs from a specific etiological risk factor to a specific cognitive risk factor to a specific disorder is very unrealistic, because more than one pathway influences each disorder, and more than one disorder is influenced by a given pathway (Pennington, 2006). But a careful dissection of a single pathway, as has been done with dyslexia, can lead to major advances.

Table 6.2 summarizes the research on RD.

DIAGNOSIS AND TREATMENT

Presenting Symptoms

The key symptoms in dyslexia are difficulty in learning to read and spell, often with relatively better performance in arithmetic. Because some dyslexic children like to read or have good reading comprehension, it is important to ask specifically about reading aloud and learning phonics—two aspects of reading with which virtually all such children have trouble. Similarly, a report of good performance on weekly spelling tests should be followed by a question to determine the quality of spontaneous spelling, as some dyslexic children will work hard to memorize the spelling list, but not spell even simple words correctly in their usual writing. Parents or teachers may also report slow reading or writing speed, letter and number reversals, problems in memorizing basic math facts, and unusual reading and spelling errors. These dyslexic errors are discussed below under "Behavioral Observations."

TABLE 6.2. Research Summary Table: RD

Definition	• Poor word recognition skill relative to age or ability expectations. • Exclusionary criteria include uncorrected sensory deficits, inadequate instruction, acquired neurological insults, and ID.
Epidemiology	• Prevalence is approximately 9%, depending on diagnostic cutoff. • Slightly more males than females are affected (approximately 1.5:1), but many more males are referred for services.
Etiology	• Work in behavioral genetics suggests a multifactorial etiology with substantial genetic effects. • There are replicated linkage sites on chromosomes 1p, 2p, 3, 6p, 15q, 18p, and Xq. • Researchers have identified four candidate genes: one on chromosome 3 (ROBO1), two on 6p (DCDC2, KIAA0319), and one on 15q (DYX1C1). All four genes are believed to be involved in prenatal brain development processes, such as neural migration and axon path finding. • Little is known about specific environmental risk factors, but they may include home language/literacy environment and instructional quality.
Brain bases	• Postmortem analyses show ectopias in a variety of brain regions, consistent with failures of neural migration and thus with the action of the candidate genes. • There are structural differences in perisylvian language areas, including regions of temporal and parietal lobes and the inferior frontal gyrus (IFG). • The most commonly reported functional differences are reduced activation of left-hemisphere occipitotemporal and temporoparietal regions, and increased activation of the left IFG (Broca's area). • There is evidence for structural and functional differences in the cerebellum, but the theoretical implications of these findings are not yet well understood.
Neuropsychology	• The word recognition deficit arises primarily from difficulties with phonological coding, or translating letter strings into their corresponding sound sequences. • Phonological coding difficulties arise from underlying deficits in phonological representations. Phonological processing difficulties are particularly evident on phoneme awareness tasks. • There are often subtler problems on a wide range of oral language tasks, including semantics and syntax. • Multiple-deficit models of RD explain the largest amount of variance in RD symptoms. • Although sensory problems (visual, auditory, and other) may be correlated with dyslexia, they do not appear to be causal.

Parents or teachers may also report some of the associated language difficulties previously discussed.

Finally and most importantly, the initial referral may be prompted not by these kinds of cognitive symptoms, but by emotional or physical symptoms, such as anxiety or depression, reluctance to go to school, or headaches and stomachaches. It is important to find out whether such symptoms occur all the time or only on school days. Even if they happen all the time, the root cause could be dyslexia because of the failures (and fear of failure) that children with dyslexia experience.

History

Most children with dyslexia do not have high-risk events in their prenatal or perinatal histories; nor do they have clear delays in early developmental milestones, although mild speech delays and articulation problems are present in some histories. Three aspects of the history are particularly informative—family history, school history, and reading and language history.

Because familial risk is substantial in dyslexia, it is important to take a careful history of reading, spelling, and related language problems in the child's first- and second-degree relatives. Parents will not necessarily know whether they or their relatives have dyslexia, but they are usually able to report accurately on reading and spelling problems, as well as problems with articulation, name finding, and verbal memory for such things as phone numbers and addresses. Parents with a dyslexic history will also often report extreme difficulty learning a foreign language. It is a fairly common clinical experience to discover a parent's or relative's dyslexia in the course of the dyslexic child's evaluation.

In terms of school history, dyslexic difficulties should be evident by first or second grade, and may be present by kindergarten as problems with learning the alphabet, letter names, or other prereading skills. It is very unlikely that reading problems with an abrupt later onset are due to developmental dyslexia; acquired etiologies need to be considered in this situation.

If the child is an adolescent when first referred, the preschool and early elementary school histories may not be readily available, and the presenting symptoms may have changed. The teen may now like to read, though more slowly than other adolescents, and the main complaints may involve poor performance on timed reading tests or difficulty in completing homework.

Behavioral Observations

When a clinician is evaluating a child for dyslexia, a wealth of information will emerge from the administration of reading and spelling tasks. First, it is important to get a sense of how the child feels about reading. Many children with dyslexia will comment that they do not like reading or will appear embarrassed or reluctant when asked to read aloud. Second, the evaluator should pay careful attention to the kinds of reading tasks that are most difficult for the child. Reading weaknesses are often more apparent on timed than on untimed tests, and so it is important to include a timed test of paragraph-level reading, which is likely to be most sensitive.

Other important behavioral observations to emerge from testing come from analysis of a child's specific reading and spelling errors. There are four main kinds of reading errors to look for: dysfluency, errors on function words, visual errors (whole-word guesses), and lexicalizations when reading nonwords. (Spelling errors will be discussed shortly). Dyslexic children are usually slow and halting in their oral reading, because their automatic decoding skills are weak. However, dysfluency may not be evident in older children and adolescents with dyslexia, who have overlearned a large, automatic reading vocabulary.

By "function word errors," we mean substitutions on "little" words, such as articles and prepositions. Children with dyslexia will frequently interchange "a" and "the" and misread prepositions. The significance of function word errors is that a dyslexic child is working hard to decode the content words in the sentence and is relying more on context than a typical reader would to identify function words. Function word errors are puzzling to parents and teachers, who remark that if the child can read the big words, why can he or she not read the little words?

By "visual errors," we mean substitutions on content words that are based on a superficial visual similarity to the target word (e.g., "car" for "cat"). The significance of these errors is that the child is using visual similarity rather than the full phonological code to name the word, and so again these errors are reflective of a phonological coding or "phonics" problem. "Lexicalization errors" in reading nonwords are misreadings of nonwords as real words, usually ones that are visually similar to the targets (e.g., "boy" for "bim"). The significance of these errors is essentially the same as that of visual errors: Lacking good phonological coding skills, the child assimilates the target to whatever other schema is available for word recognition.

In assessing spelling errors, the evaluator should mainly examine the proportion of errors that are not phonetically accurate (i.e., dysphonetic), especially errors in which consonants have been added, omitted, or substituted (e.g., "exetive" for "executive"). Dyslexic children are also weaker at spelling vowels, but typical developmental acquisition of vowel correspondences is more protracted, and so many young children without RD make vowel errors. In the groups without RD that we have studied, the mean rates of phonologically accurate (with regard to consonants) errors have been about 70% for children ages 8–12 and about 80% for adolescents and adults (Pennington, Lefly, Van Orden, Bookman, & Smith, 1987). As a rough guide, a phonological accuracy rate for consonant sequences lower than 60% in children and 70% in adolescents and adults would be suggestive of dyslexic difficulties.

The so-called "reversal errors" in reading and spelling are the final group of errors to mention. Although earlier accounts described reversal errors as the hallmarks of dyslexia, their rate of occurrence in dyslexia is actually quite low, and many dyslexic individuals who do not make such errors (Liberman, Shankweiler, Orlando, Harris, & Berti, 1971). Nonetheless, the presence of reversal errors in patients 9 years old or older is of some potential diagnostic significance, as typical readers virtually never make such errors past age 9. By a reversal error, we mean substituting a visually similar letter in reading or spelling (e.g., "bog" for "dog"). These errors most typically involve confusions of "b" and "d." Vellutino (1979) has convincingly argued that the basis of many such reversal errors is linguistic rather than visual; "b" and "d" are phonetically as well as visually similar.

Finally, it is valuable to look for subtle language difficulties that are characteristic of dyslexia. For instance, some children are unusually quiet because they have word-finding and verbal formulation problems. Such difficulties can often be observed on the Verbal subtests of the Wechsler tests or in spontaneous speech.

Case Presentations

Case Presentation 1

Background. Liam is a 7-year-old second grader. His parents have sought an evaluation because his progress in reading and spelling has been slow, in spite of extra help. This year, he has become increasingly frustrated with homework. Completing it takes him between 1 and 2 hours a night, although his teacher suggests that the amount of work assigned should take approximately 30 minutes. Liam's frustration often leads to angry and tearful confrontations with his parents that end with his refusing to do any more work. This fall, he has complained frequently of not wanting to go to school, particularly on days when his homework is not completed, and his parents note that they have had to "bribe him" to get in the car some mornings.

Liam's prenatal, birth, and early developmental histories are unremarkable. He was a sociable and happy child who was well liked in preschool. However, his parents noted that he was slower to learn his letters than his older sister was; when they asked his kindergarten teacher about it, she said that Liam was just not "developmentally ready." In first grade, he was placed in the weakest reading group, and part way through the year, his teacher nominated him for extra help. Twice a week, he arrived at school a half hour early, and a fifth-grade student sat with him to practice reading.

Liam also received private reading tutoring in the summer between first and second grades. Now, in second grade, Liam remains in the weakest reading group; his reading is slow and error-prone, and his spelling seems very poor. His parents have been encouraging him to read at home for practice, but he is reluctant to do so, and they are hesitant to push him and evoke still more conflict. Liam has had trouble learning the days of the week and still gets them confused. Although his math skills had seemed strong initially, he is now struggling to memorize basic math facts.

Liam's father reports no history of school difficulties. He is a college graduate and works in sales. Liam's mother is a college graduate who does not work outside the home. Although she reports that school went well for her overall, she had a sister who repeated first grade because of difficulty learning to read. Liam's mother also notes that her own spelling is "atrocious" and that she had great difficulty with Spanish class in high school.

A summary of Liam's diagnostic testing is found in Table 6.3.

Discussion. Liam's history is highly suggestive of dyslexia. Although his early development was normal, problems with reading and spelling were evident from first grade onward, and his parents detected subtler reading-related difficulties even in kindergarten. Both the age of onset and the persistence of Liam's problems are noteworthy. There is a family history of reading difficulty on the mother's side, with the mother's own weaknesses in spelling and learning a foreign language indicating a mild phonological processing deficit. Liam's problems in learning math facts and the days of the week suggest weaknesses in verbal memory. His parents' rating of his reading history on the Learning and Behavior Questionnaire does a good job of capturing his dyslexic history. The fact that Liam's current behavior problems did not emerge until after he had already experienced 2 years of school difficulty suggests that they are secondary to his reading problem rather than symptoms of an additional, comorbid disorder. However, the current evaluation has also included an assessment for ADHD, which is appropriate in any case where dyslexia is suspected.

Several aspects of Liam's pattern of test results support a diagnosis of dyslexia: (1) his very low (2nd percentile) Fluency score on the GORT-4, which is discrepantly poor relative to both his age and his Verbal IQ; (2) overall weaker scores for reading and spelling than for math (with the exception of WJ III Math Fluency, discussed further below); (3) poor performance in decoding nonsense words relative to reading real words; (4) weaker scores on timed than untimed tests of single-word reading; and (5) evidence of phonological processing weaknesses, particularly on the Phoneme Reversal and Nonword Repetition subtests of the CTOPP. In addition, Liam displays a profile on the WISC-IV common to children with dyslexia. Although this profile is not diagnostic, many children with dyslexia obtain

TABLE 6.3. Test Summary, Case 1 (Liam)

Construct	Standard score/ cutoff
General intelligence	
WISC-IV Full Scale IQ	90
Crystallized intelligence	93
WISC-IV Verbal Comprehension Index	
Similarities	9
Vocabulary	9
Comprehension	8
Fluid intelligence	102
WISC-IV Perceptual Reasoning Index	
Block Design	9
Picture Concepts	12
Matrix Reasoning	10
WISC-IV Working Memory Index[a]	88
Digit Span	8
Letter–Number Sequencing	8
WISC-IV Processing Speed Index[b]	85
Coding	6
Symbol Search	9
Academic	
Reading	
History	
Learning and Behavior Quest. Reading History items	< 55
Word recognition	
WJ III Letter Word ID	95
TOWRE Sight Word Efficiency	82
Phonological coding	
WJ III Word Attack	88
TOWRE Phonemic Decoding Efficiency	79
Paragraph fluency	
GORT-4 Fluency	70
Reading comprehension	
GORT-4 Comprehension	90
Math	
WJ III Math Fluency	81
WJ III Calculation	94
WJ III Applied Problems	106

(continued)

TABLE 6.3. *(continued)*

Construct	Standard score/ cutoff
Spelling	
WJ III Spelling	83
Oral language	
Phonological awareness[c]	
CTOPP Elision	90
CTOPP Phoneme Reversal	80
Verbal memory	
CTOPP Nonword Repetition	80
WRAML Sentence Memory	85
WRAML Story Memory	100
Verbal processing speed	
CTOPP Rapid Naming Composite	88
Attention and hyperactivity–impulsivity	
Gordon omission errors	110
Gordon commission errors	90
ADHD Rating Scale–IV Inattention	
Parent	2/9
Teacher	2/9
ADHD Rating Scale–IV Hyperactivity–Impulsivity	
Parent	0/9
Teacher	2/9

Note. WISC-IV, Wechsler Intelligence Scale for Children—Fourth Edition; WJ III, Woodcock–Johnson III Tests of Achievement; TOWRE, Test of Word Reading Efficiency; GORT-4: Gray Oral Reading Test—Fourth Edition; CTOPP, Comprehensive Test of Phonological Processing; WRAML, Wide Range Assessment of Memory and Learning; Gordon, Gordon Diagnostic System.
[a]See also Oral language—Verbal memory.
[b]See also Oral language—Verbal processing speed, and Academics—Math—WJ III Math Fluency.
[c]See also Verbal memory—CTOPP Nonword Repetition for another test of phonological processing.

weaker scores on both the Working Memory Index and the Processing Speed Index, with the former probably relating to phonological impairment and the latter to a second deficit in processing speed. In addition, Liam's Verbal Comprehension Index is slightly weaker than his Perceptual Reasoning Index, although both are in the average range. It is important to note that many children with impairing RD can nonetheless obtain average-range scores on some reading measures, particularly untimed tests of single-word reading, and particularly when (like Liam) they have already received some intervention.

Qualitative observations of Liam's performance also support the current diagnosis. He has made multiple whole-word guesses (e.g., "carried" for "covered" and "bars" for "boards"), as well as lexicalization errors on nonwords (e.g., "few" for "faw" and "bike" for "bice"). He has made a number of dysphonetic spelling errors, such as "gragsu" for "garage." He has performed poorly on most tests of verbal memory, with the exception of the WRAML story. However, Liam has earned an average score on this subtest primarily by remembering the gist of the stories, despite his inability to recall specific details (such as names of people or particular amounts of money). Liam's low score on WJ III Math Fluency probably reflects both a more general processing speed deficit and a weakness in memorizing math facts related to his poor verbal memory.

Because of the high comorbidity between dyslexia and ADHD, it is important to assess for difficulties with attention or impulsivity in any child with RD. Liam's early history is not indicative of ADHD; the current parent and teacher ratings of ADHD symptoms are in the normal range; he has performed adequately on the Gordon Diagnostic System; and behavioral observations during testing are not suggestive of an attentional disorder. Liam's current conflict with his parents is more likely to be a secondary consequence of his reading failure than symptomatic of a second disorder. Conflict centering around homework and reading should diminish as appropriate treatment for Liam's dyslexia is put in place.

Case Presentation 2

Background. Sydney is a 10-year-old girl who is entering fifth grade. Sydney has been diagnosed with an anxiety disorder, and her parents wonder whether a learning disorder may be contributing to her anxiety about school. Her parents have sought an evaluation because she is having trouble in reading, spelling, and math.

Sydney's birth and early development history appear to have been normal. Her father reports that he had problems learning to read, but he is college-educated and has a professional career. Sydney's mother does not report any academic difficulties. She is also college-educated and has a professional career. Sydney's parents first became concerned about her academic progress when her kindergarten teacher reported that she was slow to learn the sounds of letters and had more difficulty learning to read than other children in the classroom. Sydney's parents sought out private reading tutoring for her over the summer months between kindergarten and first grade. In first and second grades, Sydney's teachers did not express too much concern about her reading, but they noted that her reading fluency continued to be slow and suggested that her parents practice reading with her at home. It was difficult for Sydney's parents to follow through on this recommendation, because Sydney was resistant to reading. In third and fourth grades, Sydney's teachers became more concerned about her reading, because she was continuing to fall behind her peers. She began receiving extra reading tutoring at school. Sydney also had difficulty remembering the addition, subtraction, and multiplication math facts. During these years, Sydney's mood and anxiety became problematic for the family. She would get angry and upset very easily, and would scream self-belittling statements (e.g., "I'm too stupid!") when attempting to complete homework. At the beginning of her fourth-grade year, Sydney's parents consulted with a child psychiatrist, who prescribed Zoloft. According to her parents, this medication has improved Sydney's sleep, mood, and anxiety, although homework continues to be very frustrating for her. Moreover, her parents remain concerned about her academic progress, which seems modest despite the fact that she is a bright girl. Her teacher has noted that her academic skills are pretty much at grade level, but she has difficulty getting motivated to do her schoolwork and seems worried and anxious.

A summary of Sydney's diagnostic testing is found in Table 6.4.

Discussion. The diagnostic issues in this case are subtle because of Sydney's high verbal abilities. Children with high verbal abilities are less likely to be referred for a dyslexia evaluation because they are at or near grade-level performance in reading, even though their reading scores are far below IQ expectations. It is noteworthy that this referral came following Sydney's fourth-grade year, which is about the time when children move from "learning to read" (fluent decoding of words) to "reading to learn" (using reading to gain knowledge). Children with dyslexia whose decoding abilities remain behind grade expectations will have difficulty garnering the required information from texts. Children who were not referred at earlier ages may come to clinical attention at about fourth grade, because their learning is being hindered by their weak reading skills.

Although Sydney has concurrent symptoms of anxiety and mood difficulties, her difficulties with reading, spelling, and math facts are all suggestive of dyslexia. The fact that Sydney has difficulty getting started with schoolwork and is easily frustrated by her work is sometimes indicative of attention difficulties, so these symptoms have also been assessed in the evaluation.

In terms of history, her father's self-reported difficulties with learning to read, the early onset of Sydney's difficulties with learning letter sounds in kindergarten, and the persistence of Sydney's difficulties with reading and spelling are notable. The reading history questions from the Learning and Behavior Questionnaire capture these aspects of Sydney's early development.

The main behavioral observations of Sydney's test performance include dysphonetic spelling errors (e.g., "beilile" for "believe"), lexicalization errors

TABLE 6.4. Test Summary, Case 2 (Sydney)

Construct	Standard score/ cutoff
General intelligence	
WISC-IV Full Scale IQ	108
Crystallized intelligence	
WISC-IV Verbal Comprehension Index	119
Similarities	14
Vocabulary	12
Comprehension	14
Fluid intelligence	
WISC-IV Perceptual Reasoning Index	106
Block Design	8
Picture Concepts	11
Matrix Reasoning	14
WISC-IV Working Memory Index[a]	107
Digit Span	11
Letter–Number Sequencing	12
WISC-IV Processing Speed Index[b]	83
Coding	6
Symbol Search	8
Academic	
Reading	
History	
Learning and Behavior Quest. Reading History items	78
Word recognition	
WJ III Letter Word ID	95
TOWRE Sight Word Efficiency	84
Phonological coding	
WJ III Word Attack	91
TOWRE Phonemic Decoding Efficiency	86
Paragraph fluency	
GORT-4 Fluency	95
Reading comprehension	
GORT-4 Comprehension	120
Math	
WJ III Math Fluency	87
WJ III Calculation	108
WJ III Applied Problems	106

(continued)

TABLE 6.4. *(continued)*

Construct	Standard score/ cutoff
Spelling	
WJ III Spelling	88
Written expression	
WIAT Written Expression	102
Oral language	
Phonological awareness[c]	
CTOPP Elision	90
CTOPP Phoneme Reversal	85
Verbal memory	
CTOPP Nonword Repetition	90
WRAML Sentence Memory	90
WRAML Story Memory	120
Verbal processing speed	
CTOPP Rapid Naming Composite	82
Attention and hyperactivity–impulsivity	
Gordon omission errors	120
Gordon commission errors	115
ADHD Rating Scale–IV Inattention	
Parent	3/9
Teacher	4/9
ADHD Rating Scale–IV Hyperactivity–Impulsivity	
Parent	0/9
Teacher	0/9

Note. WIAT, Wechsler Individual Achievement Test. For other abbreviations, see Table 6.3.
[a]1See also Oral language—Verbal memory.
[b]See also Oral language—Verbal processing speed, and Academics—Math—WJ III Math Fluency.
[c]See also Verbal memory—CTOPP Nonword Repetition for another test of phonological processing.

of nonwords (e.g., "snake" for "snirk"), and dysfluencies. All of these errors are consistent with a diagnosis of dyslexia. Sydney's attention was quite focused in the one-on-one testing setting, and she was highly motivated to perform well. Similarly, parent and teacher reports on the ADHD Rating Scale–IV do not indicate clinically significant difficulties with attention.

The test results confirm a diagnosis of dyslexia via several converging patterns of evidence. First, on the WISC-IV, the Processing Speed Index is significantly depressed relative to Sydney's other Index scores. As discussed in this chapter, processing speed is a cognitive risk factor for dyslexia. Converging evidence for Sydney's slow processing speed can be seen on the CTOPP Rapid Naming Composite and the WJ III Math Fluency subtest. Poor verbal working memory is another cognitive risk factor for dyslexia. Although Sydney's Working Memory Index score is in the average range, she does show weaknesses on other, more demanding tests of verbal working memory, such as the CTOPP Nonword Repetition test and the WRAML Sentence Memory test. Sydney's WRAML Sentence Memory score is particularly notable, given the contrast with her very strong score on the WRAML Story Memory. The WRAML Story Memory subtest does not require the child to repeat the information verbatim, as the Sentence Memory subtest does, but simply to remember the concepts. Hence Sydney's high Story Memory score is consistent with her high Verbal IQ score on the WISC-IV.

As mentioned earlier in the chapter, phonological awareness tasks are predictive of reading ability. Consistent with this expectation, Sydney shows weaknesses on the CTOPP Elision and Phoneme Reversal tasks. Despite Sydney's strong Verbal IQ and supplemental reading tutoring, she continues to score considerably below expectations based on her Verbal IQ, although some of her scores are not too far below grade level. Sydney's word recognition and phonological coding scores show a typical pattern, in which her scores on the untimed versions of these tests (WJ III Letter Word and Word Attack) are better than her scores on the timed analogues of these tests (TOWRE Sight Word Efficiency and Phonemic Decoding Efficiency). Sydney also shows weaknesses on the GORT-4 Fluency test. Children with dyslexia often have particular difficulty with fluent reading even if they have learned the necessary decoding skills. In Sydney's case, she also has a processing speed weakness, which further contributes to her difficulties with reading fluency.

Despite Sydney's reading difficulties, she has scored very well on the GORT-4 Comprehension test. Although this might seem surprising, the GORT-4 Comprehension questions can often be answered correctly by children with strong inferencing abilities. In Sydney's case, her strong GORT-4 Comprehension score is more reflective of her strong Verbal IQ than of her reading skill per se. One might expect Sydney's strong Verbal IQ also to be reflected in her written language scores, but on the WIAT Written Expression test, her score falls below her verbal abilities. This discrepancy reflects the fact that writing is effortful for her. Even though she has many good ideas, she has made several errors in spelling, punctuation, and capitalization.

This evaluation has also included an assessment of Sydney's current socioemotional functioning, although these test scores are not included in Table 6.4. On the Child Behavior Checklist, she shows a clinical elevation on the Somatic Complaints subscale, which is consistent with her anxiety disorder diagnosis. On the Multidimensional Anxiety Scale for Children, Sydney showed a clinical elevation in the Social Anxiety domain, including concerns about performance fears and humiliation. Children with dyslexia, especially bright children, sometimes experience anxiety and poor self-esteem that result from their frustration with reading. They compare themselves to their peers and feel that they are less bright because of their particular difficulty with reading. In Sydney's case, she seems to have a particular vulnerability for anxiety, which is exacerbated by her RD.

In summary, Sydney's dyslexia diagnosis explains the referral concerns regarding her progress with reading and spelling. Her dyslexia diagnosis also explains her difficulties with math. Although dyslexia is a language-based disorder, it can affect math performance via verbal short-term memory weaknesses, which make it difficult to learn and retrieve basic math facts. The observation that Sydney is slow to get started with her work is partly explained by her slow processing speed, but she has the additional complicating factor of the anxiety she experiences, which may slow her down even further. It will be important for Sydney's parents and teachers to understand the nature of her RD and its associated cognitive weaknesses, as well as how her RD contributes to her anxiety disorder.

Treatment

A number of empirically supported interventions have been developed for RD. The development of successful treatments has benefited from our understanding of the neuropsychology of RD, and the best interventions directly target phonological coding, phoneme awareness, and reading fluency. A review of specific commercially available programs is beyond the scope of this chapter; the reader is referred to Shaywitz (2003) for further information.

A number of studies (Bradley & Bryant, 1983; Cunningham, 1990; Lundberg, Frost, & Petersen, 1988; Wise, Ring, & Olson, 1999) have demonstrated that phoneme awareness training promotes later reading skill. However, when phoneme awareness training alone is compared to phoneme awareness plus direct reading instruction (e.g., letter–sound training, practice in reading connected text), research has consistently found stronger effects for the integrated treatment (Bradley & Bryant, 1983; Cunningham, 1990; National Reading Panel, 2000). One carefully controlled study (Hatcher, Hulme, & Ellis, 1994) identified 7-year-old children experiencing early reading failure and randomly assigned them to one of four conditions: phonological training only (both rhyme and phoneme awareness), reading training only (including explicit phonics teaching), reading plus phonological training, and control. Immediately after training and at the 9-month follow-up, the group receiving reading plus phonological training showed the largest gains on all reading measures. In contrast, the phonological-training-only group showed the greatest gains on the phoneme awareness measures themselves. So these results showed that extensive training in phoneme awareness promotes phoneme awareness, but the effects transfer to reading better when intervention also includes direct reading instruction. A meta-analysis (Swanson, 1999) of 92 treatment studies reached similar conclusions, and also found that the children's IQs and the severity of their reading problems affected treatment outcomes (i.e., children with higher IQs and less severe problems benefited more from treatment).

It is not terribly surprising that the best intervention for reading failure includes reading instruction. Hatcher, Hulme, and Snowling (2004) reported a second important finding: phonological awareness training provided an additional boost, over and above the benefits of reading instruction alone (see also Ball & Blachman, 1991; Byrne & Fielding-Barnsley, 1989; National Reading Panel, 2000). A recent study (Hatcher et al., 2004) demonstrated that the added effect of phoneme awareness training may be specific to children at risk for RD. These researchers implemented a highly structured, phonics-based reading program in 20 "reception" classrooms (for children ages 4–5) in England. Some classes additionally received phoneme awareness instruction. Children who scored in the bottom third on prereading measures at study entry were considered at risk for reading failure. At-risk children showed differential effects of instruction, with the best effects for the program that included phoneme awareness training. In contrast, the typically developing children experienced no additional boost of phoneme awareness training over and above the phonics program. Presumably, the phoneme awareness training helped the at-risk children develop the skills they needed to benefit most from reading instruction, while the typically developing children may have been able to infer the necessary skills without explicit instruction. A separate but related phenomenon is that, compared to eventual good readers, young children who will later be diagnosed with RD have deficits not only in their absolute levels of phoneme awareness skill, but also in the slower rate at which they respond to phoneme awareness training (Byrne, Fielding-Barnsley, & Ashley, 2000). It is important to note that the added benefit of phoneme awareness training over and above direct reading instruction may not generalize to older struggling readers (Alexander & Slinger-Constant, 2004; Wise, Ring, & Olson, 2000).

A limitation of many early treatment studies is that the dependent measures included word-reading accuracy but not reading fluency. More recent studies have begun to investigate the impact of intervention on fluency (see Alexander & Slinger-Constant, 2004, and Torgesen, 2005, for recent reviews). These studies have generally found that slow reading is more difficult to remediate than inaccurate reading. However, difficulties with reading fluency appear preventable when intervention is begun early enough. For example, Torgesen et al. (2001) administered a treatment integrating phoneme awareness, phonological coding, and reading connected text to children experiencing reading failure. The treatment remediated deficits in single-word reading accuracy, word-reading accuracy in context, and text comprehension, but not reading fluency. It is important to note that roughly half of instructional time was spent in reading connected text, generally considered an appropriate intervention for fluency difficulties (Shaywitz, 2003). However, it is still possible that more attention to reading speed in particular would have produced a different pattern of results. This possibility is made somewhat less likely by the contrasting results of prevention studies (Torgesen et al., 2001; Torgesen, Wagner, Rashotte, & Herron, 2003). When a similar intervention was administered to kindergarten and first-grade children most at risk of reading failure, it effectively promoted both accuracy and fluency up to a year later. Torgesen (2005) has suggested that once children have experienced several years of reading failure, they have accumulated dramatically less practice in reading than their typically developing peers (Cunningham & Stanovich, 1998). Even if their word-reading accuracy deficit is largely remediated, these long-standing differences in print exposure make it difficult or impossible for them to "close the gap" on their peers in reading fluency.

In summary, numerous studies have demonstrated that combined instruction in phoneme awareness, phonological coding, and reading connected text is effective in treating word-reading accuracy difficulties in RD (National Reading Panel, 2000; Torgesen, 2005). The criteria for establishing a particular treatment as empirically supported are reviewed in Chapter 14. We can be confident of the effectiveness of this approach to treating RD, because positive results have been replicated by multiple research teams whose studies met the important criteria for treatment validation (presence of a control group, random assignment, and comparison to a control condition of equal intensity).

Studies with children as young as 4 years old demonstrate that there is no need to wait for students to experience years of reading failure to begin intervention. On the contrary, some of the most promising results have been obtained in prevention studies. We speculate that such an approach should be effective not just in promoting reading accuracy and fluency, but also in preventing the correlated psychosocial problems secondary to school failure.

These lessons have prompted a new approach to reading instruction in the public schools, called "response to intervention" (RTI). In this approach, empirically validated methods of reading instruction begin in kindergarten, and children's progress is monitored frequently with brief, teacher-administered assessments (of letter name and sound knowledge, phoneme awareness, phonological coding, reading fluency, and reading comprehension). Children who are making below-average progress are given more intensive intervention; if they still fail to respond to intervention, they are evaluated individually and may be given individual instruction. RTI, properly implemented, appears to be a promising way to reduce the number of children who develop RD. However, there is currently little empirical evidence that as currently practiced, it is an effective treatment for RD (Swanson, 2008).

Unfortunately, in some implementations, a response-to-intervention approach to reading is being coupled with significantly reduced cognitive testing by school psychologists of children with learning problems (Boada, Riddle, & Pennington, 2008). This reduced emphasis on testing runs the risk of not identifying children with RD and other learning disorders described in this book, such as LI, ASD, ADHD, and ID. Such children need early interventions, but of a different sort. Chapter 14 discusses the important topic of integrating science and practice in ways that will best serve *all* children with learning disorders.

Table 6.5 summarizes clinical issues in RD.

TABLE 6.5. Clinical Summary Table: RD

Defining symptoms	• Slow and/or inaccurate single-word recognition and poor spelling in the absence of a known cause (such as uncorrected vision or hearing problems, brain injury, or ID).
Common comorbidities	• RD is comorbid with ADHD and with other developmental language disorders (LI and SSD). There are elevated rates of internalizing problems, particularly in girls, that appear to be secondary to school failure.
Developmental history	• Reading problems typically appear by first or second grade. Difficulty in learning letter names may have been noted in kindergarten or earlier. • Early development should have been fairly typical, though there may have been subtle oral language difficulties. • Verbal memory weaknesses (problems in learning math facts, addresses and phone numbers, or names and dates). • In older children or adolescents, poor reading comprehension, difficulty getting through schoolwork, or problems in learning a foreign language.
Diagnosis	• Poor performance on standardized reading and/or spelling tests relative to age or ability expectations. • Typically, poorer performance on timed than untimed reading tests and on reading nonwords compared to real words. • Characteristic error pattern, including whole-word guesses, lexicalizations, and dysphonetic spelling errors. • IQ testing and medical history rule out exclusionary conditions.
Prognosis	• With adequate intervention, dyslexic children can learn to read quite well. Many go on to enjoy reading, though they may remain slow readers and poor spellers for their whole lives. • Underlying cognitive–linguistic weaknesses in verbal memory or phonological representations are likely to persist, but need not be impairing if the individual learns compensatory strategies (e.g., writing down names and phone numbers). • A relatively high IQ is an important protective factor. Bright children with dyslexia are more likely to have future educational and occupational success.
Treatment	• Direct literacy instruction that includes a highly structured, phonics-based approach as well as fluency training. • Particularly in young children, it is valuable to include some targeted phoneme awareness training (though always in combination with direct reading instruction). • Appropriate accommodations may include extended time for testing, access to a spell checker, or books on tape. • Intervention should be begun as early as possible, since some reading difficulties (e.g., poor fluency) are easier to prevent than to remediate.

CHAPTER 7

Speech and Language Disorders

WITH ROBIN L. PETERSON AND LAUREN M. MCGRATH

HISTORY

Leonard (2000) has provided a history of speech sound disorder (SSD) and language impairment (LI), which is briefly summarized here. The first case report of a child with limited speech was published by Gall in 1822; many other case reports followed, spurred in part by advances in understanding acquired aphasia (hence the term "congenital aphasia" for such developmental cases). The children in these case reports had extremely limited speech output, despite apparently normal language comprehension and nonverbal intelligence. Later labels for these children included "developmental aphasia" and "developmental dysphasia." Eventually, this neurological terminology was dropped in favor of terms like "developmental language disorder" or "specific language impairment" or just "language impairment" (LI), which is the term used here because of questions about how specific the problems are to language. The definitions of these latter categories excluded children who had an acquired aphasia or other identifiable cause for their language problem. Thus these definitions focused on children with an *idiopathic* problem in language development, including speech production. Other changes in current conceptions of LI and SSD have included (1) an increasing awareness that such children have other language problems besides limited speech output, such as grammatical deficits; and (2) an increased emphasis on subtypes, such as receptive and expressive LI.

DEFINITION

Like definitions of RD, current definitions of SSD and LI all have two parts: (1) a diagnostic threshold; and (2) a list of exclusionary conditions, which usually include a peripheral sensory impairment (e.g., deafness), a peripheral deficit in the vocal apparatus, acquired neurological insults, environmental deprivation, and other more severe developmental disorders (e.g., ID and ASD). Setting a diagnostic threshold for these disorders on what are essentially continua is inevitably somewhat arbitrary, as has been discussed repeatedly in other chapters. For LI, a further issue is whether the diagnostic threshold should be relative to age or IQ expectations for the particular ability involved.

Traditional definitions of LI have required that the language deficit be significantly below the child's nonverbal IQ level; this means that many children's language problems will not fit the definition, even though their language is significantly below age expectations, and even though these problems are interfering with everyday functioning. Besides excluding some children from services, IQ discrepancy definitions face a fundamental logical problem. As discussed in Chapter 6, measures of IQ, even nonverbal IQ, are moderately correlated with measures of language, but we do not fully understand the causal basis of this correlation. IQ could influence language development, language development could influence IQ, or both could be related to a third variable. Just as we have argued for RD, children with age, but not IQ, discrepancies in language development may be the children with the most severe cases of LI, and they are likely to have the same underlying cognitive deficits as children who meet the IQ discrepancy definition.

There is now an emerging research literature on the external validity of the distinction between age and IQ discrepancy definitions of LI, which does not support the validity of this distinction (Bishop, 1997). Researchers may still want to use IQ discrepancy to identify the "purest" cases, but retaining this distinction for clinical purposes seems hard to justify if the same treatments are efficacious for children with and without IQ discrepancies.

The definition of SSD, unlike RD or LI, has always emphasized age discrepancy rather than IQ discrepancy (although ID is sometimes an exclusionary criterion, along with the same exclusionary criteria used for RD and LI). Children are considered to have SSD if they substitute or omit sounds from words more than same-age peers and if these speech production errors interfere with the intelligibility of their speech. In other words, their speech errors must be developmentally atypical and must cause impairment.

EPIDEMIOLOGY AND COMORBIDITIES

Prevalence rates for LI range from about 5% to 8%. In Shriberg, Tomblin, and McSweeny's (1999) study, the prevalence was 8.1%, with a male–female ratio of 1.25:1. Just as was true for RD and SSD, this ratio is higher in referred samples, about 3:1 (Smith et al., 2001). Besides its comorbidities with RD and SSD, LI is comorbid with ADHD (Beitchman, Hood, & Inglis, 1990).

The prevalence of SSD in a recent epidemiological sample was 3.8%, with a male–female ratio of 1.5:1 (Shriberg et al., 1999). In five earlier epidemiological samples reviewed by Shriberg et al. (1999), prevalence ranged from 2% to 13% (mean = 8.2%), and the male–female ratio ranged from 1.5:1 to 2.4:1 (mean = 1.8). As is the case for RD, gender ratios for SSD are higher in referred samples. This study also found that about a third of children with SSD had LI.

ETIOLOGY[1]

Genetic Findings

One striking example of the role of genes in language development comes from the KE family. About half the members of this family are affected with a general speech and language impairment, which most notably affects expressive language and articulation. Pedigree analysis revealed that the inheritance pattern was consistent with a single-gene, autosomal dominant trait (Lai, Fisher, Hurst, Vargha-Khadem, & Monaco, 2001). The gene responsible for this disorder was eventually localized to the long arm of chromosome 7 in the 7q31 region and subsequently identified as the FOXP2 gene (Lewis, Cox, & Byard, 1993; Vargha-Khadem et al., 1998). The simple Mendelian transmission of this disorder in the KE family is a unique example; it is not representative of the larger population of individuals with speech and language disorders (Bartlett et al., 2002).

Analysis of LI outside the KE family indicates that though the disorder is significantly heritable, its etiology is typically more consistent with a complex disease model, in which multiple etiological risk factors (genetic and environmental) interact to produce an eventual phenotype. Genomewide scans of multiple families affected by LI have not identified FOXP2 as a candidate gene. Instead, significant linkage has been reported to 13q21 (with a variety of language phenotypes), 16q (with a phonological memory phenotype), and 19q (again with a variety of phenotypes) (Bartlett et al., 2002; SLI Consortium, 2002, 2004). Because LI is comorbid with RD, we

---

[1]For a description of genetic technical terms, see Box 1.1 in Chapter 1.

might expect some genetic overlap. Yet none of these LI loci overlap with those identified for RD, although it is notable that some of the positive linkage results with LI individuals used reading phenotypes (Bartlett et al., 2002; SLI Consortium, 2004). At this point, it is unclear whether the lack of overlap between RD and LI risk loci is due to a lack of power or is a true null finding.

The cause of SSD outside the KE family also appears consistent with the complex disease model, and we are accumulating knowledge about specific genetic risk factors involved. Again, the FOXP2 gene does not appear to be implicated in most cases, though mutations in this gene may play a role in the development of SSD in a small minority of cases—notably, among individuals who appear to fit a verbal apraxia subtype (MacDermot et al., 2005). Two independent studies have investigated whether SSD shows linkage to known RD risk loci, because the disorders are frequently comorbid (S. D. Smith, Pennington, Boada, & Shriberg, 2005; C. M. Stein et al., 2004). These studies reported significant linkage of SSD to chromosomes 3p12–q13 (where ROBO1 is located), 6p22 (where DCDC2 and KIAA0319 are located), and 15q21 (where DYX1C1 is located). Recent attempts to replicate the 6p22 and 15q21 loci in an independent sample with SSD have been partially successful. There is preliminary evidence of replication of the 6p22 locus (S. Iyengar, personal communication, September 8, 2006). There is also evidence for a possible replication of the 15q21 locus, although these results are ambiguous, because the linkage peak is closer to genes associated with ASD and Prader–Willi/Angelman syndrome than to the region associated with dyslexia/SSD (Stein et al., 2006).

That SSD and RD appear to share genetic risk factors is consistent with the fact that these disorders are comorbid and are both associated with impairments in phonological processing. However, the failure (to date) to find clear evidence for shared genetic risk factors for LI and RD is quite puzzling: Not only are these disorders comorbid, but they also overlap at the symptom, neuropsychological, and brain levels. Furthermore, longitudinal studies have demonstrated that children with early LI are at much higher risk for later RD than are children with isolated SSD—a finding suggesting that the overlap between RD and SSD is partly due to the third variable of LI (Bishop & Adams, 1990). Thus a goal of future research will be to identify shared etiological risk factors for RD and LI, and to clarify the etiological relationship of all three disorders.

Etiological Interactions

The heritability of LI and SSD is significantly less than 100%—a factor that points to the importance of environmental variables in their development. Such variables are likely to include the home language environment (especially for LI), as well as environmental events that have a more direct effect on biology (e.g., lead poisoning or head injury). Unfortunately, few studies investigating main effects of such environmental variables on language development have used genetically sensitive designs. In addition to main effects of environment, it is likely that the disorders considered here are influenced by G × E interactions.

A recent study in our lab used measures of the home language/literacy environment to investigate G × E interactions in a sample of children with SSD and their siblings (McGrath et al., 2007). We tested for such interactions at the two SSD/RD linkage peaks with the strongest evidence of linkage to speech phenotypes, 6p22 and 15q21. The interactions were tested with speech, language, and preliteracy phenotypes. Results showed four significant and trend-level G × E interactions at both the 6p22 and 15q21 locations across several phenotypes and home environmental measures. The direction of the interactions was such that in relatively enriched environments, genetic risk factors substantially influenced the phenotype, while in less optimal environments, genetic risk factors had less influence on phenotype. This directionality of the interactions is consistent with the bioecological model of G × E interactions (Bronfenbrenner & Ceci, 1994). This work is preliminary, because these linkage-based methods are a step away from the ideal of using identified risk alleles to test for such interactions (e.g., Caspi et al., 2002, 2003). As molecular genetic studies identify specific risk alleles for SSD and LI, the field will be able to more rigorously test etiological models that include G × E interactions.

BRAIN MECHANISMS[2]

Structural Findings

Evidence for structural abnormalities in the brains of individuals with LI has come from postmortem studies and MRI. To date, there is little research on the neuroanatomy of SSD. Interpretation of the LI results is complicated by the facts that definitions of the disorders vary across studies, and that many studies have not adequately addressed the question of comorbidity.

MRI studies have suggested that reduced or reversed planum temporale asymmetry (in contrast to the typical pattern of a left > right asymmetry) is indeed more likely to be associated with LI than with RD. In one study that directly compared children with RD to children with LI, only the group with LI had symmetrical plana temporale (Leonard et al., 2002).

Another brain region that has garnered attention in the LI literature is one discussed in Chapter 6 for RD: the IFG, which includes Broca's area,

---

[2]For a description of neuroanatomical technical terms, see Box 1.2 in Chapter 1.

long known as a critical region for language production. This structure also shows a leftward asymmetry in most typically developing individuals, whereas studies have reported reduced or reversed asymmetry in LI (De Fosse et al., 2004; Gauger, Lombardino, & Leonard, 1997). De Fosse et al. (2004) found that reduced leftward asymmetry was correlated with lower verbal IQ. As reviewed earlier, findings for RD have been similar. Thus it is possible that IFG abnormalities confer risk for both LI and RD.

LI has also been associated with more widespread neural differences across frontal, temporal, parietal, and subcortical regions (Bishop & Snowling, 2004). Furthermore, there have been some reports of total cerebral volume reduction in LI (Leonard et al., 2002; Trauner, Wulfeck, Tallal, & Hesselink, 2000), and one study found that cerebral volume was correlated with measures of LI, such as oral comprehension (Leonard et al., 2001).

In summary, like the structural findings in RD, structural studies of LI have most often implicated left-hemisphere perisylvian regions involved in language, though findings are by no means limited to these regions. The commonalities in structural findings for LI and RD are likely to be both meaningful (because some brain differences are probably shared by the disorders) and artifactual (because studies have not carefully controlled for comorbidity). Future studies should compare children who have only one of the disorders, both disorders, or neither (controls).

We are not aware of any studies that have specifically examined neuroanatomical correlates of SSD, using a precisely defined phenotype. However, in-depth study of KE family members has produced findings that could help guide future research. Their speech difficulty is often described as a verbal apraxia, which implies that their articulation difficulties arise from impairments in sequencing oral–motor movements. It is possible that verbal apraxia is a subtype of SSD that is etiologically distinct from a more common, phonologically based subtype. MRI findings in the KE family indicated bilateral abnormalities in the basal ganglia, especially the caudate nucleus, as well as in the left IFG and premotor areas of affected family members (Watkins et al., 2002). Left caudate volume was correlated with performance on a task of oral praxis, suggesting that this brain region in particular may relate to affected family members' articulation difficulties.

Functional Findings

A smaller body of literature has investigated brain function in LI than in RD, and, again, there is almost no work on SSD. As in the anatomical literature, the comorbidity of these disorders has rarely been carefully addressed.

One PET study compared brain activation in two affected members of the KE family to four typical controls (Vargha-Khadem et al., 1998). The nature of the task used (word repetition minus a baseline articulation condition) meant that the results may relate more to the family members' LI than to their speech difficulties. Affected family members showed aberrant activation patterns (some overactivation and some underactivation) across a widely distributed set of left-hemisphere sites, including the IFG, angular gyrus, motor and premotor areas, and caudate nucleus.

Two more recent studies have used fMRI to examine brain function in LI outside the KE family. Hugdahl et al. (2004) used a passive listening task that activated bilateral superior temporal gyrus and middle temporal gyrus in control subjects. Activation for five individuals with LI (all from one Finnish family) was similar to that for the control group, but smaller and weaker, particularly in the superior temporal sulcus and middle temporal gyrus. Using a verbal working memory task, another research group found that children with LI tended to have reduced activation across a number of left-hemisphere sites, including the IFG, parietal regions, and the precentral sulcus (Weismer, Plante, Jones, & Tomblin, 2005). One of the most exciting findings from this study involved a correlational analysis of the extent to which groups tended to coactivate different brain regions (possibly relating to their degree of anatomical connectivity). Compared to the control group, the group with LI showed less coactivation between the superior temporal gyrus and IFG (in the perisylvian language loop), but more extraperisylvian coactivation. Unfortunately, however, this study did not equate in-scanner performance across groups.

Summary

Taken together, the structural and functional neuroimaging literatures in LI are beginning to implicate many of the brain regions involved in skilled language use—notably including the superior temporal gyrus, IFG, and temporoparietal regions. To date, we have virtually no knowledge of the brain bases of SSD.

NEUROPSYCHOLOGY

Language Impairment

A challenge to researchers studying the neuropsychology of LI has been the heterogeneity of the phenotype. At the symptomatic level, children's primary difficulties can range from expressive syntax to receptive vocabulary. However, efforts to delineate reliable subtypes of LI have not met with great success, partly because subtypes based on symptom descriptions do not show adequate longitudinal stability (Bishop, 1997). The search for a core underlying deficit in LI has led to three competing proposals: the extended optional infinitive hypothesis, the phonological memory hypothesis, and the auditory hypothesis. These hypotheses differ importantly in the specificity of the proposed impairment, and each is reviewed very briefly below.

We believe that current evidence best supports the phonological memory hypothesis. However, even this hypothesis is clearly incomplete, probably because any single core deficit will probably be inadequate to account for the full LI phenotype (Pennington, 2006).

Of the three hypotheses, the extended optional infinitive proposal of Rice, Wexler, and Cleave (1995) is the most specific; it posits that the core deficit in LI lies in the acquisition of a particular aspect of syntax. Evidence for this hypothesis comes from the fact that children with LI make characteristic errors in their expressive language. In English, they most notably have difficulties with the past tense, often substituting an unmarked form for a marked one (e.g., "He walk there" in place of "He walked there"). This kind of error is made by typically developing children early in language acquisition, but children with LI tend to use unmarked (or infinitive) forms much longer than even younger typically developing children matched for overall language skill do. Despite the elegance of this proposal, it faces two major challenges in trying to account for all cases of LI. First, it does not adequately explain the cross-linguistic data, which have shown that the syntactic forms causing the most difficulty for children with LI vary with their perceptual salience in different languages (Leonard, 1995). Thus, in English, the past tense may be problematic in part because its marker ("-ed") is brief and often unstressed. Second, this proposal fails to explain why children with LI perform poorly on a wide range of language tasks, including those that do not require syntactic competence (Bishop, 1997). The value of this marker may be in its persistence with age, making it an important endophenotype for genetic studies.

The phonological memory hypothesis of LI holds that the core deficit lies in the ability to hold phonological forms in working memory (Gathercole & Baddeley, 1990a). Phonological memory is most often measured by asking children to repeat spoken lists of real words, such as numbers (digit span), or individual pseudowords (nonword repetition). This proposal is theoretically attractive, because work with brain-damaged adults, second-language learners, and typically developing children has converged in highlighting a role for phonological memory in language learning, particularly vocabulary acquisition (Baddeley, Gathercole, & Papagno, 1998). Furthermore, a recent computational model demonstrated that phonological deficits caused impairments in learning syntax (Joanisse & Seidenberg, 2003). Phonological memory impairment does appear to be a robust endophenotype for LI. Phonological memory deficits are heritable, and are correlated significantly with degree of language difficulty in individuals with LI (Bishop et al., 1999a). Furthermore, phonological memory deficits persist even in individuals whose broader language problems have resolved (Stothard, Snowling, Bishop, Chipchase, & Kaplan, 1998). However, the phonological memory hypothesis is unlikely to account fully for LI, because children with RD and SSD both also show phonological memory deficits, often in the face of spared broader language function. To account for this pattern of findings, Bishop and Snowling (2004) proposed a 2 × 2 classification for developmental language disorders, based on the presence or absence of (1) phonological deficits and (2) broader language deficits (including problems with semantics and syntax). According to this scheme, RD is associated with phonological deficits only, while LI is associated with deficits on both dimensions. Because broader language deficits are the defining symptom in LI, however, this classification scheme remains descriptive. A neuropsychological theory will have to specify the cognitive components that underlie these deficits.

Finally, the auditory hypothesis of LI is the least specific, because it posits that a nonlinguistic, sensory impairment leads to both phonological and broader language difficulties in LI. This hypothesis was developed in the 1970s by Tallal and colleagues, and in more recent years has been extended to RD, as discussed in Chapter 6. Early studies demonstrated that children with LI had specific difficulty discriminating rapidly presented nonspeech sounds (Tallal & Percy, 1973b), which presumably led to problems in processing certain aspects of the speech stream. However, later studies have found that despite group differences, many children with LI do not have auditory deficits, whereas many typically developing children do (Bishop, Carlyon, Deeks, & Bishop, 1999b). Furthermore, there is little evidence that the auditory impairments described in these studies are heritable (Bishop et al., 1999a). Since LI is partly heritable, this finding is problematic for the argument that deficits in the discrimination of rapid auditory stimuli are the sole cause of the disorder. However, it remains possible that auditory deficits of an environmental etiology significantly complicate language development in children already at genetic risk for LI (Bishop et al., 1999a).

Speech Sound Disorder

SSD was originally considered a disorder of generating oral–motor programs, and children with speech sound impairments were said to have "functional articulation disorder" (Bishop, 1997). However, a careful analysis of error patterns has rendered a pure motor deficit unlikely as a full explanation for the disorder. For example, children with SSD sometimes produce a sound correctly in one context but incorrectly in another. If children were unable to execute particular motor programs, then we might expect that most of their errors would take the form of phonetic distortions arising from an approximation of that motor program. However, the most common errors in children with SSD are substitutions of phonemes, not distortions (Leonard, 1995). Furthermore, a growing body of research is demonstrating that children with SSD show deficits on a range of phonological tasks, including phoneme awareness and phonological memory (Bird & Bishop, 1992; Kenney, Barac-Cikoja, Finnegan, Jeffries, & Ludlow, 2006; Leitao, Hogben,

& Fletcher, 1997; Raitano et al., 2004). Though it remains possible that a subgroup of children have SSD primarily because of motor impairments, it now seems likely that the majority of children with SSD have a type of language disorder that primarily affects phonological development. Thus there is a puzzle to be resolved: If RD, LI, and SSD are all associated with phonological impairments, why is their overlap not complete? One possibility is that phonological deficits are a shared risk factor for all three disorders, with additional risk factors specific to each disorder (Pennington, 2006). For example, work in our laboratory showed that RD and SSD were associated with similar deficits in phoneme awareness and phonological memory, but that only RD was additionally associated with impairments in rapid naming (Raitano et al., 2004).

Table 7.1 summarizes the research on LI and SSD.

TABLE 7.1. Research Summary Table: LI and SSD

Definition	• Poor language (LI) or speech articulation (SSD) skill relative to age expectations. • Exclusionary criteria include deafness, peripheral deficit in the vocal apparatus, acquired neurological insults, ID, and ASD.
Epidemiology	• Prevalence of LI: 5–8%. • Prevalence of SSD: 2–13%. • Both disorders affect slightly more males than females (approximately 1.5:1)
Etiology	• Both disorders are partially genetic. LI: Linkage to chromosomes 13q, 16q, and 19q. SSD: Linkage to chromosomes 3, 6p, and 15q. • Possible environmental risk–protective factors include home language and literacy environment. • Preliminary evidence for bioecological G × E interactions (genetic risk has a larger effect in enriched environments).
Brain bases	• LI: Anatomical differences in perisylvian regions, including reduced asymmetry of plana temporale and IFG. Evidence for widespread anatomical differences, including reduced cerebral volume. Functional differences (primarily underactivation) in bilateral temporal lobes, left IFG, and other sites during language and listening tasks. • SSD: Little research.
Neuropsychology	• LI: Poor grammar development, particularly past-tense acquisition. Characteristic zero-marking errors in past-tense production (e.g., "walk" for "walked"). Persistent phonological processing deficits, particularly in phonological memory. • SSD: Phonological processing deficits, including in phonological awareness and phonological memory. A subset of children have poor oral–motor development.

DIAGNOSIS AND TREATMENT

Presenting Symptoms

The presenting symptoms in LI vary with the age at which a child comes in for evaluation. In school-age children, school difficulty is likely to be the key complaint. Because so many children with LI also have RD, many of the presenting symptoms are likely to be similar to those described in Chapter 6. However, most (but not all) children with LI will be experiencing difficulties across the curriculum, because so much teaching and learning depend on linguistic communication. In a younger child, concern is more likely to involve language development itself. Parents will note that the child cannot talk or comprehend as well as peers or siblings can. In both older and younger children, adults may comment that the child cannot follow verbal directions, has immature grammar, or will not listen to a story for an appropriate length of time.

As with dyslexia, there will be some cases of LI in which presenting symptoms appear primarily emotional or behavioral. There may be conflict centering around homework, or stomachaches on school mornings. A child may appear "tuned out" in the classroom and may not do what is asked of him or her. In some children, these symptoms will reflect the second disorder of ADHD, but other children with LI appear inattentive because of poor language comprehension. Thus it is important to learn whether a child is also experiencing lapses in attention, difficulties with organization, or hyperactivity that cannot be explained by weak language skills. Some children with LI will be extremely frustrated by their difficulty in communicating, which in turn can lead to social problems. For example, a child who is teased on the playground and cannot generate a quick verbal retort may well hit or shove other children instead. Some children may present with a degree of emotional rigidity, manifesting as distress with departures from normal routine. Verbal explanations of what to expect are of limited use to children with significant language difficulties, and thus these children may compensate with overreliance on established routines.

Presenting symptoms in SSD are straightforward and easily observed by parents or other adults in a child's life. The child has difficulty speaking clearly, so that he or she is not well understood by strangers. In more extreme cases, even siblings or parents may struggle to understand what the child is trying to say. Some children will compensate by shortening and simplifying their utterances, so their overall expressive language will appear delayed. (Of course, poor expressive language can also reflect comorbid LI.) Children's frustration with their difficulty may be manifested in any number of ways—reluctance to repeat themselves, a quiet presentation with strangers, or attempts to use alternative means of communication (such as showing instead of saying). Children with SSD are more likely to come in for evaluation in preschool or earlier than at school age, and so school difficulty is unlikely to be a key presenting symptom.

History

The most relevant history for LI concerns early language development. Typically, all of a child's language milestones were delayed, particularly for expressive language. Thus the child will have been late to produce single words, to combine two words, and to speak in full sentences. Parents and teachers will have noticed that the child's grammar sounds immature. Errors in verb conjugation, pronouns, and word order persist long after peers have mastered these skills. Often children with LI have comorbid SSD and thus a history of articulation difficulty, so it is important to establish whether early language difficulties were limited to articulation or extended to other aspects of language development. Parents will often note that strangers understood little of what the child said. There may have been particular difficulty learning terms related to time, sequencing, or directionality (e.g., "yesterday–tomorrow," "before–after," "left–right").

When a child has a history of significant language delay, both ASD and ID may be considered for differential diagnosis, so it is important to learn about early social and nonverbal development. Children with LI may develop social problems secondary to communication difficulties, but early social development should have been fairly typical. As a baby or toddler, a child with LI would have shown interest in others, made adequate eye contact, and engaged in spontaneous imitation. Similarly, in a child with LI and not ID, early nonverbal skills should have been reasonably intact, and there would not be a history of major delays in motor milestones or learning to solve puzzles, for example.

The most relevant history for SSD concerns early speech development. Once a child begins talking, he or she is extremely difficult to understand because of the large numbers of sound substitutions and omissions. The child may be perceived as talking in "baby talk." Expressive language milestones were often delayed, but in a child with isolated SSD, receptive language development should have been fairly typical. This history can be difficult to ascertain, however, since expressive language is much more readily observable by parents. Some children with SSD have broader oral–motor difficulties, which will be evident in the history as early difficulties with feeding, swallowing, or drooling.

As are other disorders considered in this book, both LI and SSD are partly heritable, and thus the history of the child's biological family is relevant. Sometimes there is a positive family history that the parents do not believe is genetically based, because the family has developed an alternative explanation. For example, substantial cognitive delays will sometimes be attributed to a difficult birth, or speech delays to a physical problem (such as a large tongue or tight frenulum, which attaches the tongue to the floor of the mouth). It is important not to accept such explanations at face value, but to recognize that they may represent (partly or fully incorrect) attempts to understand a genetically influenced disorder.

Behavioral Observations

Children with any speech or language disorder often present as quiet or reluctant to speak. Typically, these children have had several years' experience learning that strangers cannot understand them very well and that their attempts to communicate will be unsuccessful. It may be helpful during the initial conversation with a child for a parent to be present and to act as "translator" if necessary. The examiner can also select a conversational topic for which there is more likely to be shared understanding, such as objects present in the room or a special logo on the child's shirt or shoes.

Once the child feels comfortable, he or she will provide numerous language samples, so it is important to listen carefully. Does the child speak in full sentences? Does he or she fail to conjugate verbs or make other grammatical errors? Children with LI often make word-finding errors, or have trouble coming up with the specific words they want to say. Such errors may be manifested as "groping" for a word, or by simply talking around concepts that cannot be named. Some children will make frank paraphasic errors, substituting one word or nonword for another. For example, one young child with LI responded, "Cow," when asked, "What animal goes 'meow'?" This error probably resulted from a combination of a semantic relationship between "cat" and "cow" (both are familiar animals), as well as a phonological similarity to the word the child had most recently heard ("meow"). Behavioral observation can provide rich information about receptive language as well. Some children frequently ask for clarification or appear confused after lengthy directions, or they may repeat directions to themselves while performing the task. Others will never ask for repetition, but will simply act in ways indicating that they have misunderstood the examiner. For any task with complex instructions, it is particularly important to ensure that children understand what they are to do, so that their abilities can be accurately assessed.

SSD is easily observed by parents, and should be fairly apparent to the examiner as well. In conversational speech, a child will make sound omission and/or substitution errors, and will be difficult to understand. The examiner may perceive that the child is talking rapidly, which probably relates to the examiner's own reduced comprehension (just as we often believe that people speaking languages other than our own speak very fast). Young children with severely reduced intelligibility will often resort to other means of communicating, such as getting up out of their chairs to show an evaluator what they mean. Children with SSD vary in their willingness to repeat themselves and in their frustration about not being understood. If a child has made multiple attempts to communicate something, and the examiner cannot understand him or her, it may be useful to say, "Let's ask your mom about that at the break."

Case Presentations

Case Presentation 3

Background. Megan is a 9-year-old third grader. Her parents have sought this evaluation because they are concerned about her progress in reading, reading comprehension, and math. Homework is very difficult, and often takes Megan more than twice as long as it is supposed to, although she is typically cooperative and attentive to the task at hand. Megan has had particular difficulty with a reading program in which she is required to read a book for homework and answer comprehension questions about it the next day at school. Megan often cannot answer any of the questions accurately, even though she is reading books 1–2 years below grade level. Megan herself has explained how difficult this task can be, saying, "Sometimes everybody else is on the last question and I'm still on the first one, so I just sit there and cry because I'm so frustrated."

Megan's birth history includes some risk factors. Delivery was difficult and required suction and forceps. Although her parents did not recall the specific Apgar scores, they were thought to be somewhat low, and Megan required supplemental oxygen for several hours. Nonetheless, she was thought to be ready for discharge at 3 days old, at which time she developed a fever. This illness required a week-long hospitalization with intravenous antibiotic treatment. Early motor milestones were achieved at the expected ages, but language development was somewhat delayed. According to Megan's parents, strangers could not understand anything she said until she was 3, because her articulation and expressive language were poor; however, she appeared to understand what was said to her. Megan did receive some speech therapy for articulation difficulties when she was in preschool. Although Megan is now quite chatty and can be well understood by strangers, her parents continue to have some concerns about her language development. They have commented that she cannot follow multistep directions and often has trouble coming up with the specific words she wants to say. In addition, she has a lisp when producing the /s/ sound.

Megan had trouble learning letters in preschool, and she has always been in the weakest reading group in her class. She received extra help from the reading specialist at school in first and second grades, and her parents have also pursued some private tutoring. Her spelling is quite poor, and she has always struggled to memorize her math facts. More recently, her parents have become concerned that she is having difficulty mastering new math concepts and solving math word problems.

Megan's father received speech therapy for articulation difficulties when he was 3 and 4 years old, but has not reported having any problems in school. He graduated from college and works as an administrator for a nonprofit organization. Megan's mother does not report any specific speech, language, or reading difficulties, but notes that school was a "struggle," by which she means that she received B's and C's despite working very hard. She completed a 2-year college degree. Before her children were born, she worked as an administrative assistant. For the last 10 years, she has run a home day care business.

Megan's diagnostic testing is summarized in Table 7.2.

Discussion. Megan's history is similar to that of children with RD. However, several aspects of her presentation indicate that her language difficulties are broader than typically seen in children with classic dyslexia alone and are therefore consistent with a diagnosis of LI. Although children with RD alone sometimes have subtle expressive language problems as preschoolers, Megan's early difficulties in this area were quite significant, to the point that strangers could not understand her. In addition to early history, current complaints are indicative of a more general language disorder. Her parents have noticed that Megan has substantial difficulty with word finding (coming up with the specific words she wants to say), as well as understanding complex language (e.g., multistep directions). Many children with LI also have articulation weaknesses. Compared to weaknesses in vocabulary or grammar, articulation difficulties are more likely to be noticed by parents or teachers and to result in referral to a speech–language pathologist. Megan has probably had difficulties in all three areas from an early age, though her early treatment focused primarily on articulation.

Megan's test results support a diagnosis of LI. Perhaps most notable is the very large (>2 *SD*s) split between her scores on the Verbal Comprehension Index and the Perceptual Reasoning Index of the WISC-IV. Although her nonverbal reasoning abilities are quite solid, her ability to use language to think and reason is only marginally better than that of many children with ID. Because of this large split, WISC-IV testing has been followed up with formal tests of language ability, such as the CELF-4 and the PPVT-4. The CELF-4 includes a number of subtests measuring expressive and receptive vocabulary and syntax as well as verbal working memory, and Megan has obtained below-average scores on this test. She has particular difficulty in generating sentences with correct grammatical form. Her score on the PPVT-4, a receptive vocabulary test that requires no verbal output from the

TABLE 7.2. Test Summary, Case 3 (Megan)

Construct	Standard Score/ cutoff
General intelligence	
WISC-IV Full Scale IQ	88
Crystallized intelligence[a]	
WISC-V *Verbal Comprehension Index*	75
Similarities	6
Vocabulary	6
Comprehension	5
Fluid intelligence	
WISC-IV *Perceptual Reasoning Index*	108
Block Design	13
Picture Concepts	10
Matrix Reasoning	11
WISC-IV Working Memory Index[b]	80
Digit Span	6
Letter–Number Sequencing	7
WISC-IV Processing Speed Index[c]	100
Coding	8
Symbol Search	12
Academic	
Reading	
History	
Learning and Behavior Quest. Reading History Items	60
Word recognition	
WJ III Letter Word ID	86
TOWRE Sight Word Efficiency	84
Phonological coding	
WJ III Word Attack	91
TOWRE Phonemic Decoding Efficiency	73
Paragraph fluency	
GORT-4 Fluency	70
Reading comprehension	
GORT-4 Comprehension	70
Math	
WJ III Math Fluency	101
WJ III Calculation	106
WJ III Applied Problems	110

(continued)

TABLE 7.2. (continued)

Construct	Standard Score/ cutoff
Written expression	
WIAT Written Expression	79
Spelling	
WJ III Spelling	87
Oral Language	
General	
CELF-4 Core Language	79
Semantics	
PPVT-4	93
Phonological awareness[d]	
CTOPP Elision	90
CTOPP Phoneme Reversal	75
Verbal memory	
WRAML Sentence Memory	80
WRAML Story Memory	85
CTOPP Nonword Repetition	80
Verbal processing speed	
CTOPP Rapid Naming Composite	94
Attention and hyperactivity–impulsivity	
ADHD Rating Scale–IV Inattention	
Parent	0/9
Teacher	0/9
ADHD Rating Scale–IV Hyperactivity–Impulsivity	
Parent	0/9
Teacher	1/9

Note. WISC-IV, Wechsler Intelligence Scale for Children—Fourth Edition; WJ III, Woodcock–Johnson III Tests of Achievement; TOWRE, Test of Word Reading Efficiency; GORT-4, Gray Oral Reading Test—Fourth Edition; PPVT-4, Peabody Picture Vocabulary Test, Fourth Edition; CELF-4, Clinical Evaluation of Language Fundamentals—Fourth Edition; CTOPP, Comprehensive Test of Phonological Processing; WRAML, Wide Range Assessment of Memory and Learning.
[a]See also Oral language—Semantics.
[b]See also Oral language—Verbal memory.
[c]See also Oral language—Verbal processing speed, and Academics—Math—WJ III Math Fluency.
[d]See also Verbal memory—CTOPP Nonword Repetition for another test of phonological processing.

child, is at the lower end of the average range. Relatively spared receptive vocabulary is common in children with LI, particularly if they have been exposed to good language models in the home. Like most children with LI, Megan has a weakness in verbal short-term memory. This difficulty is evident in her scores on the Working Memory Index of the WISC-IV, the Sentence Memory subtest of the WRAML, and the Nonword Repetition subtest of the CTOPP. Verbal short-term memory impairment probably contributes to her inability to follow multistep directions and can create quite a liability in the classroom setting.

Several qualitative observations also support the LI diagnosis. Megan's verbal responses on the WISC-IV were often vague and poorly organized. For example, when asked to define "hat," Megan said, "It's when it's hot outside and your mom says you're going to get a sunburn, so you put your hat on." She demonstrated word-finding difficulties in the testing situation. As one example, she described a woman she knows as "a girl, but she's old." Furthermore, when retelling the WRAML story, Megan made statements such as "The girl had her thing." She often appeared confused when complex directions were presented, and on a few occasions asked the examiner to "please talk again" (meaning to repeat the instructions).

Like most children with LI, Megan clearly has a very significant reading problem, which merits the additional diagnosis of dyslexia. Megan demonstrates the classic difficulties of a child with dyslexia, including weaknesses in word-level reading and spelling, more pronounced difficulty on timed than untimed reading tests, and difficulty with phonological processing. It is notable that Megan's reading comprehension (as measured by the GORT-4) is more impaired than would be expected in a child of her age with dyslexia alone. Her poor reading comprehension is a product of difficulties with both decoding and oral language comprehension. Although Megan's parents have been concerned about her math skills, her scores on tests of math achievement are commensurate with both her age and her nonverbal reasoning abilities. Real-world difficulties with math may arise from her language difficulties in several ways. First, new math concepts are often explained to children in complex language, which may be hard for Megan to follow. Similarly, she is likely to have difficulty in reading and understanding word problems. Finally, like other children with verbal memory weaknesses, she is likely to struggle to memorize math facts.

Given Megan's slightly risky birth history, one question is whether her difficulties could be the results of an acquired brain injury, such as damage caused by hypoxia. Overall, current results suggest that Megan's learning difficulties are more likely to have a developmental than an acquired origin. First, her pattern of performance is not characteristic of children with early-acquired neurological insults; such children often show a general low-level cognitive depression, along with relatively stronger verbal than nonverbal abilities. In fact, fluid intelligence and processing speed—the very domains most likely to be affected by an acquired insult—represent strengths for Megan. Second, there is at least some family history of speech and language difficulties.

As all children who visit our clinic are, Megan has been screened for attentional difficulties. Parent and teacher questionnaire responses are all in the normal range, and neither early history nor observations are consistent with ADHD. In fact, the parents' report suggests that attention is an area of strength for Megan, given that she is able to attend for several hours to homework that must feel extremely difficult and tedious for her.

Case Presentation 4

Background. Gabriel is a 5-year-old boy who will be starting kindergarten in a few months. His pediatrician has referred him for this assessment because of concerns about his speech development. Gabriel was a late talker, and his speech has always sounded immature, but his parents had assumed he would grow out of this "baby talk." However, at his 5-year-old well-child visit, his pediatrician noted that Gabriel's continuing struggle with articulation makes him difficult to understand, and suggested a more complete evaluation.

Gabriel's prenatal and birth histories are uncomplicated. Early motor milestones were met as expected, but his speech–language development was somewhat delayed. He first said single words at 21 months, first combined two words at 2 years, and did not speak in short sentences until he was nearly 3 years old. When Gabriel first began talking, strangers could not comprehend him, and even his parents understood him only about 75% of the time. Despite these delays, his parents always thought that his receptive language was fairly good. They remembered that he responded to his name by 6 months, understood several words by 9 months (e.g., "nose," "doggie"), and could follow a simple instruction by the time he began to walk (e.g., "Bring me the book"). Gabriel had a history of regular ear infections as a toddler, which led to placement of tubes at age 2 years, and his parents wonder whether this aspect of his history is related to his current difficulties. According to his pediatrician, however, Gabriel's hearing is normal.

Gabriel has attended preschool for the last 2 years. On the paperwork she filled out for this evaluation, his teacher wrote, "Gabriel is a bright, sweet little boy who is a delight to teach. I hope his speech improves soon, because it is difficult for me and the other children to understand him." Gabriel gets along well with his peers and is regularly invited over for play dates.

Gabriel's mother notes that she had some speech difficulties herself, and she attributes these to having "a tongue that was too big for my mouth."

She recalls that she said "cimanon" for "cinnamon" and could not pronounce the /r/ sound until she was in third grade. Although her speech has
since normalized, she notes that she sometimes has difficulty pronouncing
unfamiliar words. She graduated from college and nursing school and works
as a cardiac nurse. Gabriel's father reports no history of speech or learning
problems. He has a master's degree and works as a geographer.

Gabriel's diagnostic testing is summarized in Table 7.3.

Discussion. Gabriel's history and current presentation are consistent
with SSD. Although children with SSD are at risk for additional disorders of
language development, including LI and later RD, Gabriel appears to have
an isolated case of SSD. He does not currently have a broader LI, and his
early literacy skills are developing nicely. However, his academic progress
should be monitored closely, and a fuller evaluation of the question of RD
will have to wait a year or two, until he is older and has been exposed to
more formal literacy instruction.

On the Goldman–Fristoe Test of Articulation, a single-word elicitation
test, Gabriel consistently distorted the /r/, /l/, and /s/ sounds. In addition, he
substituted /f/ for "th" (e.g., "fum" for "thumb") and had difficulty pronouncing most consonant blends (e.g., "sk" for "skw" as in "squirrel," and
"fw" for "kr" as in "Christmas"). In conversational speech, Gabriel made
multiple sound substitutions (e.g., "tat" for "cat") and omission errors (e.g.,
"boom" for "broom"), which reduced his intelligibility. Gabriel's score on
the Goldman–Fristoe is clearly discrepant from measures of nearly all his
other cognitive/intellectual abilities, most of which fall in the high-average
to above-average range, and warrant a course of speech therapy. In addition to articulation weaknesses, the defining symptom of SSD, Gabriel has
also demonstrated a deficit in verbal short-term memory, a cognitive risk
factor for the disorder. Verbal short-term memory difficulties are evident on
the CTOPP Nonword Repetition and WRAML Sentence Memory tasks. In
addition, his somewhat lower score on the Syntax composite of the TOLD-
P:3 is due entirely to a poor score on the Sentence Imitation subtest, which
is very similar to the WRAML Sentence Memory task. For example, asked
to repeat the sentence "Yesterday my aunt forgot her lunch," Gabriel said,
"Yesterday her aunt will get her lunch."

Although Gabriel was a late talker, his current broader language skill,
as measured by formal testing, is good. It seems likely that his early language delays primarily reflected difficulties with speech development. Children whose early language delays are limited to expressive language have
a better prognosis than children with both expressive and receptive delays,
and his parents' report places Gabriel in the former group. Although his
parents are concerned about possible effects of his early ear infections, little
research to date supports a causal link to long-lasting speech–language diffi-

TABLE 7.3. Test Summary, Case 4 (Gabriel)

Construct	Standard score/ cut-off
General intelligence	
WPPSI-III Full Scale IQ	119
Crystallized intelligence[a]	
WPPSI-III Verbal IQ	110
Information	13
Vocabulary	11
Word Reasoning	12
Fluid intelligence	
WPPSI-III Performance IQ	121
Block Design	14
Matrix Reasoning	13
Picture Concepts	13
WPPSI-III Processing Speed Index[b]	113
Symbol Search	13
Coding	12
Academic	
Reading	
Word recognition	
WJ III Letter Word ID	110
Phonological coding	
WJ III Word Attack	120
Math	
WJ III Calculation	121
WJ III Applied Problems	117
Spelling	
WJ III Spelling	110
Oral language	
Speech	
Goldman–Fristoe Test of Articulation	74
Semantics	
PPVT-4	119
TOLD-P:3 Semantics Composite	112
Syntax	
TOLD-P:3 Syntax Composite	93

(continued)

TABLE 7.3. (continued)

Construct	Standard score/ cut-off
Phonological awareness[c]	
CTOPP Elision	105
CTOPP Blending	110
CTOPP Sound Matching	105
Verbal memory	
WRAML Sentence Memory	80
WRAML Story Memory	105
CTOPP Nonword Repetition	80
Verbal processing speed	
CTOPP Rapid Naming Composite	111
Attention and hyperactivity–impulsivity	
ADHD Rating Scale–IV Inattention	
Parent	1/9
Teacher	0/9
ADHD Rating Scale–IV Hyperactivity–Impulsivity	
Parent	0/9
Teacher	2/9

Note. WPPSI-III, Wechsler Preschool and Primary Scale of Intelligence—Third Edition; TOLD-P:3, Test of Language Development—Primary: Third Edition. For other abbreviations, see Table 7.2.
[a]See also Oral language—Semantics.
[b]See also Oral language—Verbal processing speed.
[c]See also Verbal memory—CTOPP Nonword Repetition for another test of phonological processing.

culties. Ear infections are quite common in the general population, so many children both with and without SSD are likely to have an early history similar to Gabriel's.

Gabriel is too young to complete an in-depth academic assessment, but a brief screen of his early literacy and math skills has been conducted with the WJ III. In addition, his phonological awareness and rapid naming abilities have been assessed with the CTOPP, since these are good predictors of later reading ability. Currently, Gabriel's achievement appears commensurate with his intellectual abilities and is not a cause for concern. In terms of math, Gabriel can solve some very simple arithmetic problems, such as "2 + 2 = __." Conceptual math ability, as measured by WJ III Applied Problems, is quite solid. In terms of literacy development, Gabriel recognizes and can write capital letters and many lower-case letters, and has learned some letter sounds. Gabriel's scores on the CTOPP are similar to estimates of his verbal conceptual abilities. Thus there is not a current indication that he is likely to struggle with the process of learning to read and spell. His parents can be reassured that the majority of children with SSD do not have unusual difficulty with literacy acquisition, especially when they have strong cognitive abilities. Nonetheless, as mentioned above, Gabriel's academic progress and especially his literacy development should be monitored carefully, and appropriate intervention should be put in place quickly if difficulties arise. A brief reevaluation at the end of first grade or the beginning of second grade should be recommended, just to ensure that his reading and spelling are developing as expected.

There is a notable family history of speech difficulties through Gabriel's mother. Despite her own account of her difficulties, it is more likely that she had an underlying cognitive–linguistic liability for speech difficulty, just as Gabriel does. Although most outward signs of her early speech difficulty have resolved, a subtle residue of this liability is observable in her current difficulty with pronouncing complex unfamiliar words.

Treatment

Treatment of LI and SSD is reviewed in Leonard (2000) and in a comprehensive meta-analysis of 25 studies by Law, Garrett, and Nye (2003). There are various approaches, including imitation, modeling, focused stimulation, and milieu teaching—all of which provide children with LI or SSD targeted exposure to, and practice with, the linguistic forms in which they are deficient. In other words, these therapies provide more intensive and focused "doses" of some of the things parents and other adults naturally do to stimulate language development. Evaluation of these various approaches find gains relative either to the language of untreated controls or to untreated linguistic forms in the children's repertoires. Such interventions have also been shown to increase the rate of language development and to transfer to spontaneous speech. In the Law et al. (2003) meta-analysis, the most reliable treatment effects were for children with speech and expressive vocabulary problems, but not for children with receptive language problems.

Despite these optimistic findings from research on the treatment of SSD and LI, there are some caveats. Just as is true in psychotherapy outcome studies, many forms of speech and language therapy appear to work, but all to about an equal extent (see a meta-analysis by Nye, Foster, & Seaman, 1987). Hence the treatments provided by clinicians using different approaches may nonetheless have some common elements, but these have not been clearly delineated. Moreover, in the Law et al. (2003) meta-analysis, no significant differences were found between trained parents and clinicians as deliverers of interventions. A second caveat is that long term follow-up studies of treated children find that initial severity of LI (or SSD) predicts language outcome, but duration of treatment does not (Aram & Nation, 1980; Bishop & Edmundson, 1987). Although these were not treatment studies per se, since the treatments were those that would ordinarily occur in community settings, it is still concerning that there is no evidence of a dose–response relation for duration of treatment. Moreover, since there is a wide range of normal variation in speech and language development in young children, some of those identified as having SSD or LI and given treatment would probably have developed normally anyway. Other children have more persisting problems; the critical question is how much treatment helps those children.

Thus, although these treatments for LI and SSD have received some research support, they do not yet meet all standards for well-established empirically supported treatments (see Chapter 14 for a more detailed discussion of these criteria). In general, it is difficult for behavioral treatments to meet these standards; however, the field would benefit from more studies that meet all of the "gold standards" for treatment evaluation, especially those that include comparison groups receiving equal-intensity intervention. It may also be the case that language disorders are inherently difficult to remediate, making identification of effective treatments even more difficult. We know, in fact, that available treatments do not cure LI or SSD. On average, adults treated for SSD as children still have phoneme awareness deficits and reading problems (Lewis & Freebairn, 1992). Follow-ups of children with LI into adolescence (Snowling, Bishop, & Stothard, 2000) or young adulthood (Rutter & Mahwood, 1991) find that a sizable proportion have declined in reading, IQ, language, and even social skills, compared to how they performed at younger ages. Because language skill is so important to development, it is not surprising that persisting LI would exact a greater and greater cost. Just as the social deficits in ASD deprive a child of important inputs for development, so does persisting LI.

Table 7.4 summarizes clinical issues in LI and SSD.

TABLE 7.4. Clinical Summary Table: LI and SSD

Defining symptoms	• LI: Delayed expressive and/or receptive language development in the absence of a known cause (such as deafness, brain injury, or ID). • SSD: Developmentally inappropriate inability to produce speech sounds in the absence of a known cause.
Common comorbidities	• LI and SSD are comorbid with each other, and both are comorbid with RD. LI is also comorbid with ADHD.
Developmental history	• LI: Late talker. Speech not understood by strangers. Comprehension (receptive language) often appears better than production (expressive language). Immature grammar and delayed learning of the past tense. School difficulties, particularly in literacy, but often across the curriculum. Trouble following multistep directions. Word-finding problems. Trouble learning directional ("left–right") and sequencing ("before–after") terms. Social problems may result from difficulty in communicating with peers. • SSD: Speech is difficult to understand, particularly for strangers. Speech may sound "babyish," or the child may be described as "tongue-tied." May be a late talker. Some children have other oral–motor difficulties (e.g., drooling, trouble chewing or swallowing, etc.).
Diagnosis	• LI: History of impairing language delay plus poor performance (i.e., < 10th percentile for age) on standardized language testing (e.g., TOLD-P:3 or CELF-4). • SSD: History of impairing speech delay plus poor performance on standardized test of articulation (e.g., Goldman–Fristoe). • IQ testing and medical history rule out exclusionary conditions.
Prognosis	• LI: Except in unusually severe cases, children will eventually show reasonable mastery of their native language (speak in full sentences, learn the past tense, etc.). However, individual differences in language skill are moderately stable. Compared to same-age peers, individuals with LI have smaller vocabularies and poorer understanding of complex language. There is some evidence for a decline in nonverbal IQ over time. Academic difficulties persist, particularly in reading, writing, and learning foreign languages. • SSD: The majority of children with SSD show normalization of speech over time, though underlying phonological processing weaknesses may still be present. Educational and occupational prognoses depend largely on whether additional disorders (LI, RD) are present.
Treatment	• LI: Regular speech–language therapy focusing on specific areas of weakness (such as vocabulary or grammar development). Special education for any subject in which the child requires additional support. Appropriate accommodations provided by teachers and parents (breaking multistep directions down into smaller pieces, using visual supports whenever possible, preview and review of material, extended time for assignments and tests, etc.). • SSD: Regular speech therapy focusing on articulation skills. In severe cases, alternative means of communication may be helpful (sign language, DynaVox).

CHAPTER 8

Autism Spectrum Disorder

WITH LAUREN M. MCGRATH AND ROBIN L. PETERSON

HISTORY

One could argue that autism spectrum disorder (ASD) is the most severe syndrome covered in this book, since it disrupts very basic aspects of personhood and does so very early in development. It is also the most recently recognized learning disorder. The first descriptions of this syndrome (Asperger, 1944/1991; Kanner, 1943) were published about 60 years ago, whereas other childhood disorders, such as dyslexia and ADHD, have been discussed in the scientific literature for over a century. These two facts about ASD—its severity and its late recognition—present us with a puzzle: How did earlier generations regard people with ASD, what treatments did such people receive, what became of them? Perhaps part of the answer to this puzzle lies in what is a very recent change in social attitudes toward those with severe developmental disabilities, such as ASD and ID. Not very long ago, such individuals were considered essentially untreatable and were institutionalized very early in life.

Public awareness of ASD has increased recently because of movies (e.g., *Rain Man*) and books about high-functioning people with autism or Asperger syndrome. Several useful books are autobiographies—one by Professor Temple Grandin at Colorado State University (*Thinking in Pictures*, 1995) and another by Liane Willey (*Pretending to Be Normal*, 1999). Most recently, the autobiography by John Elder Robison (*Look Me in the Eye: My Life with Asperger's*, 2007) has received a lot of media attention. Although these portrayals are quite useful introductions to ASD, it is important to remember that most people with autism are not high-functioning. A large proportion of such individuals have ID, and about half lack speech.

ASD, like many of the other disorders considered in this book, has been a projective test for theorists; changes in conceptions of it have reflected changes in more general notions about the nature of psychopathology. As we will see later in this chapter, ASD is still one of the least well-understood learning disorders and thus still has a lot to teach us about errors in our conceptual frameworks. The term "autism" (from the Greek word *autos*, which means "self") was introduced by Bleuler (1911/1950) to describe a symptom of schizophrenia—namely, extreme self-absorption, leading to a loss of contact with external reality. (This is a somewhat ironic term to describe the syndrome of ASD, since many theorists agree that developing a self depends on relations with others, so that extreme early social isolation should lead to *less* rather than more of a self. We will return to the topic of the early development of the self when we review competing neuropsychological theories of the development of ASD.) Partly because Bleuler's term "autism" for a symptom of schizophrenia was chosen as the name for this new syndrome, the two disorders were confused (a good example of Piaget's concept of assimilation). Autism was originally considered to be just another form of childhood schizophrenia. But it is now clear that these are etiologically distinct disorders, with different developmental courses, despite some symptom overlap.

Both Kanner (1943) and Asperger (1944/1991) selected Bleuler's term "autism" to characterize the extreme lack of social awareness in the children they were describing—whether extreme social isolation without speech (the "lives in a shell" quality), or didactic and tangential speech about an obscure subject (such as vacuum cleaners or parking garages) of little interest to the listener. The title of Kanner's paper was "Autistic Disturbances of Affective Contact," and he also spoke of "extreme autistic aloneness" (p. 242). The title of Asperger's paper was Autistic "Psychopathy in Childhood." Other features of the syndrome noted by Kanner included (1) an "obsessive desire for the maintenance of sameness" (p. 245); (2) a fascination with objects; (3) mutism and other language abnormalities, such as echolalia; (4) a normal physical appearance; and (5) evidence of some preserved intellectual skills, such as a good rote memory or good performance on spatial tasks. Finally, Kanner (1943), good clinician that he was, noted a high frequency of large head circumferences among his 11 patients. As will be discussed later, one of the most consistent brain structure correlates of autism is macrocephaly (abnormally large head circumference), so Kanner was prescient in this regard.

Asperger's (1944/1991) independent description of his different sample of cases strikingly noted many of the same characteristics; the main differences were better language skills, unusual specialized interests, and somewhat greater social awareness in Asperger's cases (see discussion in Wing, 1991). Indeed, many authors regard the syndromes described by these two men as two points on the same continuum or spectrum, with one sample just happening to be higher-functioning than the other. Other experts believe that these are two distinct syndromes. As we will see, the data from family members of probands with autism strongly supports the concept of a continuum, since subclinical variants of autism reminiscent of Asperger syndrome are found in these family members. Within the autism spectrum literature, there is also an active controversy regarding whether high-functioning autism (usually defined by the absence of ID) and Asperger syndrome are the same or different conditions. Our own and others' interpretation of the current literature is that the two disorders are more alike than different (Koyama, Tachimori, Osada, Takeda, & Kurita, 2007; Rinehart, Bradshaw, Brereton, & Tonge, 2002; Thede & Coolidge, 2007), although further research is needed to resolve this issue. So research on autism provides an example of both splitting (autism from schizophrenia) and, potentially, lumping (autism with Asperger syndrome) of disorders. The lack of conceptual and diagnostic clarity is the reason for our choice of "autism spectrum disorder" (ASD) as a general term in this chapter (see the next section for further definitional considerations).

Although both Kanner (1943) and Asperger (1944/1991) believed that their syndromes were of constitutional origin (and Asperger explicitly hypothesized genetic transmission), psychoanalytic theorists (e.g., Bettelheim, 1967; Mahler, 1952) postulated a psychosocial etiology for autism. Even Kanner himself later adopted this view. The psychoanalytic view held that rejecting, so-called "refrigerator" mothers caused these children to withdraw from social interaction, and treatment focused on changing parenting. Although, as we will see later, it is possible for very extreme environmental deprivation to produce at least some of the symptoms of ASD, it is much less plausible that parental coldness could produce such a devastating developmental outcome. Indeed, these psychosocial theories of autism were based only on clinical observations, not on systematic research. Subsequent research has shown that on average, mothers of children with autism interact with their children at least as much as, if not more than, mothers of typically developing children do—most likely because they are trying to engage them (e.g., Kasari, Sigman, Mundy, & Yirmiya, 1990). Since parents of a child with atypical development almost inevitably blame themselves for the problem, these erroneous theories undoubtedly increased their guilt and suffering. This is a fairly striking example of how clinical ignorance can lead to a violation of the Hippocratic maxim: "First, do no harm."

Rimland (1964), a scientist who was also a parent of a child with autism, was among the first to argue that this disorder was neurological rather than psychosocial in origin. A neurological etiology was supported by the association of autism with maternal rubella (Chess, 1977), late-onset seizures (Schain & Yannet, 1960), and certain genetic conditions (e.g., untreated phenylketonuria). The contemporary view of ASD emphasizes its biological origin; as we will see, it is probably the most heritable of the psychopathologies considered here. Current research is focused on identifying the genetic risk factors, the neurological phenotypes, and the resulting changes in neuropsychological development. At the same time, the psychosocial environment remains very important in the development of individuals with ASD. Early interventions has shown that the deficits in social behavior found in ASD are much more malleable than was previously thought, although there is as yet no cure.

DEFINITION

In the *Diagnostic and Statistical Manual of Mental Disorders*, fourth edition, text revision (DSM-IV-TR; American Psychiatric Association, 2000), the diagnoses of autistic disorder and Asperger's disorder fall under the broader category of pervasive developmental disorders (PDDs). The other three members of this category are Rett's disorder, childhood disintegrative disorder (CDD), and a residual diagnosis, PDD not otherwise specified (PDD-NOS). All five PDDs share at least some of the classic symptoms of autism, which is traditionally defined by a triad of qualitative impairments in (1) social interaction; (2) communication; and (3) range of behavior, interests, and activities. They differ in the extent of these symptoms and in developmental course. Both Rett's disorder and CDD require regression after a period of normal development (from 5 to 30 months in Rett's and from 2 to 10 years in CDD). So in both these disorders, an apparently normal child loses developmental gains in motor, language, and social skills, and develops at least some of the classic symptoms of autism. Rett's disorder is a rare, progressive neurological disease (in which there is a deceleration in brain growth and, as a result, in head circumference); it occurs only in girls. CDD is assumed to be due to an acquired neurological insult, but in many cases the etiology is unknown. Asperger's disorder is defined by impairment in two domains of the triad: social interaction and range of behavior, interests, and activities. Although communication impairments are not required for a diagnosis, as in autistic disorder, such impairments are often present (particularly in pragmatics). In addition, for an individual to meet diagnostic criteria for Asperger's disorder, there can be no significant delay in language or cognitive development. So, by definition, Asperger's disorder in DSM-IV-TR is a less severe form of autism, without language and cognitive delays. It is worth noting that this definition is not very different from Asperger's (1944/1991) original description. Finally, PDD-NOS is reserved for cases where symptoms of autism are present but criteria for one of the other four PDDs are not met, because of either subthreshold levels of symptoms or even later onset. In sum, the definition of these five PDDs implies an autism spectrum that runs from autism proper (autistic disorder) to Asperger's disorder to PDD-NOS and includes two autistic-like syndromes with a deteriorating course.

We now describe the autistic triad in more detail. A qualitative impairment in social interaction requires at least two of four symptoms: (1) obvious impairment in the use of nonverbal behaviors (e.g., eye contact, facial expression, and gestures) to regulate social interaction; (2) failure to develop peer relations; (3) lack of spontaneous sharing of enjoyment, interests, or achievements with others; and (4) lack of emotional or social reciprocity. A marked impairment in communication requires one of four symptoms: (1) delay or lack of spoken language development, without any attempt to compensate through mime or gesture; (2) if speech is present, obvious impairment in initiating or sustaining conversation; (3) stereotyped and repetitive, or idiosyncratic, use of language; and (4) lack of spontaneous, varied pretend play. The last part of the triad—restricted, repetitive, and stereotyped patterns of behavior—requires at least one of four symptoms: (1) an encompassing preoccupation with a narrow interest; (2) rigid adherence to specific, nonfunctional rituals or routines or rituals; (3) motor stereotypies (e.g., hand flapping); and (4) persistent preoccupation with parts of objects. For the DSM-IV-TR diagnosis of autistic disorder, the onset must occur before 3 years.

These diagnostic criteria for autism have been operationalized by a standardized, semistructured parent interview, the Autism Diagnostic Interview—Revised (ADI-R; Lord, Rutter, & Le Couteur, 1994). The ADI-R has an interrater reliability of at least 90%, and both its sensitivity and specificity also exceed 90% (Lord et al., 1994). Therefore, it is the current "gold standard" for diagnosing autism, and it is this phenotype that is being used in current large collaborative molecular genetic studies of this disorder. (The term "autism" is used hereafter, as a synonym for DSM-defined autistic disorder, and as a historical term. In mentions of the full spectrum, again, "ASD" is used.) Just as is true for the other, behaviorally defined disorders considered in this book, the question of which phenotypes with which boundaries to use in such studies is a difficult issue. Perhaps a dimensional phenotype is more appropriate than a categorical one. A recent large-population twin sample found that autistic traits were normally distributed (Constantino & Todd, 2003), so a particular diagnostic threshold is somewhat arbitrary, as is true for the other disorders in this book. Perhaps there is an endophenotype that better captures what is transmitted in families, even though it is not part of the diagnostic definition. In other words, genetic studies will help refine the phenotype, and refinements in phenotype definition will inform genetic studies. As with other disorders, we should be careful not to reify current phenotype definitions.

EPIDEMIOLOGY AND COMORBIDITIES

Epidemiology

The median lifetime prevalence of autism is about 5 per 10,000 (American Psychiatric Association, 2000), although more recent studies with broader diagnostic criteria have found a higher prevalence, about 10 to 12 per 10,000 (Bryson & Smith, 1998). Most recently, two studies from the Centers for Disease Control and Prevention (CDCP) have found even higher prevalence rates—6.7 per 1,000 or 1 per 150 (Autism and Developmental Disabilities Monitoring Network, 2007). These CDCP studies were conducted 2 years apart (2000 and 2002) through health departments in several states, and utililized a review of evaluation records at multiple sources to detect diagnosed cases of ASD. Because these studies did not directly diagnose a random population sample with a "gold standard" measure such as the ADI-R, we might expect that rates would vary according to educational and child health practices in different states, and indeed they did. The highest rates in both studies were found in New Jersey (9.9 and 10.6 per 1,000, respectively), and the lowest were found in West Virginia in 2000 (4.5 per 1,000), and Alabama in 2002 (3.3 per 1,000). Although bioenvironmental risk factors (or even genetic ones) could vary across states, it seems much more likely that the state differences reflect detection differences and not true differences. Similarly, somewhat higher rates were found in groups with higher socioeconomic status, again presumably because of detection differences. Most strikingly, the rates within states were generally stable over a 6- to 7-year period, in contrast to the rate differences across states.

These CDCP results help address a recent concern that the true rates of ASD have actually increased due to greater exposure to some environmental risk factor (e.g., vaccinations). Moreover, three studies of this issue (Madsen et al., 2002; Taylor et al., 1999, 2002) found no increase in cases of ASD after the introduction of the measles, mumps, and rubella (MMR) vaccination or a difference in rates of ASD between vaccinated and unvaccinated children. Similarly, a review by the Institute of Medicine (Stratton, Gable, & McCormick, 2001) found no evidence to support the hypothesis that an organic mercury-based preservative used in some vaccines (thimerosal) is a risk factor for ASD or other developmental disorders.

The issue of diagnostic substitution is also being examined as a possible partial explanation for the increased rates of autism (Croen, Grether, Hoogstrate, & Selvin, 2002). "Diagnostic substitution" in this context refers to the growing trend for clinicians to diagnosis ASD rather than ID. Although this diagnosis may be appropriate in some cases, there is evidence that this difficult differential diagnosis can be influenced by prevailing diagnostic trends, such as the increasing social acceptance of a diagnosis of ASD compared to one of ID. Croen et al. (2002) conducted a population-based study of eight successive birth cohorts from 1987 to 1994. Across the study period, the prevalence of autism increased from 5.8 to 14.9 per 10,000, while the prevalence of ID without autism decreased from 28.8 to 19.5 per 10,000. Although this study is correlational, it may suggest a diagnostic trend that has implications for the prevalence estimates of both ASD and ID.

In sum, the best-supported explanations for what is sometimes called an "epidemic of autism" include broader criteria, better detection, and diagnostic substitution, although more research is needed on this important issue (e.g., Chakrabarti & Fombonne, 2001).

The male–female ratio in autism ranges from 3:1 to 4:1, but females with autism have lower average IQs and hence a higher rate of ID (reviewed in Klinger & Dawson, 1996). The reasons for these gender differences are unknown.

Comorbidities

ASD overlaps with ID, LI, and anxiety disorders (including obsessive–compulsive disorder). Symptoms of inattention and hyperactivity are quite common in ASD, but according to DSM-IV-TR (American Psychiatric Association, 2000), the diagnosis of any PDD precludes one of ADHD.

The comorbidity of autism with ID makes the differential diagnosis of these two syndromes very complicated, particularly in young children (e.g., Vig & Jedrysek, 1999). Although children with a primary diagnosis of autism may also have ID, children with a primary diagnosis of ID may exhibit symptoms of autism because of their cognitive delay, without having the full autism phenotype. For this reason, best-practice parameters recommend that any ASD assessment should include an assessment of cognitive ability, so that behavioral symptoms can be interpreted within the context of the child's developmental level (Ozonoff, Goodlin-Jones, & Solomon, 2005). In young children, the symptom overlap of autism and ID can be significant. For example, delays in verbal communication and symbolic play are associated with both disorders and so cannot inform the differential diagnosis. Similarly, repetitive behaviors are often seen in both disorders (Vig & Jedrysek, 1999). The most reliable symptoms for differentiating children with a primary diagnosis of autism from those with a primary diagnosis of ID are in the social realm. Because social interaction skills emerge early in development, they can be assessed even in children with delayed development. Children with autism are more likely to show impairments in social skills, such as imitation, joint attention, and eye gaze modulation (Vig & Jedrysek, 1999). In a study of home videos of first-birthday parties of children later assigned a primary diagnosis of autism or ID, Osterling, Dawson, and Munson (2002) reported that children with autism looked at others and oriented to their names less frequently than children with ID did. So, although the differential diagnosis of autism and ID is a difficult one, research suggests that developing social behaviors most reliably differentiate the two in young children.

DEVELOPMENTAL COURSE

For the vast majority of individuals with ASD, it is a lifelong developmental disability that limits independent living, but early intervention can make a difference, as will be discussed later. In a large Japanese outcome study of 197 young adults with autism, only 1% were living independently, only 27% were either employed or pursuing postsecondary education, and only half had enough language to permit verbal communication (Kobayashi, Murata, & Yoshinaga, 1992). Across a number of studies, both IQ and the presence of some communicative speech before age 5 are the best early predictors of a more favorable outcome (reviewed in Klinger & Dawson, 1996). As would be expected, romantic relationships are rare among individuals with autism and only a very few manage to marry and have children.

ETIOLOGY[1]

There are excellent recent reviews of the etiology of ASD (Bailey, Phillips, & Rutter, 1996; Rutter, 2000; Veenstra-Vander Weele & Cook, 2004); the presentation here summarizes those reviews. Genetic influences on ASD were long doubted, both by psychodynamic theorists and by geneticists, but for different reasons. As noted earlier, psychodynamic theorists postulated that autism was caused by the maternal environment. Geneticists were struck by the apparent lack of both vertical transmission and associated chromosomal anomalies (Rutter, 2000). Ironically, more recent research has documented that autism is both the most familial and possibly the most heritable of all psychiatric diagnoses, with a significant minority of cases associated with chromosomal anomalies or known genetic syndromes. The following discussion shows how research results changed the view that autism was not genetic.

---

[1] For a description of genetic technical terms, see Box 1.1 in Chapter 1.

Familiality

Because individuals with autism very rarely marry and have children, vertical transmission of the diagnosis of autism from parent to child will rarely be observed. But this fact does not exclude genetic transmission, since parents could transmit genetic risk factors without having the diagnosis themselves. Although the rate of autism in siblings (2% in earlier studies and 3% in later ones) appeared low, it was considerably higher than the population rates cited earlier. Dividing the sibling rates by the appropriate population rates, one obtains a sibling relative risk of about 20 to 60, which is considerably higher than that of other psychiatric disorders—although sibling risk will be lower when the CDCP rates are used. Using the CDCP population rates, one finds a sibling relative risk in the range of 5; this is still considerable, but closer to the sibling risk for other disorders (e.g., dyslexia and ADHD).

Recent studies have also made it clear that the behavioral phenotype that is transmitted in families of individuals with autism is broader than the specific diagnosis of autism (e.g., Piven, 1999). Hence the familial phenotype may be dimensional rather than categorical. First-degree relatives of probands with autism have increased rates of autistic symptoms such as shyness and aloofness, and pragmatic language problems, compared to control relatives (Rutter, 2000). In the Maudsley study (Bolton et al., 1994), if the phenotype was broadened to any PDD, the rate in siblings was 6% versus none in controls. Even broader phenotypes, defined by autistic symptoms and cognitive deficits, were found in 12% of relatives versus 2% of control relatives, and 20% versus 3%, respectively, depending on how stringent a cutoff was used. With continuous measures of these phenotypic features and large samples, one could test whether the familial phenotype is dimensional rather than categorical. If it is dimensional, powerful genetic methods for identifying QTLs could be employed. Several studies have also found higher rates of anxiety and depressive disorders among relatives of probands with autism. However, these disorders did not cosegregate with the "broader autism phenotype" (which is defined by social and cognitive deficits) and their rate did not increase with the severity of autism in the probands, unlike the broader autism phenotypic (Rutter, 2000). Although individuals with the broader autism phenotype had higher rates of reading and spelling problems, perhaps because of other cognitive and language problems, a specific reading and spelling problem (i.e., dyslexia) was not more common in such families; nor were ID or seizure disorders, which were increased in probands. Although more work is needed to define the broader autism phenotype, especially work using neuropsychological markers, these studies are exciting and clearly have implications for what phenotype is used in molecular studies.

Heritability

The question of heritability has necessarily been pursued through twin studies, because adoption studies of autism are less feasible. The first, now classic, twin study of autism was conducted by Folstein and Rutter (1977). The concordance rate in monozygotic (MZ) pairs (36%) was significantly greater than that found in dizygotic (DZ) pairs (0%). If the phenotype was broadened to include a cognitive or language disorder, these concordance rates became 82% and 10%, respectively. So this study provided evidence that autism is significantly heritable and that the heritable phenotype is broader than the diagnosis of autism itself, consistent with the family studies just discussed. Two subsequent studies (Bailey et al., 1995; Steffenburg et al., 1989) also found significant heritability for autism. In the Steffenburg et al. (1989) study, the MZ concordance rate was 91%, and the DZ concordance rate was 0%. The Bailey et al. (1995) study is the most methodologically sophisticated of the three, because it (1) used a total population ascertainment; (2) based diagnosis on both parent interviews and observations of each child, using standardized diagnostic instruments, the original ADI and the Autism Diagnostic Observation Schedule (ADOS); (3) excluded non-idiopathic cases (those with medical conditions and chromosomal abnormalities); and (4) assessed zygosity with blood tests. In this study, the MZ concordance rate for autism was 60% versus 5% in DZ pairs, whereas these rates rose to 90% versus 10%, respectively, when a broader phenotype of social or cognitive deficits was used. These two results confirm the two key results of the earlier Folstein and Rutter (1977) study, although the definition of the broader phenotype shifted in the later study to focus more on social abnormality. Interestingly, a similar social deficit was found in those with the broader phenotype in a follow-up of the earlier sample (Rutter, 2000). Finally, within the 16 MZ pairs concordant for autism or atypical autism in the Bailey et al. (1995) study, there were wide differences in IQ and clinical symptomatology, such that similarity within these MZ pairs for these features was no greater than that between individuals picked at random from different pairs concordant for autism. This finding argues that although the diagnosis of autism is highly heritable, there is hardly rigid genetic determinism for an exact phenotype. Instead, even with an identical genotype, epigenetic interactions and nonshared environmental influences must produce divergence in phenotypes.

Across these three twin studies of autism, one can see that the disparity between MZ and DZ concordance rates is quite large, with the MZ-DZ ratio averaging roughly 10:1. For other psychiatric disorders, such as schizophrenia, depression, and bipolar disorder, this ratio is considerably lower (between about 2:1 and 4:1). Such a marked discrepancy in MZ versus DZ concordance rates indicates that nonadditive genetic effects are operating. In the case of autism, these nonadditive effects are likely to represent "epistasis," or interactions among several different genes, rather than nonadditive effects (dominance) of a single major locus (Rutter, 2000). The large disparity between MZ and DZ concordance rates, as well as the very high MZ concordance rate for the broader phenotype, indicate a high heritability for autism. Quantitative analysis of the Bailey et al. (1995) data indicate a heritability greater than 90%, making autism one of the most heritable of psychiatric disorders. So G × E interactions may be less important in the etiology of autism than in many of the other disorders considered in this book; there are interactions in the development of autism, but they appear to be mainly among genes. There are also unknown epigenetic interactions that produce the wide phenotypic variability found within concordant MZ pairs.

Gene Locations

Three methods have been used to identify risk genes for ASD: linkage studies, chromosomal studies, and association studies. Several large, multisite molecular studies are in progress, and some results are emerging, although none are definitive as yet (see reviews by Lamb, Moore, Bailey, & Monaco, 2000; Veenstra-Vander Weele & Cook, 2004). The strongest linkage finding so far is for a locus on chromosome 7q (International Molecular Genetic Study of Autism Consortium, 1998), which has been replicated by the IMGSAC group and three other independent studies (Lamb et al., 2000). Although the location of the 7q locus varies somewhat across studies, the confidence interval for a QTL affecting a complex trait is large (as great as 25 centimorgans [cM]), given sample sizes similar to those in these studies (Lamb et al., 2000). Other replicated linkage results include loci on chromosomes 1q, 2q, 3q, 16p, 17q, and 19q (Lamb et al., 2000; Veenstra-Vander Weele & Cook, 2004).

The largest genome scan to date of autism (Szatmari et al., 2007) was recently reported by the Autism Genome Project Consortium. Nearly 1,200 families were involved in this study, which also examined copy number variations (CNVs). CNVs are submicroscopic deletions, insertions, or duplications of DNA sequences, some of which are in coding regions of genes. Szatmari et al. (2007) found a new autism linkage on chromosome 11p, and found modest linkage support for previously identified linkage regions on 2q and 7q. In addition, their CNV analysis identified the neurexin-1 gene as a possible candidate gene. Consistent with the function of other candidate genes for autism, neurexin 1 plays a role in the development of glutamate neurons. The convergence of these results suggests that further investigation of glutamate-related genes is likely to be a promising future direction.

Sebat et al. (2007) also found an association between CNVs and sporadic cases of autism (i.e., probands with no affected first-degree relative). CNVs were found in 12 of 118 (10%) of sporadic cases of autism, 2 of 77 (3%) of nonsporadic cases, and 2 of 196 (1%) of controls. These CNVs were in many different locations. If CNVs arise spontaneously in meiosis (i.e., are not present in parents), MZ pairs would share them, but DZ pairs would not. CNVs could contribute to the high heritability that is observed for autism, as well as to the large differences between MZ and DZ concordances. So CNVs are a novel genetic mechanism in autism and possibly other disorders.

A related novel mechanism is variation in human-specific gene duplications. For instance, copies of the "domain of unknown function" (DUF) 1220 are much more common in humans (~212) than in great apes (~34), and deletion of DUF 1220 domains has been found in both idiopathic ID and autism (Fortna et al., 2004).

Another promising locus on 15q11–q13 was suggested by chromosomal studies. A duplication of this region, mainly inherited from the mother, is the most frequent chromosome anomaly in ASD and is found in 1–3% of all cases. This region of chromosome 15 is also the Prader–Willi/Angelman syndrome region, and these two syndromes also involve altered numbers of the genes in this region and parental transmission effects. For instance, Angelman syndrome involves deletions of this chromosome 15 region and is associated with autism. However, this location has not been identified in whole-genome searches (Lamb et al., 2000), perhaps because of its rarity.

Association studies with candidate genes have also been attempted. Some of these investigated a GABA receptor gene located in the 15q region implicated by cytogenetic abnormalities, and others pursued serotonin receptor genes, based on the well-replicated finding of peripheral serotonin elevations in autism (discussed below). The majority of results in both cases are negative (Lamb et al., 2000), although it remains possible that these candidates may be important for a subtype of autism. There is also a recent report of an association with an allele of a homeobox gene, HOXA1 (Rodier, 2000), although subsequent studies have not replicated it (Veenstra-Vander Weele & Cook, 2004).

Other candidate genes include the RELN gene in the 7q linkage region; the neuroligin-3 (NLGN3) and neuroligin-4 (NLGN4) genes on chromosome Xq13.1 and Xp22.23, respectively; and the MECP2 gene, a mutation of which causes the X-linked Rett syndrome/Rett's disorder, discussed earlier. All four candidate genes affect early brain development. The RELN gene was first identified in a mutant mouse called "reeler" because of its unsteady gait. This gene is involved in neuronal migration and is related to human lissencephaly (smooth brain). The neurolignin gene family codes for cell adhesion proteins important for synapse formation and functions.

Deletions of neurolignin genes have been found in cases of ASD. Recently Tabuchi et al. (2007) created a transgenic mouse with a mutated version of human NLGN3, which causes increased inhibitory synaptic transmission. Behaviorally, mice with this mutation avoided a strange mouse placed in their cage and spent more time with inanimate objects. This social aversion phenotype appeared to be specific, because these mice outperformed control mice on the Morris water maze, a test of spatial memory, and were similar to controls on tests of anxiety and motor coordination. Finally, consistent with the deteriorating course found in Rett syndrome, the MECP2 gene is expressed later in early brain development and may play a stabilizing role.

The existence of several large family samples will speed the verification of these linkage and association results.

Associations with Genetic Disorders

The two strongest associations of autism with genetic disorders are with tuberous sclerosis and fragile X syndrome (FXS) (Bailey et al., 1996). Tuberous sclerosis is an autosomal dominant neurocutaneous (i.e., affecting both brain and skin) disorder, with a prevalence of about 1 per 10,000. In this disorder, there is abnormal tissue growth in the skin, brain, and other organs. Both the physical and behavioral phenotypes are quite variable. Behaviorally, the phenotype can range from normal functioning to severe problems, with the latter including severe ID, seizure disorders, and symptoms of autism. Less severe behavioral problems associated with tuberous sclerosis include learning disabilities, hyperactivity–impulsivity, aggression and uncooperative behavior (see review in Patzer & Volkmar, 1999). Across studies, there is evidence for a significant two-way association between tuberous sclerosis and autism. Rates of autism in individuals with tuberous sclerosis range between 17% and 61%, and rates of tuberous sclerosis in individuals with autism range between 0.4% and 9% (reviewed in Bailey et al., 1996, and Patzer & Volkmar, 1999). All of these rates are well beyond the chance rate, which is roughly 1 in 10 million. Since the association is strongest in persons with tuberous sclerosis who have both ID and a seizure disorder, it seems unlikely that there is a direct or specific effect of the genes that cause tuberous sclerosis on the symptoms of autism. Instead, it seems much more likely that the abnormal tissue growth (benign tumors) in tuberous sclerosis sometimes occurs in particular parts of the brain, damage to which is important for the development of autism (see Bailey et al., 1996). Nonetheless, localizing these benign brain tumors in individuals with ID and tuberous sclerosis, both with and without autism, could shed light on which brain structures (when damaged) are important in the development of autism. Indeed, one study did just that, finding that tumors in the medial temporal lobe were associated with autism (Bolton & Griffiths, 1997).

The association between FXS and autism once appeared to be much stronger than what later studies have found—probably because the earlier studies had small samples, used cytogenetic rather than DNA measures of the fragile X mutation, and used clinical rather than standardized assessments of autism (Bailey et al., 1996). In recent methodologically adequate studies, rates of autism in FXS average about 3–5%, and those of FXS in autism about 2.5–4% (Bailey et al., 1996; Patzer & Volkmar, 1999). These rates still support a significant two-way association, at least if chance is determined simply by multiplying the prevalence of autism by the prevalence of FXS (which yields a liberal chance value of 1 in 1 million). Although there is a robust two-way association relative to population base rates, it can be argued that the appropriate base rates need to be derived from populations with intellectual levels similar to those found males with FXS and males with autism, both of which fall in the ID range. For instance, the rate of FXS in unselected males with ID is about 1.9% (Sherman, 1996), which is still clearly less than the rate of FXS in males with autism, although it could still be argued that the intellectual levels might differ across the two sets of studies.

A better study would compare the rates of autism in FXS-negative and FXS-positive males matched on IQ, drawn from the same population with ID. To our knowledge, only two such studies exist (Einfeld, Maloney, & Hall, 1989; Maes, Fryns, Van Walleghem, & Van den Berghe, 1993). Both found *no* differences in the rates of autism between FXS-positive and FXS-negative males with similar levels of intellectual functioning. However, both did find higher rates of certain autistic symptoms in the FXS-positive group—specifically, gaze avoidance and hand flapping in the Einfeld et al. (1989) study, and stereotypic movements (including hand flapping, rocking, and hitting, scratching, or rubbing their own bodies), echolalia, gaze avoidance, and ritualistic behaviors in the Maes et al. (1993) study.

Further evidence has been found for an association between FXS and certain autistic features, such as stereotypies, perseveration, and avoidance of eye contact, which are found in over 80% of males with FXS (Hagerman, 1996). Moreover, FXS is somewhat distinctive among ID syndromes in exhibiting this association with autistic features, which are found less often in either Down or Williams syndrome. Lachiewicz, Spiridigliozzi, Gullion, Ransford, and Rao (1994) studied 55 boys with FXS and 57 IQ-matched controls with several behavioral questionnaires, and found that boys with FXS were four times more likely to have both tactile defensiveness and abnormal speech (perseveration and rapid speech) than were controls. A controlled study by Reiss and Freund (1992) demonstrated a unique profile of behavior within the DSM-III-R criteria for autism in males with FXS, including more difficulty with peer interactions (compared to adult interactions), more stereotypies, and more unusual nonverbal interactions compared to IQ-matched controls. Closer analysis of these autistic features in males with FXS has yielded some interesting contrasts with idiopathic autism. Cohen, Vietze, Sudhalter, Jenkins, and Brown (1989) showed that males with FXS were more sensitive to an adult's initiation of social gaze and demonstrated a subsequent greater aversion to mutual gaze than did individuals with autism but without FXS. Other studies have found that the eye contact disturbance in autism is not so much a decrease or avoidance of eye contact as it is inappropriate use of eye contact, which is probably due to deficits in joint attention. Sudhalter, Cohen, Silverman, and Wolf-Schein (1990) found that the speech of patients with FXS exhibited more perseveration of words and phrases, and less echolalia, than that of autistic patients without FXS and controls with ID.

In summary, since not all forms of ID are associated with an increased risk for autism, it appears that there is something more specific to the association between FXS and at least certain symptoms of autism. One intriguing possibility is that since both disorders are characterized by increases in brain size, unlike the microcephaly (abnormally small head circumference) that is characteristic of Down syndrome and many other forms of ID, such increases (perhaps reflecting too many connections, due to a lack of pruning) somehow lead to these shared symptoms.

Finally, about 5% of cases with behaviorally defined autism have chromosomal anomalies detectable with standard cytogenetic methods (Bailey et al., 1996), and these rates are higher if one includes submicroscopic CNVs (Sebat et al., 2007).

To sum up the findings across the three genetic associations reviewed here (tuberous sclerosis, FXS, and various chromosomal anomalies), it is clear that a sizable minority (up to about 20%) of cases of individuals diagnosed with autism will have identifiable genetic anomalies. Hence a genetic evaluation should be a standard part of the clinical workup of such individuals. It is also clear that the majority of such individuals will not have an identifiable etiology (they will fall in the idiopathic category). As progress is made in understanding the molecular genetics of idiopathic autism, this proportion will drop.

Environmental Influences

Although earlier reports implicated prenatal infections (i.e., maternal rubella; see Chess, 1977) and obstetrical complications in the etiology of autism, neither of these environmental influences have proven to be very important. On follow-up, children with congenital rubella no longer appeared autistic (Chess, 1977), and other studies of possible infectious influences have been mostly negative (see Bailey et al., 1996). With regard to obstetrical complications, the weight of evidence indicates that these are caused by genetically abnormal fetuses (e.g., with congenital malformations or with a greater familial loading for autism), rather than being etiological in themselves (see discussion in Bailey et al., 1996). Incidentally, it appears that this explanation of associated obstetrical complications has not been adequately explored in some psychopathologies (e.g., schizophrenia).

It is worth noting that extreme environmental deprivation, including decreased social stimulation, can produce a phenocopy of autism. Such a phenocopy has been found in congenital blindness (Brown, Hobson, Lee, & Stevenson, 1997; Rogers & Pennington, 1991) and in some orphans placed in minimally stimulating institutions as infants (Rutter et al., 1999). The existence of these phenocopies is very important theoretically, because it reminds us that social relatedness is not innate, but rather depends on interactions with a caregiver. Factors that strongly limit those interactions, whether environmental or genetic, can lead to the development of the symptoms of autism. In inherited autism, one key theoretical puzzle is to identify which early psychological deficits in infants who will develop autism are the ones that strongly limit their ability to participate in socializing interactions with caregivers (see discussion in Rogers & Pennington, 1991). We will consider possible answers to this puzzle in the "Neuropsychology" section, but first let us consider brain mechanisms in autism.

BRAIN MECHANISMS[2]

This section includes studies of brain structure, brain function, and neurotransmission. Although differences in each type of brain study have been found in individuals with autism, the list of well-replicated findings is very short, and the neurological cause of autism remains unknown.

Structural Findings

The best-replicated structural finding in autism is macrocephaly in about a quarter of cases. As mentioned earlier, Kanner's (1943) original case report noted enlarged head circumferences. More recently, macrocephaly has been found in structural MRI studies (Filipek, Kennedy, & Caviness, 1992; Piven et al., 1995) and in autopsy samples (reviewed in Bailey et al., 1996). What change in brain development produces this macrocephaly, and how it relates to brain function, are currently unknown. Can we exclude the experience of growing up with autism as the cause of this brain phenotype? It is likely that we can, because other examples of macrocephaly are due to changes in prenatal processes of brain development, mainly in the cortex (see Bai-

---

[2]For a description of neuroanatomical technical terms, see Box 1.2 in Chapter 1.

ley et al., 1996), such as an excess of neuronal proliferation or a failure of early neuronal elimination (apotsosis or programmed cell death). But a different mechanism appears to be operating in autism, because there is a lack of macrocephaly at birth, and it is only detectable by age 12 months (Courchesne, Carper, & Akshoomoff, 2003; Lainhart et al., 1997).

This postnatal emergence of macrocephaly is hypothesized to be due at least in part to postnatal overgrowth, which is followed by slower or arrested brain growth later in childhood (Courchesne, 2004). A recent meta-analysis of brain size reports in autism indicated that some of the mixed findings regarding macrocephaly were due to varying ages of the participants, with large brains being less common in adults (in whom brain growth may have halted abnormally early) (Redcay & Courchesne, 2005). If macrocephaly in autism were just due to a failure of experience-dependent pruning mechanisms, it would emerge later in development and not be consistent with later slowing of brain growth. So it is difficult to argue that macrocephaly in autism is just secondary to abnormal social and other experience. There is growing evidence for abnormal patterns of neural connectivity in autism, with increased local connectivity (perhaps particularly within the frontal lobes) and decreased long-range connectivity (Belmonte et al., 2004; Courchesne & Pierce, 2005). Such a pattern could be consistent with both the unusual course of brain growth and (potentially) with some aspects of the autistic phenotype (discussed below). Clearly, more work is needed to understand the brain growth and neural connectivity in autism.

More specific volume reductions have been found in frontal, basal ganglia, limbic, and cerebellar structures (Toal, Murphy, & Murphy, 2005). Volume reductions in medial temporal lobe structures, such as the hippocampus and amygdala, have also been found. Their role in memory and emotion could be theoretically important for autism. Bauman and Kemper's (1994) autopsy studies found abnormally small, densely packed neurons in these and other limbic structures, although this finding is not consistent across other autopsy studies (reviewed in Bailey et al., 1996). In addition, structural MRI studies have found reduced amygdala volumes in autism (Abell et al., 1999; Aylward et al., 1999).

Other candidate structural differences in autism have not been consistently replicated, such as the hypoplasia in the cerebellar vermis first reported by Courchesne, Yeung-Courchesne, Press, Hesselink, and Jernigan (1988) or lateral ventricular enlargement (see review in Bailey et al., 1996).

Functional Findings

The main functional findings consist of (1) a reduced P300 response to novel stimuli in event-related potential (ERP) studies (reviewed in Klinger & Dawson, 1996); (2) more variability in regional metabolic rates in PET studies, suggesting less coordinated processing across brain regions (reviewed in Bailey et al., 1996); and (3) fMRI findings of differences in the brain substrates used to process social stimuli, such as faces (Baron-Cohen et al., 1999; Bookheimer, 2000; Schultz et al., 2000). Some earlier PET studies found global hypermetabolism in groups with autism, but this result has not been replicated in several other studies (reviewed in Bailey et al., 1996).

We focus here on the fMRI studies, which indicate brain activation differences in processing social stimuli. In two studies, Schultz et al. (2000) contrasted brain activation for face versus object processing in subjects with autism and controls. Subjects saw pairs of faces and objects and had to determine whether they were same or different. In controls, the face task produced focal activation in the classical face area (the bilateral fusiform gyrus [FG], which is on the ventral surface of the occipital and adjacent temporal lobes), whereas the object task produced focal activation in the inferior temporal gyrus. In contrast, in subjects with autism, the face task did not activate the FG, but instead activated the adjacent inferior temporal gyrus. These results suggest that subjects with autism have not developed the typical specialized cortical area for face recognition, and instead process faces as if they were other objects. Although such a difference could be innate, these authors speculate that this difference is due to reduced social experience in autism. At this point, it is unclear whether these fMRI findings would generalize to individuals with high-functioning autism and to various types of face stimuli (Hadjikhani et al., 2004).

Bookheimer (2000) examined processing of facial emotion in an fMRI study. Subjects had to either match or label angry or fearful facial expressions. In controls, both tasks activated the face area (FG), and the matching task also activated the amygdala bilaterally. In contrast, in subjects with autism, neither the FG nor the amygdala activation was observed; instead, Broca's area was activated. Similar reductions in FG and amygdala activation while processing facial emotion were found by Critchley et al. (2000).

A third study (Baron-Cohen et al., 1999) examined brain activation on the Eyes task, in which a subject sees a photograph of the eye portion of a face and decides which of two descriptors (e.g., "concerned" vs. "unconcerned") best describes the mental state of the individual in the picture. The control task was identifying the gender of the individual in the same photographs. Controls specifically activated the amygdala in the mental state task, whereas the group with autism did not. Controls also exhibited more activation of the inferior frontal gyrus (IFG) and the insula, whereas the group with autism had greater activation in superior temporal gyrus. In sum, across these studies involving processing of different aspects of faces (identity, emotion, and mental state), there are converging differences in the group with autism in the FG and the amygdala. The amygdala differences are consistent with some of the structural differences discussed earlier and suggest that individuals with autism have difficulty in basic aspects of processing emotion—a topic considered in the "Neuropsychology" section.

Recently, functional neuroimaging studies of autism have focused on mirror neurons (Rizzolatti, Fogassi, & Gallese, 2006), which are equally activated by performing or observing the same action and are found in several parts of the brain, including the IFG, the superior temporal sulcus, and the inferior parietal lobule. Since mirror neurons were originally found in monkeys, it is probably too simple to equate them with the human neural substrate for imitation (since monkeys do not imitate), but they are likely to play a role in human imitation. Since imitation is known to be impaired in autism (Rogers & Pennington, 1991), mirror neurons are theoretically interesting structures to examine.

There have now been several imaging studies of mirror neurons in autism (see Williams & Waiter, 2006, for a review). Using various imaging methodologies, these studies have documented lower activations in mirror neuron regions while participants are observing another's actions, but not while they are executing the same action. These are exciting results, but they are unlikely to explain all of ASD because of the findings for other aspects of social perception and cognition reviewed here, and because the neural correlates of imitation differences in ASD specifically also extend beyond the mirror neuron system to structures like the amygdala (Ramachandran & Oberman, 2006; Williams et al., 2006; Williams & Waiter, 2006).

Neurotransmission

The topic of neurotransmission in ASD is reviewed in Bailey et al. (1996) and Patzer and Volkmar (1999); their main conclusions are summarized here. The search for neurotransmitter abnormalities in autism has been pursued for about 40 years, but with very few consistent results. Currently, there is only limited evidence of an abnormality in neurotransmission in the central nervous system, and there is not an effective neurochemical treatment for the main symptoms of autism. Investigations of the dopaminergic, noradrenergic, and opiate neuropeptide systems have not produced evidence of consistent abnormalities (Bailey et al., 1996).

The sole consistent result is elevated serotonin levels in peripheral blood (hyperserotonemia) in about a quarter of individuals with autism, which is caused by increased amounts of serotonin in platelets in the blood. However, there are not elevations of the serotonin metabolite 5-hydroxyindoleacetic acid in the cerebrospinal fluid of individuals with autism, suggesting that serotonin elevation does not extend to the central nervous system (Bailey et al., 1996). Hyperserotonemia is also found in severe ID, raising the possibility that this neurochemical abnormality is related to ID rather than to autism. However, there are reports of hyperserotonemia in ID-negative relatives of individuals with autism (Bailey et al., 1996), suggesting some specificity. The finding of hyperserotonemia prompted an attempt to treat autism neurochemically, with a serotonin antagonist, fenfluramine, which lowers platelet levels of serotonin. However, a multicenter treatment study of fenfluramine did not produce clear positive results, so fenfluramine is not an empirically validated treatment for autism (Campbell, 1988). In sum, we still do not understand the etiological significance (if any) of hyperserotonemia, the one consistent neurochemical correlate of autism.

NEUROPSYCHOLOGY

As implied in Table 5.2, there is not as clear-cut a cognitive profile for ASD as there is for the other main learning disorders discussed in this book, for which cognitive testing is much more helpful in making the diagnosis. The main neuropsychological deficits in ASD are in social cognition, though these appear to cause cognitive and language deficits (including ID, LI, and executive deficits), as we discuss in more detail below. As is true for the other learning disorders covered in this book, no single neuropsychological deficit has been found that is sufficient to cause ASD. Less progress has been made in testing a multiple-cognitive-deficit model of ASD than in the case of RD and ADHD. The review that follows identifies promising candidate deficits that could be tested in a multiple-deficit model of ASD.

Recent research on the neuropsychology of ASD provides an excellent example of the power of the developmental psychopathology approach. This work is interdisciplinary, and illustrates the reciprocal relation between studies of typical and atypical development. Not only has ASD research drawn on the latest theories and paradigms from studies of typical early development, but it has also become an important stimulus for these studies, as witnessed by the numerous articles on typical development of a theory of mind appearing in the recent literature. ASD research has brought the early social and cognitive accomplishments of nondisabled human infants into sharper relief, making it clearer what needs to be explained in early development and which early skills may be useful to examine in both within- and cross-species comparisons. These research accomplishments have relevance for deep and fundamental questions in psychology and philosophy. For instance, how do we become aware of other minds? What is a person, and how do infants form a concept of persons? How does the self develop? What are the cognitive requirements for intersubjectivity and later human relatedness? How are early social and cognitive development intertwined? We touch on the relevance of ASD research for these issues in the present review.

Theorizing about the nature of the primary psychological deficit in ASD has come full circle. As discussed earlier, Kanner (1943), in the original description of the autistic syndrome, suggested the possibility that autistic children were born "with an innate inability to form the usual, biologically provided affective contact with people" (p. 42). But a psychogenic hypothesis prevailed in the next two decades in psychoanalytic accounts of autism (e.g., Mahler, 1952). As evidence for an organic etiology of autism accumulated, researchers concerned with the underlying processing deficit shifted their focus to various cognitive possibilities, neglecting Kanner's original insight that the disorder might represent a primary *social* deficit of constitutional origin. Various possible primary cognitive deficits were investigated, including deficits in arousal, language, symbolic thought, memory, and cross-modal processing. However, when autistic children were compared to nonautistic children with ID who were similar in mental age, few reliable differences were found in these various cognitive processes. Even when reliable differences were found, there were other reasons why the apparent deficits in these areas were unlikely to be primary (Fein, Pennington, Markowitz, Braverman, & Waterhouse, 1986). Specifically, most of these cognitive processes develop after the onset of autistic symptoms, are theoretically inadequate to explain autistic aloofness, cannot be found in all autistic children, and may be the very cognitive abilities that depend most heavily on typical social functioning. Other reasons for regarding the social symptoms as primary in autism include (1) the dissociability of social and cognitive impairments both within and across developmentally disabled populations; (2) the special difficulty autistic children have with social stimuli; and (3) the rarity of social relatedness deficits in babies with even severe brain damage of other types, and their resistance to change in autism.

Research published subsequent to the Fein et al. (1986) review has refined our understanding of which social processes are impaired and intact in autism. Somewhat surprisingly, some early social behaviors have proved *not* to be specifically impaired in autistic children compared to controls of similar mental age. These include attachment behaviors, self-recognition, person recognition, and differential social responsiveness (reviewed in Ozonoff, Pennington, & Rogers, 1990; Rogers & Pennington, 1991).

Social processes that are clearly impaired in autism include social orienting, joint attention, imitation, face processing, theory of mind, empathy, and aspects of emotional expression (Hill & Frith, 2003; Klinger & Dawson, 1996). Some of these deficits, such as those in social orienting and joint attention, are present early in the development of the disorder (Osterling & Dawson, 1994), whereas others (i.e., theory-of-mind deficits) cannot be measured until later in development. It is currently unclear when deficits in imitation, empathy, and emotional expression appear in the development of autism. All of these social processes contribute to the typical protracted development of "intersubjectivity" (e.g., Stern, 1985; Trevarthen, 1979), which refers to the awareness of mental states (i.e., emotions, other motivations, attention, intentions, and beliefs) in both self and others, and the use of this awareness in social interactions. Almost by definition, individuals with autism are deficient in intersubjectivity. The key questions are which aspects of intersubjectivity are deficient, and what underlying neuropsychological deficits disrupt the development of these deficient aspects of intersubjectivity. For instance, very young infants share emotions with caregivers through imitative exchanges (Stern, 1985). An infant with deficits in either imitation or emotion would have trouble participating in these exchanges, and would thus miss some of the experiences necessary for the development of very early aspects of intersubjectivity. By about the end of the first year, infants share attention with caregivers (joint attention) and give evidence of some understanding of intentions (e.g., Csibra, Gergely, Biro, Koos, & Brockbank, 1999). An infant could have trouble with this part of the development of intersubjectivity because of a general or specific processing deficit, and this in turn would be expected to undermine later-developing aspects of intersubjectivity. Or selective difficulties could arise at later points in the development of intersubjectivity. The developmental dependencies among these different aspects of intersubjectivity are not completely understood, making it difficult to evaluate competing neuropsychological theories of autism.

Since a great deal of human development depends on social transmission, a child deficient in intersubjectivity would miss much of the input necessary for typical development. Since brain development depends on environmental input, as discussed earlier, this lack of input would change brain development in autism (Mundy & Neal, 2000). Some of the deficits in autism (such as in language and IQ) can be seen as secondary to this missing input. While missing this typical input, some individuals with autism may "specialize" in learning other things about the environment; this "specialization" could explain the savant skills that are sometimes found in such persons. This hypothesis would also explain why intensive early intervention can succeed in children with autism; such intervention reduces this secondary deprivation (Mundy & Neal, 2000).

A successful neuropsychological theory of autism must account not only for these impaired social processes, but also for the classic triad of symptoms (see "Definition," above) and other features of the disorder, such as the high rate of ID and the uneven profile of cognitive abilities. The hypothesized primary psychological deficit must also (1) be present before the onset of the disorder, and hence very early in development; (2) be pervasive among individuals with the disorder; and (3) be specific to autism. This is a tall order, and there is fairly good agreement among ASD researchers that no current psychological theory of autism meets all these criteria (see discussion in Bailey et al., 1996). Some of these current theories are (1) the theory-of-mind theory (Baron-Cohen, Leslie, & Frith, 1985, 1986; Baron-Cohen et al., 2000); (2) the executive theory (Ozonoff, Pennington, & Rogers, 1991; Russell, 1997; Russell, Jarrold, & Henry, 1996); (3) the praxis/imitation theory (Meltzoff & Gopnik, 1993; Rogers & Pennington, 1991); (4) the emotion theory (Hobson, 1989, 1993); (5) the empathizing–systemizing or "extreme male brain" theory (Baron-Cohen et al., 2005); and (6) the enactive mind approach (Klin, Jones, Schultz, & Volkmar, 2005). These major contending theories of the development of autism all agree that intersubjectivity is disrupted in some way, but disagree about why it is disrupted. An initial deficit in any one of these areas could conceivably derail the development of intersubjectivity and lead to deficits in the other areas.

The theory-of-mind theory holds that the initial deficit is a cognitive inability to compute second-order representations, or metarepresentations, which are necessary for pretense and understanding others' intentions and beliefs. The executive theory (Russell, 1996) posits that a deficit in action monitoring leads to a deficit in understanding others' intentions and beliefs. The praxis theory (Rogers & Pennington, 1991) holds that the initial deficit is in imitation. The emotion theory (Hobson, 1993) holds that the initial deficit is in affective contact. According to the empathizing–systemizing view, autism represents an extreme form of a typical brain-based gender difference—namely, that females tend to be higher on empathizing (responding appropriately to the mental states of living things), and males tend to be higher on systemizing (understanding the rules that govern non-living, mechanical systems) (Baron-Cohen et al., 2005). The enactive mind approach holds that from very early in development, autistic individuals have fundamentally atypical social orienting biases, perhaps as the result of an early face-processing deficit (Klin et al., 2005; Schultz, 2005). These biases lead to a cascade of atypical social experiences and ultimately, the construction of impoverished social understanding.

Although cross-sectional studies have consistently found deficits in each of the social processes emphasized by the different theories in groups with autism, we do not know which of these deficits, if any, has causal priority in the development of the intersubjectivity deficit in autism.

Each theory has significant shortcomings. Theory of mind per se does not develop until considerably after the onset of autism. In addition, deficits on theory-of-mind tasks are not found in some individuals with autism, indicating a lack of universality; moreover, they *are* found in some nonautistic populations (e.g., children with deafness, blindness, ID, and LI), indicating a lack of specificity (for a review, see Tager-Flusberg, 2001). Theory-of-mind theorists also freely admit that this theory does not account for the repetitive, stereotypic symptoms. The executive theory can plausibly explain these repetitive symptoms, but it does not as straightforwardly explain the social and communicative symptoms, which the theory-of-mind theory explains so well. Although the executive theory seems like a plausible account of the repetitive symptoms in autism, correlations between these two constructs have been hard to find in empirical studies. In addition, executive problems are not specific to autism (see discussion in Pennington & Ozonoff, 1996), and recent studies have failed to find executive deficits early in the development of ASD (Dawson et al., 2002a, 2002b; Griffith, Pennington, Wehner, & Rogers, 1999; Yerys, Hepburn, Pennington, & Rogers, 2007).

The praxis theory must explain why children with worse praxis deficits than those found in autism (such as children with cerebral palsy) do not develop autism. Deficits in praxis may nonetheless help define a subtype of ASD and contribute to the failure of speech development in this disorder (Gernsbacher, Sauder, Geye, Schweigert, & Goldsmith, 2008). So a deficit in praxis per se does not suffice as a theory of autism, but a more specific deficit in imitation or mimicry still might. The imitation theory finds support from the recent mirror neuron studies discussed earlier. For a review of imitation in both typical development and individuals with autism, see Rogers and Williams (2006). Support for the empathizing–systemizing theory comes from both the gender asymmetry in autism and the fact that even nonautistic males are more likely than nonautistic females to display certain autism-like characteristics. Although the theory posits an underlying biological mechanism (fetal androgen exposure), it remains somewhat descriptive at the neuropsychological level. It also fails to account for why many individuals with high levels of prenatal androgen exposure are not autistic.

Proponents of the enactive mind approach note that even newborn infants are predisposed to orient to human faces and voices. It is clearly true that as both children and adults, individuals with ASD demonstrate aberrant patterns of social orienting, and it makes good sense that their social learning will therefore be atypical. However, although early detection is an area motivating much current research, it is as yet unclear whether babies who will later have ASD demonstrate unusual social orienting in early infancy. Furthermore, despite exciting findings demonstrating social orienting failures (e.g., response to their own names) in later infancy among children eventually diagnosed with ASD, such difficulties are neither universal in nor specific to the disorder (Coonrod & Stone, 2005; Osterling et al., 2002). Finally, the emotion theory has not been sufficiently explored; recent theoretical analyses of emotion processing have identified components that have not been fully evaluated in ASD (e.g., mimicry).

In addition to these six theories, each of which emphasizes a single deficit, the weak central coherence theory (Frith & Happé, 1994) provided an early multiple-deficit account of the disorder. Frith and colleagues noted that the predominant theory-of-mind approach failed to account for robust aspects of the phenotype outside the classic triad. For example, in visual processing tasks, individuals with autism showed enhanced processing of specific details and reduced processing of the whole (gestalt). In linguistic tasks, these individuals paid inadequate attention to context (e.g., by pronouncing the word "tear" to rhyme with "fear" in the sentence "There was a tear in her dress") (Happé, 1997). According to the theory of weak central coherence, autism is associated with a domain-general bias toward enhanced processing of feature-level information (Happé, 2005; Plaisted,

Saksida, Alcántara, & Weisblatt, 2003). This approach most powerfully explains nondiagnostic aspects of the autistic phenotype; it was not originally designed to explain, and does not easily account for, the full range of social and communication difficulties. A benefit of weak central coherence is that it provides an account of strengths associated with the disorder, such as good performance on the WISC Block Design subtest. At the level of neural mechanism, it is currently unclear what might unite performance on such disparate tasks, though the suggestion of enhanced local connectivity and reduced global connectivity is alluring.

Notice that one aspect of developing intersubjectivity—the understanding of others' intentions—is crucial to at least two current theories of autism, the theory-of-mind and executive theories. Both of these theories assume that the robust early deficit in joint attention behaviors (e.g., Mundy, Sigman, Ungerer, & Sherman, 1986), which is found even in very young children with autism, is an early marker of a failure to understand other people's mental states, attention, and intentions (see discussion in Russell, 1996; Tager-Flusberg, 2001). This is an inference, since measures of joint attention do not directly test understanding of others' intentions. Conceivably, other underlying deficits could disrupt joint attention behaviors, such as a deficit in aspects of emotion (Mundy & Sigman, 1989). Hence it is logically possible that a young child with autism could understand another's intentions, but still not exhibit joint attention behaviors. If this were the case, it would seriously challenge both the theory-of-mind and executive theories of autism.

Thus the question of whether young children with autism understand others' intentions is crucial for testing competing theories of this disorder. Yet this particular aspect of early social cognition has not been as intensively studied in autism. A study in our lab (Carpenter, Pennington, & Rogers, 2001) used Meltzoff's unfulfilled-intentions task to examine this issue in a group of preschool children with autism compared to a control group of children with developmental disabilities, who were similar in both chronological and mental age. Meltzoff's (1995) task assesses understanding of another's intentions in an imitation context with novel objects. In his study, typically developing 18-month-old infants were as likely to perform a target action on an object (e.g., pulling two halves of a dumbbell apart) regardless of whether they saw an experimenter perform this action successfully (target condition) or just saw the experimenter attempt this action but fail (intention condition). Moreover, these infants performed the target action significantly more often in these two conditions than in either of two control conditions: a baseline condition with no demonstration, or a manipulation condition in which the experimenter performed an unrelated action on the object. The fact that infants in the intention condition produced the target action instead of what the experimenter actually did indicates that they understood the intention.

The Carpenter et al. (2001) study used this paradigm, but added an end-state condition (in which subjects saw the transformed object, without any actions being performed on it). Both groups of infants (those with autism and those with other developmental disabilities) gave evidence of understanding intentions, because there were not significant differences between the target and intention conditions in either group, whereas there were significant differences between the intention and baseline conditions in both groups. There were also no between-group differences. Although the pattern of results suggested a slightly less mature understanding of intention in the group with autism, they nonetheless had a much more marked deficit in joint attention.

These results suggest that the early, robust joint attention deficit in children with autism may *not* reflect a deficit in one aspect of intersubjectivity: understanding others' intentions. Moreover, a similar null result on Meltzoff's task has been found in another study of young children with autism (Aldridge, Stone, Sweeney, & Bower, 2000). In addition, null results on a different measure of understanding intentions were found in an older sample of children (Russell & Hill, 2001). Finally, another study in our lab (Rutherford, Pennington, & Rogers, 2006) found that perception of animacy, arguably a prerequisite for understanding intentions, was essentially intact in young children with autism.

If children with autism understand animacy and others' intentions (at least their intentions toward objects), then both the executive and theory-of-mind theories can be rejected. The theory-of-mind theory requires a deficit in some or most aspects of understanding mental states that appears earlier in typical development than the understanding of false belief. If young children with autism understand the important mental state of intentions, then they are not globally impaired in mental state understanding per se, and perhaps their later problems with false belief have a different explanation. For the executive theory to work, it must derive problems in understanding mental states from executive dysfunction (Russell, 1996); otherwise, executive dysfunction only straightforwardly explains the third part of the autism symptom triad, restricted and repetitive activities. This means that some other deficit, possibly in some aspect of emotion, must underlie the earlier and later social deficits.

Recent work on automatic aspects of emotion processing in autism, including mimicry of emotional expressions (McIntosh, Reichmann-Decker, Winkielman, & Wilbarger, 2006; Moody & McIntosh, 2006), finds deficits, whereas earlier studies of offline, nonautomatic emotion processing often did not. Mimicry is the unconscious and automatic copying of another's gestures and is an important component of interpersonal synchrony, so an early deficit in mimicry could undermine social understanding.

In summary, although we now have a much better understanding of what is impaired and intact in the development of social cognition in people with autism, much more remains to be done to determine (1) why the development of intersubjectivity is disrupted in this disorder, (2) what secondary effects this lack of intersubjectivity produces, and (3) what interventions may compensate for these problems.

Table 8.1 summarizes the research on ASD.

DIAGNOSIS AND TREATMENT

Currently, the diagnosis of autism and Asperger syndrome is based primarily on symptoms and history. To date, a definitive neuropsychological test profile for either disorder does not exist, in part because typical neuropsychological test batteries do not evaluate social cognition. There are cognitive test profiles that would be consistent with either disorder, however, and cognitive testing is important to identify strengths and weaknesses in children whose everyday performance may present a confusing picture of their underlying abilities.

Presenting Symptoms

Children with ASD are often referred for failure to meet language and motor milestones in the preschool years. A loss of speech or other developmental attainments is particularly telling, though only true in a minority of cases. In addition, other important symptoms may be mentioned. These include reduced social engagement; reduced or unusual play behavior; nonsocial attachments (e.g., to pieces of string); odd communication (echoing, making up words, mixing up pronouns); motor rituals (rocking, spinning, hand flapping); unusual or repetitive interests (e.g., in timetables, calendars, meteorology, and astronomy); unusual responses to sensory stimuli; and preserved or enhanced areas of function, such as precocious reading or excellent rote memory.

History

Symptoms of ASD are typically recognized early in development, usually by the toddler years, although children with higher-functioning autism or Asperger syndrome may not be referred until later school age. At about 1 year of age, initiation of joint attention and consistent response to name are two behaviors that reliably discriminate typically developing children from children with ASD. During the toddler years, parents often report having to work hard to engage their child in social games and interactions. The child may show reduced or unusual nonverbal communication, such as reduced eye contact, inappropriate facial expressions, and reduced gesture use. Lan-

TABLE 8.1. Research Summary Table: ASD

Definition	• Autism requires qualitative impairments in (1) social interaction; (2) communication; and (3) range of behavior, interests, and activities.
	• Asperger syndrome requires qualitative impairments in social interaction and range of behavior, interests, and activities. By definition, a child with Asperger syndrome cannot have a delay in language or cognitive development.
Epidemiology	• Prevalence is 0.05%–1%, depending on the stringency of the diagnostic criteria.
	• Male–female ratio ranges from 3:1 to 4:1, but females with autism have lower average IQs.
Etiology	• One of the most heritable psychiatric diagnoses (heritability > .90), with a significant minority of cases associated with chromosomal anomalies or known genetic syndromes.
	• The broader autism phenotype, characterized by social and cognitive deficits, runs in families.
	• The best-replicated linkage finding to date is on 7q.
	• Several candidate genes have been proposed, one of which has led to a possible mouse model for autism. The model is a transgenic mouse with a mutated version of human neuroligin-3 (NLGN3).
	• Contrary to early reports, prenatal infections and obstetrical complications have *not* proven to be very important in the etiology of autism.
Brain bases	• Macrocephaly is evident in a substantial minority of cases, particularly children.
	• There is now good evidence that early macrocephaly is due to an abnormal growth pattern. At birth, the brain is normally sized. There is then rapid overgrowth in the first years of life, followed by an unusually early cessation of brain growth.
	• The main functional findings are (1) a reduced P300 response to novel stimuli in ERP studies; (2) more variability in regional metabolic rates in PET studies, suggesting less coordinated processing across brain regions; (3) differences in the brain substrates (fusiform gyrus [FG] and amygdala) used to process social stimuli, such as faces; and (4) lower activations in mirror neuron regions while observing another's actions, but not while executing the same action.
Neuropsychology	• Primary deficits in social cognition, including impairment in social orienting, joint attention, face processing, imitation, theory of mind, empathy, and aspects of emotional expression.
	• There is a growing consensus among researchers that a multiple-deficit account will be necessary to explain the full autism phenotype.

guage milestones may be delayed (although this is not true for Asperger syndrome), and language may have an odd or repetitive quality. Behavioral outbursts that are triggered by attempts to change a routine or transition to a different activity are common. During preschool, the child's social and play difficulties become more apparent, because the child has consistent opportunities to interact with same-age peers. The child may have limited skills in pretend play and may prefer parallel or solitary play activities to cooperative play. He or she may also fixate on certain toys/activities/interests to the exclusion of others. In later school years, social difficulties continue to be an area of weakness, especially in maintaining reciprocal conversations and establishing and maintaining friendships.

Behavioral Observations

Evaluating a child with ASD places a heavier than usual burden on the examiner, because the very nature of the disorder can prevent the child from forming any relationship with the examiner, or significantly disrupt this relationship. It may be very difficult to complete some procedures; thus behavioral observations will play a greater role in the diagnostic formulation. These are usually abundant and clinically rich. For instance, a child may bring a "pet rock" to the session, repetitively sniff pencil shavings or Magic Markers, or ask, "Is the test manual asking me questions?" These rare but highly deviant behaviors provide a great deal of diagnostic information.

The examiner should look for any of the unusual behaviors discussed previously. The examiner should also bear in mind that children with ASD are poor at adapting to new situations, and so the examining situation itself is likely to be particularly stressful and elicit unusual behaviors. We have seen autistic children who read everything in sight as a way of coping with this anxiety, as well as children whose reactions become even more rigid and ritualized in this new situation. Behavioral observations during neuropsychological testing can also provide converging evidence for a diagnosis by identifying executive deficits and particular cognitive styles that are characteristic of ASD, such as cognitive inflexibility or overfocusing on details in visual–spatial or other tasks.

Case Presentations

Case Presentation 5

Background. Logan is a 7-year-old boy who is currently in second grade. Logan has been referred for an evaluation because of speech–language delays, social difficulties, and behavior problems (including intense outbursts).

There is a family history of speech–language delays and social difficulties. Logan's father reports that he has difficulty making friends and tends to avoid large social gatherings. He works as a computer programmer. Logan's paternal cousin had a speech–language delay, but did not experience additional developmental delays. Logan's prenatal and birth histories were uncomplicated. Logan's parents first became concerned about his development when he was a toddler, because he showed motor and language milestone delays. He did not walk independently until he was 18 months old. His first words emerged when he was about 1 year old, but he remained in the single-word stage until he was about 2½ years old. At this time, his parents sought an evaluation through the state's early intervention program. This evaluation described delays in his speech–language, cognitive, motor, socioemotional, and daily living skills. He began receiving in-home speech–language therapy and occupational therapy. When Logan turned 3 years, he was enrolled in an integrated preschool with special education support. Since that time, Logan has continued to be enrolled in self-contained special education classrooms that provide speech–language and occupational therapy support services. He also continues to receive private speech–language and occupational therapy.

According to Logan's parents, it was difficult when he was a toddler to know what items he was requesting, and he would often "melt down" if he did not receive the desired item. To solve this problem, they taught him to point to indicate his requests when he was about a year old. Although Logan would point to indicate his requests, he very rarely pointed to direct his parents' attention to items. Despite Logan's language delays, his parents do not remember him using any gestures besides pointing to communicate. To get his parents' attention, he would bring interesting items to them, but he tended to be more focused on the object than on the social interaction. Logan's parents also describe his language as unusual at times. As a preschooler, he would get his pronouns mixed up—for instance, saying "Help you" when he meant "Help me." He also repeats phrases and sentences from his favorite movies at unusual times.

Logan's parents' concerns about his social skills did not emerge until he entered preschool, although they report in retrospect that Logan was less socially engaged than their younger daughter. They recall having to work hard to get him to smile as an infant. When Logan was a toddler, his parents felt that he did not know his name because he would not always respond to their calls. They worked on Logan's eye contact when he was a toddler and felt that it improved. When Logan was excited about something, he would laugh and flap his hands. His parents thought (and still think) that this hand-flapping behavior was very unusual.

Logan has had a very difficult time establishing and maintaining friendships. He has particular difficulty playing cooperatively with other children; he prefers to engage in solitary or parallel play. He enjoys lining up his toys, and he becomes very upset if someone disturbs them. This rigidity makes it difficult for him to play with other children. Logan also does not engage in pretend play with his toys, preferring instead to crash his favorite toys (trains) together.

Behaviorally, Logan began having intense temper tantrums when he was a toddler. His tantrums were usually triggered by transitions or disruption in Logan's routine or agenda. Logan's parents described that he could get "stuck" on an idea or a play activity, and it was very difficult for him to make the transition to another activity even when they provided warnings. Currently, Logan continues to have difficulty with transitions and disruptions in his routine. He likes certain daily routines to be completed in a precise order. If his routine or agenda is disrupted, he will often have aggressive behavioral outbursts. Logan's parents also describe him as a child who becomes "obsessed" with items. Currently, he plays with trains to the exclusion of other play materials.

Logan's diagnostic testing is summarized in Table 8.2.

Discussion. Logan's persistent difficulties with social interactions, his verbal and nonverbal communication delays, and his behavioral rigidity are all suggestive of ASD. Several specific behaviors reported in the parent interview are also highly suggestive of this diagnosis. First, Logan did not spontaneously learn to point. Once his parents had taught him to point, he did not use this gesture to initiate joint attention. Logan also showed an inconsistent response to his name, which led his parents to believe that he did not know his own name. Both of these indicators are highly indicative of ASD.

When the examiner first met Logan, he did not respond to her greeting, but he willingly came to the table and demonstrated interest in the materials. During the testing session, he frequently insisted on continuing with an activity in the manner he initiated. If he was interrupted, he became visibly upset. The examiner was able to help him make transitions between tasks by providing ample warnings and structure via visual schedules. Logan's manipulation of the testing materials revealed considerable difficulties with fine motor control. Additional behavioral observations were obtained during administration of the ADOS—Module 3, a semistructured, play-based interview that provides a series of social situations within which a range of social and communicative behaviors should occur. During the ADOS, Logan had considerable difficulty sustaining social interactions. He did not join in with a play script that the examiner initiated; instead, he reverted to functional play by himself. Although he seemed to enjoy the activities of the ADOS, he did not share this enjoyment with the examiner. He showed limited gesture use and eye contact. Although Logan generated spontaneous utterances, his language also included immediate echoes of the examiner's language and delayed echoes from his favorite movies. He also tended to get

TABLE 8.2. Test Summary, Case 5 (Logan)

Construct	Standard score/cutoff
General intelligence	
WISC-IV Full Scale IQ	50
Crystallized intelligence[a]	
WISC-IV-Verbal Comprehension Index	57
Similarities	1
Vocabulary	3
Comprehension	4
Fluid intelligence	
WISC-IV-Perceptual Reasoning Index	57
Block Design	5
Picture Concepts	1
Matrix Reasoning	3
WISC-IV Working Memory Index[b]	71
Digit Span	6
Letter–Number Sequencing	4
WISC-IV Processing Speed Index[c]	50
Coding	1
Symbol Search	1
Adaptive behavior	
Vineland-II Adaptive Behavior Composite	68
Academic	
Reading	
History	
Learning and Behavior Quest. Reading History items	60
Word recognition	
WJ III Letter Word ID	70
TOWRE Sight Word Efficiency	65
Phonological coding	
WJ III Word Attack	72
TOWRE Phonemic Decoding Efficiency	73
Math	
WJ III Math Fluency	56
WJ III Calculation	70
WJ III Applied Problems	68
Spelling	
WJ III Spelling	60
Oral Language	
General	
CELF-4 Core Language	52

(continued)

TABLE 8.2. *(continued)*

Construct	Standard score/cutoff
Semantics	
PPVT-4	59
Verbal memory	
WRAML Sentence Memory	75
WRAML Story Memory	65
CTOPP Nonword Repetition	78
Executive functions	
Inhibition	
D-KEFS Color–Word Interference—Inhibition condition	52
Generating	
D-KEFS Verbal Fluency—Letter Fluency condition	55
Set shifting	
WCST (perseverative errors)	48
D-KEFS Trail Making—Number–Letter Switching condition	50
Attention and hyperactivity–impulsivity	
ADHD Rating Scale–IV Inattention	
Parent	4/9
Teacher	5/9
ADHD Rating Scale–IV Hyperactivity–Impulsivity	
Parent	2/9
Teacher	3/9
Visual–spatial	
Rey–Osterrieth Complex Figure Test	55
Beery–Buktenica Test of Visual–Motor Integration	46
Social communication	
SCQ	21/40 (cutoff = 15)
ADOS—Module 3	
Communication	6 (cutoff = 3)
Reciprocal Social Interaction	10 (cutoff = 6)

Notes. WISC-IV, Wechsler Intelligence Scale for Children—Fourth Edition; WJ III: Woodcock–Johnson III Tests of Achievement; Vineland-II, Vineland Adaptive Behavior Scales, Second Edition; TOWRE, Test of Word Reading Efficiency; PPVT-4, Peabody Picture Vocabulary Test—Fourth Edition; CELF-4, Clinical Evaluation of Language Fundamentals—Fourth Edition; CTOPP, Comprehensive Test of Phonological Processing; WRAML, Wide Range Assessment of Memory and Learning; D-KEFS, Delis–Kaplan Executive Function System; WCST, Wisconsin Card Sorting Test; ADOS, Autism Diagnostic Observation Schedule; SCQ, Social Communication Questionnaire.
[a]See also Oral language—Semantics.
[b]See also Oral language—Verbal memory.
[c]See also Academics—Math—WJ III Math Fluency.

"stuck" on certain topics or ideas and mentioned them several times. For example, he moved a chair in the testing room and then told the examiner several times not to move the chair when he left the room. Logan's difficulties in social communication during the ADOS are consistent with his parents' report on the SCQ, which assesses social, communication, and play behaviors and special interests, and helps determine whether an individual's developmental history is consistent with ASD.

Logan's WISC-IV Full Scale IQ score and his adaptive behavior score on the Vineland-II are consistent with ID. The fact that Logan's adaptive behavior score is considerably stronger than his IQ estimate probably reflects the fact that he has benefited from the interventions and supports he has received through his school and privately. On the WISC-IV, Logan shows some scatter among and within his Index scores. His strongest score is on the Working Memory Index. As previously described, Logan likes to echo language and so is fairly adept at repeating back information verbatim, such as on the Digit Span task and on a related subtest, WRAML Sentence Memory. Logan did have difficulty reversing the order on the backward condition of the Digit Span subtest. For each item, he repeated it forward initially, but he was able to reverse the order if prompted. Although this violated standard administration procedures, his performance with prompts was felt to be a more accurate assessment of his abilities, because his tendency to get "stuck" on a certain procedure was hindering his performance. This tendency for Logan to get "stuck" was also apparent on the Symbol Search and Matrix Reasoning subtests, where he fell into a response set of choosing the leftmost items on the page. Logan also got "stuck" in response sets during the executive function tests in this battery. Most notably, on the WSCT, Logan perseverated on matching by color for the whole task and only completed one category.

Another pattern evident in the Verbal Comprehension Index and Perceptual Reasoning Index of the WISC-IV is that Logan has particular difficulty with abstract reasoning, consistent with his ID. For example, the Similarities subtest requires a higher degree of abstraction than the other subtests of the Verbal Comprehension Index. Logan was not able to answer any of these items correctly. Logan also struggled with the visual analogue of the Similarities subtest, the Picture Concepts subtest of the Perceptual Reasoning Index.

Logan continues to show significant fine motor delays, despite occupational therapy interventions. These fine motor delays have probably affected his performance on timed written tests of this battery (e.g., the WISC-IV Processing Speed Index subtests, WJ III Math Fluency) and on tests requiring precise visual–motor integration (e.g., the Beery–Buktenica Test of Visual–Motor Integration, the Rey–Osterrieth Complex Figure Test). Above and beyond these fine motor difficulties, Logan showed a tendency to overfocus on the details to the detriment of the gestalt on both of the visual–spatial tests. This strategy was fairly generalized, as it also characterized his recall on the WRAML Story Memory subtest.

Overall, Logan's academic skills are on par with his cognitive abilities. He shows a relative strength in tasks requiring rote skills, such as word decoding and simple mathematical computations, compared to more integrative and abstract tasks.

Ratings from Logan's parents and teachers on the ADHD Rating Scale-IV indicate some difficulties with inattention, although they do not meet the symptom criteria for an ADHD diagnosis. Further interview has indicated that these symptoms are closely related to Logan's behavioral rigidity, which causes him to be distracted and have difficulty following directions.

In summary, Logan is a child with ID, but his social difficulties and behavioral rigidity cannot be entirely explained by this diagnosis. He also meets DSM-IV-TR criteria for autistic disorder, based on converging evidence from his developmental history, testing results, and clinical observations during the ADOS.

Case Presentation 6

Background. Sam is a 9-year-old boy who is currently in fourth grade. Sam has been referred for an evaluation because of concerns about his social development and his difficulty in adapting to transitions and changes in routine.

Sam's family history is positive for anxiety disorder and depression. His prenatal and birth histories were uncomplicated. According to his parents, his early development was typical to advanced, and he met his language and motor milestones within developmental expectations. Sam's parents observed that his language development seemed particularly advanced, because his vocabulary was quite large by the time he was about 1½ years old. However, the parents reported that his eye contact was limited during his toddler years and his facial expression did not always seem appropriate to particular situations. For example, Sam's parents described him as very caring and affectionate, but if somebody in his family was hurt or sad, he might not notice and smile instead of expressing concern. Sam was very interested in the world around him and he would point out items to his parents, but he did not check back to see whether they were looking at the item with him. Sam would play simple back-and-forth social games, like peekaboo, but he tired of these games quickly and would wander off to play by himself. Sam's response to his name was also inconsistent when he was a toddler. If he was engrossed in an activity, his parents would need to work to get his attention, but other times he would respond immediately.

Sam's parents' first concerns emerged when he was about 2 years old. He began exhibiting severe temper tantrums that occurred almost daily and lasted for about 30 minutes. These tantrums were usually triggered when Sam's routine changed or when he did not get what he wanted. Even as a toddler, Sam would latch onto certain routines and then insist that his parents follow them. For example, at bedtime, he always requested the same two books to be read to him. If his parents attempted to expand his repertoire, he would get very upset. Currently, Sam continues to have difficulty with transitions and changes in his routine. Although he now throws tantrums only rarely (about once every 6 months), his parents note that he can have "meltdowns" when something unexpected occurs.

In terms of Sam's academic history, Sam's preschool and kindergarten teachers reported that he excelled academically but that they had concerns about his social development and rigidity. He did not show much interest in other children and typically played alone. He had difficulty playing with other children because he wanted to be "in charge." For example, he liked to line up cars, and then he would tell the children which cars to play with, what road to take, and so on. Currently, Sam continues to excel academically, but his social difficulties and rigidity have continued into grade school. His parents describe that he struggles to make and sustain friendships. Sam has a current interest in *Star Wars*, which provides a point of connection with other children, but Sam gets frustrated when the children do not want to play *Star Wars* according to his rules. He likes to use the action figurines to act out the scenes of the movies exactly. He does not like it if children want to pretend or add to the script he has in mind.

In terms of communication with peers, Sam often does not respond to other children's attempts to initiate conversations, and he does not ask questions of other children. Sam sometimes makes socially inappropriate comments to his peers that isolate him further. For example, when a child gets an answer wrong in class, he may say, "Anybody should know that." His parents are puzzled by these statements, because he is not mean or rude to children in other contexts. With adults, Sam sometimes does not understand power hierarchies, and he relates to his parents and teachers as if they were his peers. Sam's conversations with adults tend to be less stilted than with peers, especially if he is permitted to talk about his interest in *Star Wars*. Nevertheless, his parents indicate that these conversations are often one-sided, with Sam providing information that he has already told them. They find it difficult to interrupt and redirect him when he is talking about *Star Wars*. They can usually move him off the topic for a couple of minutes, but then he brings the topic back up again. If Sam's parents initiate a conversation that is not about his interest, they find that he is less willing to participate in the conversation.

Although *Star Wars* is Sam's current interest, he has a history of restricted interests in dinosaurs, cars, and trains. According to his parents, all of these interests have been unusually intense, even though the topics have been age-appropriate. For example, regarding *Star Wars*, Sam will only

read books about *Star Wars*, even though his parents have tried to interest
him in other science fiction novels. He plays primarily with *Star Wars* action
figures, watches the movies repeatedly, and prefers to talk about *Star Wars*.
His parents find that his interest in *Star Wars* limits his exposure to other
age-appropriate topics and toys.

Sam's diagnostic testing is summarized in Table 8.3.

Discussion. Sam's persistent difficulties with reciprocal social and play
interactions, his difficulty with transitions, and his restricted special interests are all suggestive of ASD. Sam has not shown any delays in his language
development, so the diagnosis of Asperger syndrome is the most appropriate. Although Sam has not exhibited delays in his structural and semantic
language development, he does show pragmatic difficulties, which are often
associated with Asperger syndrome. Children who are high-functioning like
Sam are often *not* referred for an evaluation, because they can perform well
in an academic setting. They are often seen as bright children whose social
awkwardness is attributable to their high cognitive abilities. In addition, these
children typically interact better with adults than with their peers, because
adults are generally more patient with one-sided conversations about their
special interests and with their presentation as "little professors." Moreover,
if a child does receive a diagnosis of Asperger syndrome, often teachers and
family members in the child's life are disbelieving of the diagnosis, because
they associate ASD exclusively with the lowest-functioning individuals. As
such, a family and child can feel unsupported in implementing the interventions that are necessary for the child's optimal development.

Sam's initial presentation was somewhat unusual. He was standing in
the waiting room watching the clock and did not orient when the examiner
greeted his mother. He did orient when the examiner explicitly called his
name. At a later testing session, he asked whether he would be working
in the same room as before, and then went ahead to wait in the room by
himself while the examiner spoke to his mother. As in Logan's case, additional behavioral observations were obtained during administration of the
ADOS—Module 3. During the ADOS, Sam showed deficits in his nonverbal
and verbal social-communicative behaviors. In the nonverbal realm, his eye
contact and repertoire of facial expressions were limited. He made an occa-
sional smile, but otherwise his affect was notably restricted. His gesture use
was also limited to contexts in which gestures were prompted (e.g., "Show
me" and "Tell me").

In regard to Sam's verbal communication style, his voice quality was
loud and high-pitched. His language also had a pedantic quality because
of his repeated use of particular phrases (e.g., "Actually"). In fact, speaking with Sam was like talking to a "little professor," because he related to
the examiner like a peer (e.g., suggesting ways to increase the efficiency of

TABLE 8.3. Test Summary, Case 6 (Sam)

Construct	Standard score/cutoff
General Intelligence	
WISC-IV Full Scale IQ	125
Crystallized intelligence	
WISC-IV Verbal Comprehension Index	124
Similarities	13
Vocabulary	16
Comprehension	13
Fluid intelligence	
WISC-IV Perceptual Reasoning Index	131
Block Design	17
Picture Concepts	15
Matrix Reasoning	13
WISC-IV Working Memory Index[a]	102
Digit Span	12
Letter–Number Sequencing	9
WISC-IV Processing Speed Index[b]	115
Coding	12
Symbol Search	13
Adaptive behavior	
SIB-R	105
Academic	
Reading	
History	
Learning and Behavior Quest. Reading History items	110
Word recognition	
WJ III Letter Word ID	112
TOWRE Sight Word Efficiency	115
Phonological Coding	
WJ III Word Attack	111
TOWRE Phonemic Decoding Efficiency	117
Paragraph fluency	
GORT-4 Fluency	125
Reading comprehension	
GORT-4 Comprehension	115
Math	
WJ III Math Fluency	110
WJ III Calculation	121
WJ III Applied Problems	116

(continued)

TABLE 8.3. *(continued)*

Construct	Standard score/cutoff
Written expression	
WIAT Written Expression	90
Spelling	
WJ III Spelling	122
Oral language	
Verbal memory	
WRAML Sentence Memory	100
WRAML Story Memory	105
CTOPP Nonword Repetition	101
Executive functions	
Inhibition	
Gordon commission errors	105
D-KEFS Color–Word Interference—Inhibition condition	115
Set shifting	
WCST (perseverative errors)	65
D-KEFS Trail Making—Number–	
Letter Switching Condition	112
Attention and Hyperactivity–impulsivity	
Gordon omission errors	100
ADHD Rating Scale–IV Inattention	
Parent	3/9
Teacher	2/9
ADHD Rating Scale–IV Hyperactivity–impulsivity	
Parent	1/9
Teacher	1/9
Visual–spatial	
Rey–Osterrieth Complex Figure Test	82
Beery–Buktenica Test of Visual–Motor Integration	85
Social communication	
SCQ	18/40 (cutoff = 15)
ADOS—Module 3	
Communication	5 (cutoff = 3)
Reciprocal Social Interaction	8 (cutoff = 6)

Note. SIB-R, Scales of Independent Behavior—Revised; WIAT, Wechsler Individual Achievement Test; GORT-4, Gray Oral Reading Test—Fourth Edition; Gordon, Gordon Diagnostic System. For other abbreviations, see Table 8.2.
[a]See also Oral language—Verbal memory.
[b]See also Academics—Math—WJ III Math Fluency.

the testing) and because he had such a high level of verbal expression and comprehension. Nevertheless, despite these strong verbal skills, Sam had marked difficulty with reciprocal conversations. He was very interested in talking about *Star Wars*, but when the examiner pressed for conversations about other topics, Sam did not respond. A nice strength for Sam, however, was that he was socially motivated to participate in conversations, albeit about his own topics. He also made verbal bids for the examiner's attention (e.g., "Look"), but these verbalizations were not integrated with eye contact or facial expressions.

Sam's play was notably poor, especially given his strong cognitive scores, discussed below. He mostly exhibited functional play, such as putting items in the pockets of characters. When the examiner tried to engage him in a reciprocal play interaction, he interrupted and redirected the play toward his own interests.

Sam also showed limited insight into typical social relationships and feelings. When asked what makes him feel certain feelings, he referred to his video games (e.g., he feels sad when he can't complete a level). His understanding of relationships also appears limited. When asked about his friends, he said that he could not remember whether he and another boy are friends; when asked about why people get married when they are older, he said it is because they can have cake.

Sam's Full Scale IQ score on the WISC-IV falls in the superior range, consistent with teacher reports that Sam is a bright boy who excels at academic work. His Index scores do show some scatter. His scores on the Verbal Comprehension and Perceptual Reasoning Index are both in the superior range, while his score on the Processing Speed Index is in the high-average range, and his score on the Working Memory Index is in the average range. These scores suggest that verbal rote memory may be an area of relative weakness for Sam. Behavioral observations of Sam's performance during the Similarities and Block Design test are possibly the most important for diagnostic formulation. On the Similarities subtest, Sam had difficulty deriving the global rule that related the two items together. He had trouble switching from a more detailed strategy (e.g., which letters the words have in common) to a more global strategy, but once he was able to accomplish this switch, he was able to answer the more difficult items correctly. During the Block Design subtest, Sam stated that he was going to make his pattern different, not the same—consistent with observations that he often pursues his own agenda. It was difficult to move him away from this agenda, but once this was done, he was able to complete some of the most difficult patterns. Together, these observations reveal a quality of cognitive inflexibility that is often characteristic of ASD. This weakness also emerged on the WCST, in which Sam was able to complete the color and form categories, but could not make the transition to sorting by number. His perseverative errors on this test placed him at the first percentile. It is important to note that Sam's fluid intelligence scores are quite discrepant from his score on the WCST. Although his abstract problem-solving abilities are above average, he has difficulty using these reasoning abilities in an unstructured task where social feedback is necessary for solving the problem. This pattern suggests that Sam's rigidity and social difficulties will interfere with his ability to make full use of his abstract problem-solving abilities in some contexts.

A second cognitive style is evident from Sam's scores on the WRAML Story Memory, the Beery–Buktenica Test of Visual–Motor Integration, and the Rey–Osterrieth Complex Figure Test. On each of these tests, Sam tended to overfocus on details. On the Beery and the Rey, his copies were very detail-oriented, but they often lost the gestalt in the midst of the details. His recall of the Rey was severely fractionated, indicating that he encoded the design in isolated fragments. The same pattern was evident on the WRAML Story Memory. On the delayed recall, Sam remembered several details about the story, but he did not recall the global thematic elements. This tendency to overfocus on details is a cognitive style characteristic of Asperger syndrome.

Sam's scores on the academic tests are consistent with his strong academic performance in school. He did show one weakness on the WIAT Written Expression subtest: His story lacked coherence and was overly focused on details. One academic demand that is often difficult for children with Asperger syndrome is writing essays, especially creative writing. Constructing an essay requires a child to stay focused on a topic and provide relevant details. It is likely to be difficult for Sam to write about topics outside of his special interests, just as it is difficult for him to talk about such topics.

This assessment battery includes an assessment for symptoms of inattention and hyperactivity–impulsivity, which are often present in children with Asperger syndrome. Although DSM-IV-TR precludes a diagnosis of ADHD when a PDD is also present, these symptoms can be treated medically or behaviorally if they are impairing. In Sam's case, he does not seem to be experiencing clinically significant ADHD symptoms at this time. It is also important to include a socioemotional screen for secondary features of internalizing disorders. For example, children with Asperger syndrome often have anxieties about making friends and being bullied. As these children approach adolescence, they are at increased risk for mood and anxiety problems, especially as they become more sensitive to not "fitting in" socially. Sam does not show secondary mood or anxiety difficulties at this time, but these symptoms should continue to be monitored.

In summary, Sam's persistent social difficulties, restricted interests, and difficulty with change and transitions are consistent with a diagnosis of Asperger syndrome. This diagnosis is primarily based on Sam's history and observations of his social-communicative behaviors during testing, although converging evidence has been obtained from the testing results. Although Sam has excelled on most of the tests, he shows some cognitive inflexibility and a tendency to overfocus on details, both of which are consistent with Asperger syndrome.

Treatment

ASD changes development more pervasively than any disorder considered in this book, even ID. Language, cognitive, and social development all depend on many thousands of hours of learning, which strengthen connections in the relevant neural networks. Since children with ASD have missed much of this natural learning, it would be very surprising if a neurochemical intervention could abruptly reverse their symptoms. However, intensive early interventions targeting these areas of development have been more successful in reversing some autistic symptoms.

As mentioned earlier, there are no proven pharmacological treatments for the main symptoms of ASD, although medications can be helpful with associated symptoms, such as attention problems, aggressive or self-injurious behavior, and seizures. For instance, methylphenidate (Ritalin) can help with attention problems, and standard anticonvulsants are used to control seizures.

The most efficacious current treatments are psychosocial, involving intensive early intervention, although more rigorous research is needed to evaluate what aspects of these psychosocial treatments are helpful (see National Research Council, 2001). The short-term goals of these intensive early interventions are to improve social and language skills and to reduce behaviors that interfere with learning. The long-term goals are to promote adaptive and vocational skills. As reviewed earlier, a wide range of adult outcomes are found among individuals with ASD from a need for complete custodial care to independent living. It is currently unknown to what extent intensive early interventions improve adult outcome.

One of the first evaluations of an intensive early intervention program was the report by Lovaas (1987) on a 2-year, 40-hour-per-week program of behavior modification, which actively included parents. This intervention appeared to produce dramatic improvement, in that nearly half of the children in the treatment program obtained normal IQ scores and successfully completed first grade in a standard classroom, whereas none of the control children had either outcome. Later follow-ups of these samples (McEachin, Smith, & Lovaas, 1993) have found that about half of the treated children have continued to succeed in a normal classroom, compared to almost none of the controls. However, this study has been criticized because there was not random assignment of cases to the treatment and control conditions, and because no data on behavior (including symptoms of autism) were reported.

Nonetheless, at least some aspects of this approach appear to be useful, and have influenced other early intervention programs. Some of these (e.g., Ozonoff & Cathcart, 1998; Rogers, 1998) have focused more explicitly on teaching the deficient social skills reviewed earlier, such as imitation.

Dawson and Osterling (1997) reviewed eight different university-based early intervention programs for children with autism. Upon entry into these programs, all children exhibited ID, with a mean IQ below 55. After treatment, there was an average IQ gain of 23 points, and half the children were successfully placed in regular elementary school classrooms. These authors identified several common elements across these different programs: (1) a curriculum focused on attention, imitation, communication, social and play skills; (2) a highly structured teaching environment, with a low student-to-staff ratio; (3) strategies for generalizing skills to a wide range of contexts; (4) a predictable and routine daily schedule; (5) a functional rather than aversive approach to problem behaviors; (6) emphasis on skills needed for the transition to a regular classroom; and (7) a high level of family involvement. There have also been recent advances in the early identification of ASD (Cox et al., 1999), making even earlier interventions feasible. A later review (National Research Council, 2001) examined 10 such programs, which were either developmental or behavioral in their theoretical orientation, and came to conclusions similar to those of Dawson and Osterling (1997).

Nonetheless, despite considerable progress in developing early treatments for ASD, we still lack a rigorous treatment study with random assignment of individuals to treatment conditions. The work of Lovaas and colleagues suggests that the gains from early intervention are maintained years later, but more rigorous evidence is needed on that point as well. In addition, more research is needed comparing particular treatments to each other, to tease apart the active components of the interventions. So, according to the guidelines for establishing a particular treatment as effective (which are discussed further in Chapter 14), these psychosocial interventions currently have Level II evidence and could probably reach Level I with additional research studies.

Table 8.4 summarizes clinical issues in ASD.

TABLE 8.4. Clinical Summary Table: ASD

Defining symptoms	• Often referred because of failure to meet language and motor milestones. • Other important symptoms include reduced social engagement; reduced or unusual play behavior; odd communication (echoing, making up words, mixing up pronouns); motor rituals (rocking, spinning, hand flapping); and unusual or repetitive interests.
Common comorbidities	• Children with autism are at increased risk of having ID. Attention problems are also common in children with autism. • Adolescents and adults with high-functioning autism and Asperger syndrome are at increased risk for internalizing disorders, particularly if they are sensitive to social failure.
Developmental history	• Autism: In toddlerhood, delayed language and motor milestones, rigidity about routines and rituals, reduced initiation of joint attention, reduced gesture use, odd language, inconsistent response to name, reduced social engagement, reduced eye contact, facial expression not always appropriate. In preschool, limited pretend play, limited cooperative play, preference for parallel or solitary play activities. May fixate on certain toys/activities/interests. In later school years, social difficulties, including initiating and maintaining conversations and initiating and maintaining peer friendships. • Asperger syndrome: Similar to above, except that language milestones are met within typical limits or even earlier.
Diagnosis	• For autism, impairment must be present in three domains: social, communication, and stereotyped interests/repetitive behaviors. • For Asperger syndrome, cognitive and language delays must *not* be present, although pragmatic difficulties are common. • Diagnosis is based on developmental history (e.g., ADI-R, parent interview) and current social and communication behaviors (e.g., ADOS, play observations). • Behavioral observations during testing can provide converging evidence for a diagnosis by identifying executive deficits and particular cognitive styles characteristic of ASD (e.g., cognitive inflexibility, overfocusing on details).
Prognosis	• Higher IQ and the presence of some communicative speech before age 5 are the best early predictors of a more favorable developmental course.
Treatment	• No proven pharmacological treatments for the main autistic symptoms, but medications can be helpful in treating associated symptoms, such as attention problems, aggressive or self-injurious behavior, and seizures. • The most efficacious current treatments are psychosocial, involving intensive early intervention. • Effective psychosocial interventions often include the following elements: (1) a curriculum focused on attention, imitation, communication, social, and play skills; (2) a highly structured teaching environment, with a low student-to-staff ratio; (3) strategies for generalizing skills to a wide range of contexts; (4) a predictable and routine daily schedule; (5) a functional rather than aversive approach to problem behaviors; (6) emphasis on skills needed for the transition to a regular classroom; and (7) a high level of family involvement.

CHAPTER 9

Attention-Deficit/ Hyperactivity Disorder

WITH LAUREN M. MCGRATH AND ROBIN L. PETERSON

HISTORY

A syndrome involving hyperactivity in children was first described over 160 years ago by a German physician, Heinrich Hoffmann (1845), who wrote a humorous poem describing the antics of "fidgety Phil who couldn't sit still." Somewhat later, Still (1902) described the main problem in this syndrome as a deficiency in "volitional inhibition" or "a defect in moral control." Barkley (1996) points out that Still (1902) recognized several features of attention-deficit/hyperactivity disorder (ADHD) that have been validated by contemporary research: (1) It overlaps with oppositional and conduct problems; (2) it is familial; (3) it is cofamilial with conduct problems and alcoholism; (4) there is a male predominance of about 3:1; and (5) it may also be caused by an acquired brain injury. As we will also see, problems with inhibition continue to be central to current conceptions of ADHD, although much more is now known about the brain bases of these problems.

Whether there is brain dysfunction in ADHD, and how to characterize it if there is, have been confusing and controversial issues in the history of ADHD research. The notion of childhood hyperactivity as a brain disorder was also promoted by Strauss and Lehtinen (1947), based on similarities with the behavior of children who had suffered brain damage because of encephalitis. Unfortunately, this analogy led to some muddled terminology, whereby children with hyperactivity were described as having "minimal brain damage" or "minimal brain dysfunction." These terms are misleading for several reasons: (1) The large majority of children with ADHD have a developmental disorder, not acquired brain damage; (2) the damage or dysfunction to the brain implied in these labels was not documented directly, but was only inferred from behavioral symptoms that could have had many different causes; (3) many children with acquired brain damage do not have hyperactivity (Rutter & Quinton, 1977); and (4) these terms were vague and overinclusive, and thus impeded progress in delineating distinct neuropsychological syndromes affecting learning and behavior in childhood.

As we will see, there is now much more direct evidence that ADHD is a specific kind of brain dysfunction caused mainly by genetic differences. Although ADHD is now more clearly defined and better understood than it once was, it remains a somewhat broad diagnosis. Researchers are making progress in testing the validity of ADHD subtypes, including those in DSM-IV-TR and those defined by comorbidities. As will be discussed later, this research supports the validity of two of the three DSM-IV-TR subtypes of ADHD (inattentive and combined), but questions the validity of the hyperactive–impulsive subtype.

DEFINITION

DSM-IV-TR (American Psychiatric Association, 2000) defines ADHD with two distinct but correlated dimensions of symptoms: those involving *inattention* (e.g., making careless mistakes and not paying close attention to details; forgetfulness; difficulty in organizing tasks and activities; and failure to begin or complete tasks that require sustained mental effort) and those involving *hyperactivity–impulsivity* (e.g., excessive fidgeting, locomotion, or talking; interrupting or intruding in conversations, games, and other situations). With two dimensions, there are thus three possible subtypes of ADHD: inattentive, hyperactive–impulsive, and combined. Someone who meets the diagnostic cutoff (six of nine symptoms) for a single dimension qualifies for that subtype; someone who meets this cutoff on both dimensions qualifies for the combined subtype. Additional requirements for the diagnosis are that the symptoms (1) cause a clinically significant impairment in adaptive functioning; (2) are inconsistent with developmental level (e.g., not just secondary to ID); (3) have been present for at least 6 months, with an onset of some symptoms before age 7; (4) are present in two or more settings; and (5) are not better accounted for by another mental disorder (a PDD, psychosis, or a mood, anxiety, dissociative, or personality disorder). Again, there is better empirical support for the construct validity of the inattentive and combined subtypes than for the hyperactive–impulsive subtype.

EPIDEMIOLOGY AND COMORBIDITIES

Epidemiology

ADHD is one of the most common chronic disorders of childhood, with a 6-month prevalence of 3–5% among school-age children, according to epidemiological studies (U.S. Department of Health and Human Services [DHHS], 1999). Of course, prevalence depends on definition, and definitions vary in how pervasive they require the ADHD symptoms to be. In a careful epidemiological study that required pervasiveness across three different reporters (a parent, a teacher, and a physician), the prevalence was only 1.2% (Spreen, Tupper, Risser, Tuckko, & Edgell, 1984). Male–female ratios in referred samples have been reported to be as high as 9:1, but an epidemiological study found a ratio of 3:1 (Szatmari, Offord, & Boyle, 1989). Thus, as in other disorders, such as RD, males are more likely to be referred than females. Because much of the research on ADHD has relied on referred samples, we know less about ADHD in females than in males. Recent work has demonstrated that the diagnosis of ADHD is valid in both genders, and that the external correlates of the diagnosis are quite similar across genders (Hartung, Freidman Crawford, Willcutt, & Pennington, 2008; Hartung et al., 2002).

ADHD has been found across socioeconomic levels and cultures. There are higher rates of ADHD in lower-income populations, but these rate differences appear to be due to comorbid conditions, such as conduct disorder (see review in Barkley, 1996). In contrast, there is a consistently higher rate of ADHD as defined by teacher ratings in African American children than in European American children; this cannot be explained by socioeconomic status, and it is also found in some but not all studies when ADHD is defined by parent ratings (Samuel et al., 1997). More work is needed to understand this ethnic group difference in rates of ADHD and to test whether it is a valid diagnosis in African American children.

Roughly comparable rates of ADHD have been found in studies in the United States, Japan, and India, with a somewhat higher rate in Germany (Barkley, 1996). There can be dramatic differences in prevalence even between very similar cultures (i.e., the United States and the United Kingdom). Such differences appear to be due to variations in diagnostic criteria and practice (SGR, 1999), rather than representing true differences in prevalence.

In terms of natural history, the age of onset is usually in early childhood, with a peak "age of onset" between ages 3 and 4 (Palfrey, Levine, Walker, & Sullivan, 1985; DHHS, 1999). Retrospective clinical reports from mothers suggest that symptoms of ADHD may appear earlier, even *in utero*. It is becoming clearer that ADHD is a chronic disorder across the lifespan (Gittelman, Mannuzza, Shenker, & Gonagura, 1985), and that many of the tasks of adult development are disrupted by ADHD, because sustained effort, planning, and organization are central to many adult responsibilities.

Comorbidities

Over half of children who meet diagnostic criteria for ADHD qualify for a comorbid diagnosis (Biederman et al., 1992). The list of comorbid disorders includes conduct disorder, depression, anxiety, Tourette syndrome, dyslexia, and bipolar disorder. Moreover, children with ASD, schizophrenia, and ID frequently exhibit the symptoms of ADHD, although DSM-IV-TR stipulates that their more serious primary diagnoses exclude an ADHD diagnosis. More research is needed to understand the basis of these comorbidities and to define purer subtypes of ADHD.

ETIOLOGY[1]

Although the exact etiology of ADHD is still unknown, we know more about its etiology and pathogenesis than we do for many other behaviorally defined disorders. Thus ADHD represents a fairly clear success story for a neuroscience approach to understanding developmental disorders. In this section, we review genetic and environmental influences on ADHD, and evidence for G × E interactions in the etiology of ADHD.

Familiality

The rate of ADHD in families of male probands with ADHD has been found to be over seven times the rate of the disorder in nonpsychiatric control families (Biederman, Faraone, Keenan, Knee, & Tsuang, 1990); later studies reported a similar increase in risk among relatives of female probands (Faraone et al., 1992; Faraone, Biederman, Keenan, & Tsuang, 1991).

Heritability

A meta-analysis of over 20 twin studies of ADHD found a mean heritability of .76, with the remaining variance accounted for by nonshared environment (Faraone, Spencer, Aleardi, Pagano, & Biederman, 2004). These results indicate that the substantial familiality of ADHD is almost entirely due to genetic influences, but, as discussed below, they do not take into account possible G × E interactions. If present, such interactions will be included

---

[1] For a description of genetic technical terms, see Box 1.1 in Chapter 1.

as heritability, or the main effects of genes, in a simple genetic model. A heritability of .76 means that ADHD is one of the more heritable complex behavioral disorders—more heritable than RD or major depression.

Although extreme scores on both the defining dimensions of ADHD, inattention and hyperactivity–impulsivity, are moderately heritable, this appears *not* to be the case for the latter dimension once the correlation between the two dimensions is accounted for (Willcutt, Pennington, & DeFries, 2000). That is, extreme scores on the inattention dimension are moderately heritable, regardless of the level of hyperactive–impulsive symptoms in the proband (i.e., both the inattentive and combined subtypes of ADHD are moderately heritable). However, extreme scores on the hyperactivity–impulsivity dimension were *not* significantly heritable (heritability = .08) when probands did not also have extreme scores on inattention. These results suggest that the etiology of the hyperactivity–impulsivity subtype is largely nongenetic and differs from the etiology of the other two subtypes.

Gene Locations

Efforts to identify specific genes influencing ADHD illustrate the potential power of the candidate gene/association approach. This approach usually depends on a hypothesis derived from an understanding of the neurobiology of the disorder. We know that the primary drug used to treat ADHD, methylphenidate (Ritalin), is a dopamine agonist, and that it achieves this effect by blocking the dopamine transporter, a receptor on the presynaptic neuron involved in the reuptake of dopamine in the synapse. Hence blocking reuptake increases the dopamine available in the synapse. Since receptors are coded for by genes, a gene for a dopamine transporter or genes for other dopamine receptors are reasonable candidate genes in ADHD.

Hence molecular genetic research on ADHD has focused on dopamine genes and some other neurotransmitter genes (reviewed in Faraone et al., 2005). Replicated associations with ADHD have been found for variants of genes for the following: a dopamine transporter (DAT1); an enzyme that acts on dopamine (dopamine-beta-hydroxylase—DBH); two dopamine receptors (DRD4 and DRD5); the serotonin transporter (5-HTT); a serotonin receptor (HTRIB); and two norepinephrine receptors (ADRA 2A and ADRA 2C). Besides these genes involved in neurotransmission, there is also a replicated association with a gene for synaptosomal-associated protein (SNAP-25); this protein is widely expressed in the cortex. As reviewed by Faraone et al. (2005), the odds of these associations are all less than 1.5, meaning that each increases risk for ADHD by less than 50%. Since the sibling risk (lambda) is about 700% and appears to be mostly genetic, we can see that most of the genetic variance in ADHD is not accounted for by these associations, even in combination.

Linkage scans of ADHD (also reviewed by Faraone et al., 2005) have been less successful so far than association studies, and only one replicated risk locus has been identified, on 17p11. Because of the heterogeneity of the ADHD phenotype (DSM-IV-TR subtypes, as well as potential subtypes defined by comorbidities or neuropsychological deficits), linkage scans targeting more specific ADHD phenotypes or endophenotypes may be more successful.

Other possible explanations for some of the unaccounted-for genetic variance in ADHD are G × E interactions. We review this topic after we consider environmental risk factors for ADHD.

Environmental Influences

There are several known bioenvironmental correlates of ADHD, including low birth weight, maternal smoking during pregnancy, fetal alcohol exposure, environmental lead, and pediatric head injury (see Barkley, 1996). However, exposure to these bioenvironmental risk factors is not randomly assigned, so is important to test for gene–environment (G-E) correlations before concluding that there is an environmental main effect. The environmental risk for ADHD posed by maternal smoking and low birth weight cannot be explained by a G-E correlation (e.g., Thapar et al., 2003). Moreover, maternal smoking and low birth weight are the two best-replicated environmental risk factors for ADHD.

We do not have evidence that the social environment in general, or parenting practices in particular, can directly cause ADHD. At the same time, there is no doubt that the social environment influences the course of ADHD—especially whether ADHD develops into another disruptive behavior disorder, such as conduct disorder.

G × E Interactions

Studies of possible G x E interactions in ADHD have focused on replicated risk alleles of dopamine genes and bioenvironmental risk factors (e.g., maternal smoking and drinking during pregnancy). To date, there have been four such studies (Brookes et al., 2006; Kahn, Khoury, Nichols, & Lanphear, 2003; Neuman et al., 2007; Seeger, Schloss, Schmidt, Ruter-Jungfleisch, & Henn, 2004). Two of these studies found a G × E interaction between maternal smoking and the DAT1 gene, but for different risk alleles of that gene (the 10-repeat allele in Kahn et al., 2003, and the 9-repeat allele in Neuman et al., 2007). Brookes et al. (2006) found a G × E interaction between prenatal alcohol exposure and a common DAT1 haplotype (distinct from the DAT1 risk alleles that demonstrated an interaction in the Kahn et al. and Neuman et al. studies). Finally, Seeger et al. (2004) found an interaction between the DRD4 7-repeat risk allele and season of birth. More research is needed to test these initial G × E findings for ADHD, and to test others.

BRAIN MECHANISMS[2]

The hypothesis of frontal lobe dysfunction in ADHD has been advanced by several researchers from the 1970s onward (Gualtieri & Hicks, 1985; Mattes, 1989; Pontius, 1973; Rosenthal & Allen, 1978; Stamm & Kreder, 1979; Zametkin & Rapoport, 1986), based on the observation that frontal lesions in both experimental animals and human patients sometimes produce hyperactivity, distractibility, or impulsivity, alone or in combination (Fuster, 1989; Levin, Eisenberg, & Benton, 1991; Stuss & Benson, 1986). Of course, lesions in other parts of the brain can also produce these symptoms. In what follows, we review evidence that supports frontostriatal dysfunction in ADHD.

Structural Studies

Hynd et al. (1990), using MRI scans, found an absence of the usual right > left frontal asymmetry in children with ADHD. They compared children with ADHD to both children with dyslexia and controls; the frontal finding was present in both clinical groups, but did not differentiate between them, even though the dyslexic group was selected not to include children with ADHD. This lack of frontal asymmetry in ADHD has been replicated in two other studies (Castellanos et al., 1996; Filipek et al., 1997). Abnormalities of caudate volume have also been found across numerous studies of ADHD (Castellanos et al., 1996; Filipek et al., 1997; Hynd et al., 1993; Mataro, Garcia-Sanchez, Junque, Estevez-Gonzalez, & Pujol, 1997). In addition, the globus pallidus has been found to be significantly smaller in those with ADHD (Aylward et al., 1996; Castellanos et al., 1996; Singer et al., 1993). These structural studies support developmental differences in frontostriatal structures known to be important in action selection.

The hypothesis that these structural differences were related to deficits in action selection was tested in a study by Casey et al. (1997). They correlated performance on three separate inhibition tasks with measures of prefrontal cortex and basal ganglia volume. The three inhibition tasks, which tapped response inhibition at different stages of attentional processing, were

---

[2]For a description of neuroanatomical technical terms, see Box 1.2 in Chapter 1.

all impaired in the children with ADHD as compared to controls. Furthermore, prefrontal cortex, caudate, and globus pallidus volumes correlated significantly with task performance. Of course, this correlation does not prove cause. Such a finding could be a *result* or just a *correlate* of ADHD.

Brain structure differences in ADHD are not found exclusively in the prefrontal cortex and basal ganglia. In addition, decreased areas in different regions of the corpus callosum have been observed in several studies (Baumgardner et al., 1996; Castellanos et al., 1996; Giedd et al., 1994; Hynd et al., 1991; Semrud-Clikeman et al., 1994), as well as smaller total cerebral volume and a smaller cerebellum (Castellanos et al., 1996).

Functional Studies

In terms of brain function, electrophysiological measures have supported the hypothesis of central nervous system underarousal in at least a subgroup of hyperactive children (Ferguson & Rappaport, 1983). Likewise, Lou, Henricksen, and Bruhn (1984) found decreased regional cerebral blood flow to the frontal lobes in children with ADHD; this flow increased after the children received Ritalin. Ritalin treatment also decreased blood flow to the motor cortex and primary sensory cortex, "suggesting an inhibition of function of these structures, seen clinically as less distractibility and decreased motor activity during treatment" (Lou et al., 1984, p. 829). These investigators replicated this result in an expanded sample (Lou, Henriksen, Bruhn, Borner, & Nielsen, 1989); in this second report, they emphasized the basal ganglia as the locus of reduced blood flow in ADHD. Zametkin et al. (1990) used PET scanning to study the parents of children with ADHD, who as a group had residual type of attention deficit disorder as defined in DSM-III. They found an overall reduction in cerebral glucose utilization, particularly in right frontal areas, but increased utilization in posterior medial orbital areas. A second study by this group (Zametkin et al., 1993) investigating teenagers with ADHD replicated some but not all of those findings. This second study found significant reductions in the ADHD group in normalized glucose metabolism in 6 of 60 brain regions, including the left anterior frontal lobe. Metabolism in that region correlated inversely with ADHD symptom severity across the combined sample of patients and controls. Since hyperfrontality of blood flow is characteristic of the normal brain, hypofrontality in ADHD could explain the low central arousal found in the electrophysiological studies.

Other studies have demonstrated decreased blood flow in subjects with ADHD, both in prefrontal regions and the striatum (Amen, Paldi, & Thisted, 1993). An fMRI study has demonstrated similar results, showing hypoperfusion in the right caudate nucleus, which was ameliorated after methylphenidate treatment (Teicher et al., 1996).

More recently, fMRI has been used in over 20 studies to investigate brain activation differences in groups with ADHD in response to the demands of a variety of cognitive control tasks, including several that are well-replicated neuropsychological markers of ADHD, such as go/no-go tasks and the Stroop task (see review in Durston & Konrad, 2007). A deficit in frontostriatal activation is found across studies, consistent with the earlier work just reviewed. These studies have also found cerebellar activation differences consistent with the structural difference in cerebellum found by Castellanos et al. (1996).

NEUROPSYCHOLOGY

As discussed in Chapter 1, until recently the goal of neuropsychological research on a behaviorally defined disorder has been to find a single underlying core deficit that provides a parsimonious, causal explanation of the diversity of behavioral symptoms found in the disorder. Earlier reviews (Morton & Frith, 1995; Pennington & Welsh, 1995) explicated the logic of single-cognitive-deficit models of such developmental disorders as autism, dyslexia, and ADHD. Although testing these simple models was a reasonable initial strategy, it is becoming increasingly clear that a single cognitive deficit will not suffice for any of these disorders (Pennington, 2006).

We have recently tested a multiple-deficit model of the relation between ADHD and RD, which are known to share genetic risk factors. Because earlier work in our lab demonstrated that ADHD and RD both involve a deficit in processing speed (Shanahan et al., 2006), we used structural equation modeling to test whether such a deficit was shared by RD and ADHD. This study used multiple indicators of the neuropsychological and diagnostic constructs of RD and ADHD. We found that a combination of phoneme awareness, language skill, and processing speed accounted for around 80% of the variance in RD symptoms (speed and accuracy of single-word reading), and that a combination of inhibition and processing speed accounted for over 30% of the variance in inattentive and hyperactive–impulsive symptoms. In contrast, verbal working memory did not predict unique variance in either RD or ADHD symptoms. Most importantly, the shared processing speed deficit reduced the correlation between RD and ADHD symptoms to a negligible level, meaning that this shared cognitive deficit accounts for their comorbidity. In sum, a multiple-cognitive-deficit model is needed to account for RD, ADHD, and their comorbidity. Several other researchers have discussed the shortcomings of single-cognitive-deficit models of ADHD, and we next review their views.

An article by Nigg, Willcutt, Doyle, and Sonuga-Barke (2005) documents a problem for the executive function theory that is shared by other current neuropsychological theories of ADHD. This problem is that the sensitivity and specificity of any single executive deficit is not high enough to support executive dysfunction as the cause of all cases of ADHD. Across three samples, only about 50% of children with ADHD have a deficit on the most sensitive measure (stop signal reaction time), compared to 10% of controls. While nearly 80% of children with ADHD have a deficit on at least one measure executive function, the same is true of nearly 50% of controls. Given these results, Nigg et al. argue that the field should distinguish an executive dysfunction subtype of ADHD, since there is evidence that this subtype is familial, is more impairing than ADHD without executive dysfunction, and can be distinguished from other potential subtypes of ADHD (e.g., a delay aversion subtype). So this proposal assumes that we may be able to resolve the heterogeneity of ADHD into a number of different single deficit subtypes, the executive dysfunction deficit subtype being one of these.

Sonuga-Barke (2005) explicates one of the main alternatives to the executive dysfunction model of ADHD: a motivational dysfunction model, in which there is disruption in signaling of delayed reward. This delay aversion model of ADHD is supported by both human and animal data (Sagvolden, Russell, Aase, Johansen, & Farshbaf, 2005). Sonuga-Barke ties the executive dysfunction model to one frontostriatal circuit (prefrontal–dorsal neostriatum) and the delay aversion model to another (orbitofrontal–ventral striatum). Each circuit is modulated by dopamine.

Like Nigg et al. (2005), Sonuga-Barke (2005) also proposes single-neuropsychological-deficit subtypes of ADHD (specifically, an executive dysfunction subtype and a motivational deficit subtype). But Sonuga-Barke considers an important alternative to single-deficit models—namely, a dual- or even multiple-deficit model. So the critical question facing ADHD researchers is how many cases of ADHD can be explained by a single neuropsychological deficit (whether cognitive or motivational), and how many cases involve a combination of deficits.

Sergeant (2005) reviews another motivational model of ADHD: his cognitive–energetic model. This model distinguishes ongoing information processing and action selection from energetic pools that influence these cognitive processes. It proposes that the underlying deficit in ADHD is an energetic dysfunction in the regulation of activation and effort needed to optimize ongoing information processing. This model is supported by the well-replicated result that individuals with ADHD are slower and more variable in their reaction times than persons without ADHD, as well as the fact that their performance varies more than controls as a function of event rate (a faster event rate normalizes the performance of groups with ADHD). As Sergeant points out, further testing of this cognitive–energetic model requires direct measures of the hypothesized energetic pools. In the context of the issues raised by Nigg et al. (2005) and Sonuga-Barke (2005), we can ask several pertinent questions about the cognitive–energetic model. Does this model reflect a distinct single-deficit subtype of ADHD? How does this model relate to the other main motivational model of ADHD, the delay aversion model? If cognitive–energetic deficits are distinct from delay aversion and executive dysfunction in ADHD, do they interact with these latter deficits in some children with ADHD? In other words, does a cognitive–energetic deficit constitute a single-deficit subtype of ADHD, or is it one factor in a multiple-deficit model of the disorder?

In sum, an important next step in developing a neuropsychological model of ADHD is to explicitly test the validity of single-deficit subtypes of ADHD—specifically, the putative executive dysfunction, delay aversion, and cognitive–energetic deficit subtypes. Another important next step is to clarify the relationships among these three models of ADHD and to test multiple-deficit models in which the three types of deficits interact. Our work on processing speed deficits in ADHD is a step in that direction (Shanahan et al., 2006, 2007). We need to determine what proportion of individuals with ADHD have each of these three single-deficit subtypes, what proportion have combinations of these deficits, and what proportion remain unexplained by these three models taken singly or in combination.

More fundamentally, we need a stronger theoretical model of the normal behaviors that are disrupted in ADHD. In what follows, we discuss some of the requirements for such a model. A fundamental challenge for neuropsychological theories of psychopathology is how to integrate cognitive and motivational processes (Pennington, 2002). Neuroimaging studies of different disorders—from depression to ASD to ADHD to schizophrenia—find differences in an overlapping set of brain structures, including the dorsal lateral and orbital prefrontal cortices, the basal ganglia, the amygdala and other parts of the limbic system, and the cerebellum. Our theories of what these individual structures do range from very cognitive (dorsal lateral prefrontal cortex) to very motivational (amygdala) to somewhere in between (orbital prefrontal cortex). But we generally lack a theory of how interactions among these structures implement the interactions between cognition and motivation that characterize both adaptive and maladaptive behavior.

ADHD illustrates this theoretical dilemma well. As mentioned earlier, one of the earliest clinical descriptions of ADHD (Still, 1902), spoke of a deficiency in "volitional inhibition" or "a defect in moral control." Although these terms sound quaint to our modern ears, they capture the idea that motivation is inevitably an important input to the process of response selection. The nervous system always selects or inhibits candidate actions and foci of attention with reference to reinforcers, motives, and values. The symptoms of ADHD consist of maladaptive actions and foci of attention that are selected despite being inappropriate to their context. So, almost by definition, each of these symptoms represents a failure of inhibition, but just using that term does not take us very far. That is because the underlying failure may be in the cognitive system, in the motivation system, or in their interaction. All of us will make inappropriate action slips (e.g., putting the milk in the pantry instead of the refrigerator) if we are in a less than optimal cognitive state brought on by fatigue, illness, or intoxication. Conversely, all of us, given enough affective arousal, will commit impulsive actions (e.g., using angry words in an argument) in the absence of preexisting cognitive impairment. And the same is true for our focus of attention. These everyday examples also illustrate how difficult it is to separate cognition and motivation.

So it is not too surprising that both cognitive and motivational theories of ADHD have been proposed, and that neither kind of theory adequately explains all the features of ADHD or the variations across individuals with this diagnosis. One of the limitations of research on the neuropsychology of ADHD is that none of our candidate deficits, whether cognitive or motivational, has a very big effect size. Consequently, none of them by themselves account for much variance in ADHD symptoms. This could mean there are subtypes of ADHD, each with a different single deficit, or that multiple interacting deficits are involved, or that our current candidate deficits are only weak correlates of the actual underlying deficit. So far, the evidence for the first possibility is weak (e.g., Chhabildas, Pennington, & Willcutt, 2001).

Another challenge posed by neuropsychological research on ADHD, especially for prefrontal theories, is that the profile of deficits across measures of executive functions found in ADHD diverges somewhat from what has been found in children with either early-acquired prefrontal lesions or prefrontal dopamine depletion (such as that found in early-treated phenylketonuria). Children with ADHD are most consistently impaired on measures of motor inhibition (such as variants of the go/no-go task), but are not consistently impaired on measures of set shifting (like the WCST) or on other measures of inhibition (like the interference condition of the Stroop) (Willcutt et al., in press).

So it is clear that we need a better theoretical model of how cognition and motivation interact in response selection and attentional control, and of the different ways this process can go awry. Such a model would point to better measures of the neuropsychological deficits in ADHD, which could in turn be tested with a range of neuroscience methods. In what follows here, we first discuss what a better theoretical model needs to include, and then briefly discuss neural network models of the prefrontal cortex and basal ganglia that address these needs.

At a minimum, a better theoretical model of response selection, including where to focus one's attention, will need to include the following:

1. An active memory system to maintain a cognitive representation of the current context (which includes both the immediate environmental context, and a distal context composed of representations of goals and one's past experiences with similar contexts) until a response is selected and executed.
2. A motivation system that can take on different states in response to both the internal survival needs of the organism and the external context.
3. A means for reciprocal interaction between 1 and 2.
4. A computational mechanism for using the constraints provided by 1, 2, and 3 to select and execute an appropriate response.
5. A means of evaluating the success of the chosen response and generating a feedback signal that will affect the selection of the next response.

Based on current neuropsychological evidence, we can tentatively associate most of these five components with a brain region: the dorsolateral prefrontal cortex with 1; the limbic system with 2; both the orbital prefrontal cortex and the projections of brainstem nuclei with 3; and possibly the anterior cingulate gyrus with 5. Components 3 and 4 remind us that we should not think too simply about relating these components to brain structures, because they all must interact in response selection. So it is clear from this list of components that there are multiple possible reasons for such inappropriate action selection as is evident in the symptoms of ADHD. Existing theories of ADHD have mainly focused on components 1 and 2. It would be useful to design studies that test for possible deficits in 3, 4, and 5. Conceivably, ADHD could derive from a faulty interaction between components 1 and 2, or a tendency for the computational mechanism to settle too quickly into a local attractor, or a downstream deficit in error monitoring, but there is little research on these possibilities.

Work by Cohen, O'Reilly and colleagues (Cohen, 2003; Cohen & Servan-Schreiber, 1992; Frank, 2005; O'Reilly, 2003; O'Reilly, Braver, & Cohen, 1999; O'Reilly & Munakata, 2000) on computational models of prefrontal function are useful to consider in this context, although they have not been directly applied to ADHD. (In fact, to our knowledge, there has not been a connectionist model of ADHD.) Their work began by modeling how reduced dopaminergic input creates working memory deficits in models designed to simulate performance on three tasks impaired in groups with schizophrenia: the Stroop, the "AX" version of the continuous performance test, and a lexical disambiguation task (Cohen & Servan-Schreiber, 1992). These models had context units that implemented working memory for the current task context. When these context units were less active, the models, like patients with schizophrenia, were more likely to make prepotent responses. So these models included components 1 (an active memory system), 3 (the dopaminergic input), and 4 (a computational mechanism).

Subsequent models have added interactions with the hippocampus (O'Reilly et al., 1999), the basal ganglia (Frank, 2005; O'Reilly, 2003), and conflict-monitoring units on the output layer to simulate the hypothesized error-monitoring function of the anterior cingulate gyrus (Cohen, 2003). Interactions with the basal ganglia implement a dopamine-controlled gating mechanism, which updates the contents of the working memory system in response to changing reward contingencies. This model incorporates the direct and indirect pathways from the basal ganglia to the thalamus. These pathways have opposite effects on the selection and execution of candidate actions in the frontal cortex: The direct pathway facilitates them, and the indirect pathway suppresses them. Phasic changes in dopamine, in response to error feedback, regulate which pathway predominates. Frank (2005) has used this computational model to explain the implicit learning deficits found in Parkinson disease on probabilistic classification and reversal tasks. So dopamine, which is important in reward-seeking behavior, can selectively gate which information gets into the working memory system of the dorsal lateral prefrontal cortex. Other research has shown that the anterior cingulate gyrus receives noradrenergic inputs from the locus ceruleus, which might help implement a change in motivational state upon error detection (i.e., more vigilance).

These added components, including error monitoring and reward-related gating, make the newer model a much more complete one in terms of components 2 (the motivation system) and 3 (interactions between the motivation and active memory systems) in the list above. In this latest model, there is now a very dynamic interaction between motivation signals (mediated by brainstem neurotransmitter inputs) and cognitive processing in the dorsal lateral prefrontal cortex and the basal ganglia. Since there is evidence for both dopaminergic and noradrenergic deficits in ADHD, it would be very fruitful to use such a model to simulate ADHD. An important long-term goal of this and other work is to understand how the inhibition problem in ADHD compares and contrasts with the inhibition problems found in other disorders, such as schizophrenia, Tourette syndrome, and early-treated phenylketonuria. Such a model could also help us evaluate the role the right prefrontal cortex plays in ADHD, which some researchers argue is central (Aron & Poldrack, 2005).

A better theoretical understanding of how response and attentional selection goes wrong in ADHD (which may vary by subtypes of ADHD) will help guide work on animal models and behavioral and molecular genetic studies of ADHD, including the search for endophenotypes of ADHD. In turn, the results from animal models and genetic studies will help refine this neuropsychological model of ADHD.

Even though ADHD is familial and heritable, it has not been studied with high-family risk longitudinal designs. In fact, we know very little about the preschool development of ADHD. It is quite possible that some of the behavioral symptoms defining ADHD are secondary, while others are primary, or that some of the many comorbidities found in ADHD are secondary, while others identify primary subtypes of ADHD. Longitudinal designs could answer these questions, as well a providing a clearer understanding of the roles of cognition and motivation in the development of this disorder.

In sum, a better theoretical understanding of how self-regulation goes wrong in the development of ADHD (which may vary by subtypes of ADHD) will help guide work on animal models and behavioral and molecular genetic studies of ADHD, including the search for endophenotypes of ADHD. It will also inform work on the typical development of self-regulation.

Table 9.1 summarizes the research on ADHD.

DIAGNOSIS AND TREATMENT

The diagnosis of ADHD is difficult, both because of the number of confounding conditions that must be excluded, and because objective tests of ADHD are less well developed than those for dyslexia or other learning disorders. So clinicians should be duly cautious in making this diagnosis. Diagnosis is primarily based on interview and observation to establish history, current symptoms, and the pervasiveness of impairment. Although objective tests for ADHD are not well developed, testing results can often support the diagnosis by identifying underlying cognitive deficits that are often present in ADHD.

Presenting Symptoms

Because the diagnosis is based primarily on symptoms, much of the research on diagnosis has focused on developing lists of critical or primary symptoms and developing behavioral rating scales for parents and teachers that incorporate these critical symptoms. Once again, the critical symptoms described in DSM-IV-TR fall into two categories: inattention and hyperactivity–impulsivity.

Other symptoms that demonstrate an association with ADHD, but do not appear to be primary, include aggressive behavior, oppositionality, other learning disorders, depression, anxiety, social difficulties, and poor self-esteem.

History

Symptoms of ADHD are usually present from early in life. DSM-IV-TR requires that the symptoms be present by age 7 for the diagnosis to be made,

TABLE 9.1. Research Summary Table: ADHD

Definition	• DSM-IV-TR defines ADHD in terms of two distinct but correlated symptom dimensions: inattention and hyperactivity–impulsivity. • With these two dimensions, there are three possible subtypes of ADHD: inattentive, hyperactive–impulsive, and combined. • There is better empirical support for the construct validity of the inattentive and combined subtypes than for the hyperactive–impulsive subtype.
Epidemiology	• ADHD is one of the most common chronic disorders of childhood, with a 6-month prevalence of 3–5% among school-age children. • Male–female ratios in referred samples have been reported to be as high as 9:1, but one epidemiological study found a ratio of 3:1. • ADHD has been found across socioeconomic levels and cultures. • Age of onset is usually in early childhood, with a peak at ages 3–4. • ADHD is a chronic disorder across the lifespan.
Etiology	• ADHD is both familial and heritable. A meta-analysis of over 20 twin studies of ADHD found a mean heritability of .76. This large heritability estimate indicates that ADHD is one of the more heritable complex behavioral disorders. • Molecular genetic research on ADHD has focused on the candidate gene approach. Replicated associations include several dopamine genes, but also serotonin and norepinephrine genes, as well as a gene for synaptosomal-associated protein. Effect sizes for these candidate genes are modest. • There are several known bioenvironmental correlates of ADHD, including low birth weight, maternal smoking during pregnancy, fetal alcohol exposure, environmental lead, and pediatric head injury. These findings are complicated by possible G–E correlations. • There is evidence for G × E interactions in ADHD, such that genetic risk factors coupled with environmental risk factors can produce worse outcomes than either risk factor alone.
Brain bases	• There is evidence for frontostriatal dysfunction in ADHD. • Main structural findings: absence of frontal asymmetry, abnormal caudate volume, smaller globus pallidus. • Main functional findings: central nervous system underarousal, including a deficit in frontostriatal activation.
Neuropsychology	• Single-cognitive-deficit models of ADHD are not sufficient, because the sensitivity and specificity of any single deficit are too low. • Prominent neuropsychological theories of ADHD are the executive dysfunction theory and motivational deficit theories (e.g., delay aversion model, cognitive–energetic deficit model). • The next step in developing a neuropsychological model of ADHD is to clarify the relationships among these single-deficit models and to test multiple-deficit models.

and some researchers recommend an earlier age-of-onset criterion. If the symptomatic behaviors are not present before first grade, they may be secondary to reading problems and not reflective of primary ADHD. Therefore, an examiner will be more convinced by a history that includes clear examples of inattention, impulsivity, and hyperactivity in the preschool years. The one exception may be a child with the inattentive subtype of ADHD, whose difficulties with sustained attention may not become problematic until the later school grades when expectations for focus and attention increase. Such children are usually referred later for an evaluation than children with hyperactive behaviors are.

In infancy, symptoms may include a high activity level, less need for sleep, colic, frequent crying, and poor soothability—characteristics of what is often called "a difficult infant." In toddlerhood, the child with ADHD often has a low sense of danger, an unusual amount of energy, and a tendency to move from one activity to another very quickly. Parents may notice that the child wears out shoes, clothing, and toys faster than other children (Cantwell, 1975).

Children with ADHD nearly always come to clinical attention in the early school years because of the behavior management problems they pose in a classroom setting: frequent talking, getting out of their seats, difficulty in keeping their hands to themselves, and problems with finishing schoolwork. If a patient does not have a history of these and related problematic behaviors in the early school years, a diagnosis of ADHD (except for acquired causes, such as a closed head injury later in childhood) is unlikely to be correct. In later school years, organization often becomes particularly problematic for children with ADHD. They may have difficulty turning in homework on time, remembering deadlines, and using good study skills. These weaknesses may result in low grades, despite the fact that the children appear able to do the work successfully when additional structure is in place. In such cases, poor grades may be mistakenly attributed to "laziness" or "lack of motivation."

In terms of family history, the family studies previously reviewed indicate a greater risk for ADHD in children of parents who themselves had or have ADHD. Therefore, the psychiatric histories of the parents will be important diagnostic information.

Behavioral Observations

Because children with ADHD may not manifest their problematic behaviors in a novel or structured situation, the absence of ADHD symptoms in the clinician's office does not necessarily rule out the diagnosis. If such behaviors do occur, they then provide important converging evidence. Fidgetiness, poor attention, daydreaming, impulsive response style, problems persisting with difficult tasks, rushing through work, and making careless mistakes are all behaviors in the clinical setting that are consistent with the diagnosis.

Case Presentations

Case Presentation 7

Background. Elliot is an 8-year-old third grader. His parents have sought an evaluation on the advice of his teacher, who is concerned that Elliot's inability to focus during class is impeding his progress in school. The teacher has told Elliot's parents that she can't tell "whether it's a behavior problem or whether it's out of his control." Elliot rushes through classwork, often making careless mistakes or turning in half-completed papers. Although he is a good reader, his writing seems weaker than that of his peers, in terms of both handwriting and compositional skills. In addition, he has fallen behind his classmates in math "Mad Minutes." Elliot's parents are concerned that his school difficulties are leading to problems with self-esteem and peer relationships. They note that he gets few calls for play dates, and that neighborhood children seem to gravitate to his younger brother rather than to Elliot. In moments of frustration in the last year, Elliot has made comments such as "I can't do it because I'm an idiot," or "I told you I'm a stupid-head!"

Elliot's prenatal, birth, and early developmental histories are unremarkable. He was an extremely active infant and toddler, however. His mother has described an incident that occurred when Elliot was 12 months old: She heard a loud noise as he was waking from his nap, and went upstairs to discover Elliot climbing out of his crib onto a nearby dresser and repeatedly jumping from the dresser back into his crib. Although Elliot's parents had not planned to send him to preschool until he was 4, they enrolled him in a morning program when he turned 3 because his mother "was too exhausted to keep up with him all day." She notes that one of her primary criteria for choosing a preschool was how many acres of land it had, so that Elliot would have enough room to run and play. Elliot did well in a relatively unstructured preschool environment and seemed well liked by teachers and peers alike. Concerns were first raised in kindergarten, when Elliot got in trouble on several occasions because of difficulty remaining quietly seated on the school bus. His kindergarten report card stated, "Elliot is still learning to listen respectfully, and circle time has been especially challenging for him." Similar concerns continued in first and second grades. Elliot was often placed at a desk away from other children during work times and was described by teachers as "disruptive," "silly," and "loud and fast-moving." Now, in third grade, Elliot's difficulties are becoming more apparent in social interactions. He has had two playground altercations this fall that led to visits to the principal. Most recently, he shoved another child during an argument about a soccer game and was sent home for the afternoon. His mother describes him as remorseful and apologetic after the incident.

Elliot's mother reports no history of school difficulties. She is a college graduate currently working part-time as a graphic designer. Elliot's father received poor grades in several high school courses, but did better in college "because I finally decided to apply myself." He is now a successful executive. He is less concerned about Elliot than his wife is, and notes, "He's exactly like I was at that age—he just needs to grow out of it."

A summary of Elliot's diagnostic testing is found in Table 9.2.

Discussion. A diagnosis of ADHD is made primarily based on careful interview and observation to establish history and current symptoms, but neuropsychological test results can often help support the diagnosis. Elliot's case illustrates this pattern well. His early history is consistent with ADHD. He showed signs of hyperactivity even as an infant and toddler; such symptoms are often observable earlier in development than are symptoms of inattention, because maintaining a high level of focused attention is rarely expected until a child reaches school age. Elliot's school history is suggestive of difficulties with both ADHD symptom dimensions. Teacher complaints about lack of focus and difficulty in completing work relate to inattention. Most of Elliot's other behavioral difficulties (shouting out, not remaining seated, shoving another child) can be understood as resulting from impulsivity, and it is clear that his activity level remains very high. His teacher's ratings on the ADHD Rating Scale–IV place him in the clinical range (>6 symptoms) on both dimensions, whereas parent ratings on each dimension fall just under the clinical cutoff. However, his parents' verbal description of Elliot's behavior is consistent with a diagnosis of ADHD, combined type. Elliot's difficulties may be less impairing in the home than in the school setting. It is also possible that Elliot's father in particular may be underreporting some of Elliot's symptoms, because his own likely ADHD history may have increased his tolerance for inattentive and hyperactive behavior.

Although ADHD-related behaviors are not always observable in the structured one-on-one testing environment, Elliot's behavior in testing provided a number of telling observations. Compared to others his age, Elliot had difficulty persisting with difficult tasks and required a great deal of encouragement. When presented with a difficult math problem, for example, he said, "Next!" and tried to turn the page before attempting it. Elliot was also fidgety and restless, and played with any objects left out on the testing table, such as pencils or the tape recorder. He required three breaks during a 2-hour session; for each break, he typically ran down the hall, got a drink of water, and ran right back. On the morning of the final test session, Elliot

TABLE 9.2. Test Summary, Case 7 (Elliot)

Construct	Standard score/ cutoff
General intelligence	
WISC-IV Full Scale IQ	109
Crystallized intelligence	
WISC-IV *Verbal Comprehension Index*	119
Similarities	13
Vocabulary	13
Comprehension	14
Fluid intelligence	
WISC-IV *Perceptual Reasoning Index*	108
Block Design	10
Picture Concepts	13
Matrix Reasoning	11
WISC-IV Working Memory Index[a]	104
Digit Span	11
Letter–Number Sequencing	11
WISC-IV Processing Speed Index[b]	91
Coding	7
Symbol Search	10
Academic	
Reading	
History	
Learning and Behavior Quest. Reading History items	110
Word recognition	
WJ III Letter Word ID	121
Phonological coding	
WJ III Word Attack	117
Paragraph fluency	
GORT-4 Fluency	110
Reading comprehension	
GORT-4 Comprehension	115
Math	
WJ III Math Fluency	90
WJ III Calculation	114
WJ III Applied Problems	111

(continued)

TABLE 9.2. *(continued)*

Construct	Standard score/ cutoff
Written Expression	
WIAT Written Expression	86
Spelling	
WJ III Spelling	113
Oral Language	
Verbal memory	
WRAML Sentence Memory	105
WRAML Story Memory	110
Executive functions	
Inhibition	
Gordon commission errors	71
D-KEFS Color–Word Interference—Inhibition condition	115
Generating	
D-KEFS Verbal Fluency—Letter Fluency condition	90
Attention and hyperactivity–impulsivity	
Gordon omission errors	104
ADHD Rating Scale–IV Inattention	
Parent	5/9
Teacher	9/9
ADHD Rating Scale–IV Hyperactivity–impulsivity	
Parent	4/9
Teacher	8/9
Visual–spatial	
Beery–Buktenica Test of Visual–Motor Integration	83

Note. WISC-IV, Wechsler Intelligence Scale for Children—Fourth Edition; WJ III, Woodcock–Johnson III Tests of Achievement; WIAT, Wechsler Individual Achievement Test; GORT-4, Gray Oral Reading Test—Fourth Edition; WRAML, Wide Range Assessment of Memory and Learning; Gordon, Gordon Diagnostic System; DKEFS, Delis–Kaplan Executive Function System.
[a]See also Oral language—Verbal memory.
[b]See also Academics—Math—WJ III Math Fluency.

was reluctant to start and hid under the table in the waiting room until his mother convinced him to come out. He commented that he did not want to begin testing, because "Those games are too hard and boring."

Several aspects of Elliot's pattern of test results further support a diagnosis of ADHD. First, he made an unusually high number of commission errors on the Gordon Diagnostic System continuous performance test, probably reflecting his impulsive response style. Elliot was aware of many of these errors and often commented aloud on them ("Oops! I did it again"). Second, his scores on the Processing Speed Index of the WISC-IV and on WJ III Math Fluency suggest weaknesses in processing speed, a cognitive risk factor for ADHD. Although both scores fall at the lower end of the average range, they are significantly lower than estimates of either his conceptual reasoning abilities or his untimed math skills (WJ III Calculation and Applied Problems). Third, consistent with teacher report, written composition (WIAT Written Expression) represents an area of weakness for Elliot. Although his composition included a number of wonderfully creative ideas, it was poorly organized and included multiple punctuation, capitalization, and grammatical errors. Fourth, Elliot shows some evidence of executive difficulties, particularly on the D-KEFS Letter Fluency subtest (an updated version of the so-called "FAS" test). He was only able to generate three words starting with F, four with A, and four with S. Again, although this score is itself at the lower end of the average range, it is quite weak in the context of Elliot's general verbal abilities. Finally, like many children with ADHD, Elliot has poor handwriting. Fine motor and organizational difficulties probably relate to his low score on the Beery.

Many children with impairing ADHD show mixed results on neuropsychological testing, and this is true of Elliot to a degree. For example, he has done well on the D-KEFS Color–Word Interference subtest, a measure of inhibitory control. Furthermore, he does not demonstrate the verbal short-term memory weaknesses found in some individuals with ADHD. In the context of history, current functioning, and observations, however, the diagnosis of ADHD, combined type is warranted.

It is important to screen children with ADHD for dyslexia because of the high degree of comorbidity. In Elliot's case, neither history nor current test results suggest RD; in fact, reading seems to represent a strength for him and should be encouraged. Elliot does appear to be experiencing some secondary problems with self-esteem and social relationships as a result of his ADHD. His difficulties with peers appear to relate primarily to impulsivity, and like many children experiencing increasing school failure, he is developing a poor self-image. These problems should be carefully monitored as treatment for his ADHD is put in place. If they continue, behavioral intervention (e.g., with a psychologist) may be helpful.

Case Presentation 8

Background. Joan is a 14-year-old girl who is currently in eighth grade. Joan has been referred for an evaluation because of ongoing concerns about her poor performance in school. She has difficulty keeping track of her assignments, turning in her work on time, and staying on task. Her grades have begun to suffer because of these difficulties, and her parents are very concerned about her upcoming transition into high school.

Joan's birth and early development histories were uncomplicated. Her paternal uncle and his son have been diagnosed with ADHD. Joan's parents first became concerned about her academic progress in early elementary school. Her teachers reported that Joan was a slow worker and often needed to be prompted to finish her work because she was daydreaming, doodling, or staring out the window. The teachers often placed her in the front of the room to help her pay attention. Her reading skills also lagged behind those of her peers. In third grade, Joan received extra reading help in the form of a structured phonics-based reading program. This program reportedly improved her reading accuracy, although she continued to be a slow reader. Joan's academic difficulties became even more problematic in middle school because of the increasing homework demands. Her parents observed that Joan was spending much more time on her homework than her peers were. Despite this extra effort, Joan would often forget to turn in assignments that she had completed. Currently, Joan's organizational skills continue to be poor, and she still has difficulty keeping track of assignments and turning them in on time. Her teachers describe that she has ongoing difficulties with focus and attention in class; her reading speed continues to be slow; and she has difficulty with writing assignments.

Joan's diagnostic testing is summarized in Table 9.3.

Discussion. Joan's persistent difficulties with sustained attention and organization are suggestive of ADHD, particularly the inattentive subtype. In addition, Joan's early difficulties with reading acquisition and persistent fluency weaknesses may be suggestive of dyslexia. There is a family history of ADHD, and the Reading History questions from the Learning and Behavior Questionnaire capture Joan's early difficulties with reading.

During the testing sessions, Joan was motivated to do well, and she remained very focused. It is important to note that it is rare to observe clinically significant symptoms of inattention in a novel one-on-one testing situation, although these symptoms may be clinically significant in other settings. Accordingly, an interview with Joan's teacher revealed significant difficulties with sustained attention and organization, consistent with her parents' report. Ratings on the ADHD Rating Scale-IV from Joan, her parents, and

TABLE 9.3. Test Summary, Case 8 (Joan)

Construct	Standard score/ cutoff
General intelligence	
WISC-IV Full Scale IQ	101
Crystallized intelligence	
WISC-IV Verbal Comprehension Index	114
Similarities	13
Vocabulary	12
Comprehension	13
Fluid intelligence	
WISC-IV Perceptual Reasoning Index	98
Block Design	10
Picture Concepts	8
Matrix Reasoning	11
WISC-IV Working Memory Index[a]	99
Digit Span	9
Letter–Number Sequencing	11
WISC-IV Processing Speed Index[b]	83
Coding	5
Symbol Search	9
Academic	
Reading	
History	
Learning and Behavior Quest. Reading History items	66
Word recognition	
WJ III Letter Word ID	108
TOWRE Sight Word Efficiency	86
Phonological coding	
WJ III Word Attack	104
TOWRE Phonemic Decoding Efficiency	83
Paragraph fluency	
GORT-4 Fluency	90
Reading comprehension	
GORT-4 Comprehension	110

(continued)

TABLE 9.3. *(continued)*

Construct	Standard score/ cutoff
Math	
WJ III Math Fluency	87
WJ III Calculation	108
WJ III Applied Problems	110
Spelling	
WJ III Spelling	92
Written expression	
WIAT Written Expression	85
Oral Language	
Phonological awareness[c]	
CTOPP Elision	95
CTOPP Phoneme Reversal	85
Verbal processing speed	
CTOPP Rapid Naming Composite	91
Verbal memory	
CTOPP Nonword Repetition	90
WRAML Sentence Memory	95
WRAML Story Memory	110
Executive functions	
Inhibition	
Gordon commission errors	85
Generating	
D-KEFS Verbal Fluency—Letter Fluency condition	88
Attention and hyperactivity–impulsivity	
Gordon omission errors	80
ADHD Rating Scale–IV Inattention	
Parent	8/9
Teacher	7/9
Self-report	7/9
ADHD Rating Scale–IV Hyperactivity–impulsivity	
Parent	2/9
Teacher	1/9
Self-report	2/9

Note. TOWRE, Test of Word Reading Efficiency; CTOPP, Comprehensive Test of Phonological Processing. For other abbreviations, see Table 9.2.
[a]See also Oral language—Verbal memory.
[b]See also Oral language—Verbal processing speed and academics—Math–WJ III Math Fluency.
[c]See also Verbal Memory—CTOPP Nonword Repetition for another test of phonological awareness.

her teacher are all consistent in meeting the DSM-IV-TR symptom criteria for the inattentive type of ADHD. Converging evidence for this diagnosis is provided by the test results. On the Gordon Diagnostic System continuous performance test, Joan appeared to "space out" at times and missed more of the identified targets (omission errors) than 90% of children her age, suggesting great difficulty in sustaining a high level of focus. She also pressed the button when she should not have (commission errors) more than 84% of children her age. Because the Gordon is known to be somewhat insensitive in adolescents, Joan's difficulties on this subtest should be given considerable weight. In addition, Joan has obtained a low score on the Math Fluency subtest of the WJ III, although her scores on the other math subtests are consistent with expectations based on her cognitive abilities. The Math Fluency subtest is a timed test of basic math facts. Because the different math operations are intermixed (e.g., addition, subtraction, and multiplication), it requires sustained concentration as well as efficient retrieval of math facts. This subtest is often sensitive to the attention difficulties associated with ADHD and the verbal short-term memory weaknesses associated with dyslexia. Another piece of converging evidence for an ADHD diagnosis comes from Joan's WISC-IV Index scores. She shows a weakness on the Processing Speed Index, which is a cognitive risk factor for ADHD. Finally, Joan's score on the D-KEFS Verbal Fluency—Letter Fluency condition is in the low-average range. This test requires a considerable degree of organization in order to generate a large number of responses. In Joan's case, she named words with no phonological or semantic relation. Joan's poor performance on this test is inconsistent with her strong verbal conceptual skills and indicates difficulties with organization.

The other important behavioral observation during testing was that although Joan was an accurate reader, she was notably slow. Her test results suggest that she has mild dyslexia for which she has compensated to some degree. Individuals who receive early and effective interventions often become quite good at reading, although weaknesses in reading fluency, sounding out unknown words, spelling, and proofreading often remain. This profile is evident in Joan's testing results. Most notably, Joan's scores on timed tests of reading (TOWRE and GORT-4 Fluency) are much lower than her scores on untimed tests. Given's Joan's strong verbal conceptual skills, her consistently low-average to average scores on tests of spelling, phonology, verbal processing speed, and verbal short-term memory are consistent with the diagnosis of mild dyslexia.

Joan's difficulties with sustained attention, organization, and spelling make writing a very difficult task for her. On the WIAT Written Expression test, she was given 15 minutes to write about a topic, but she only used 5 minutes and was reluctant to add more. Her writing lacked a coherent organization and contained spelling errors.

Joan's diagnosis of ADHD, inattentive type, explains the referral concerns regarding sustained attention and organization. In the mass media, ADHD has come to be primarily associated with hyperactive behaviors, so parents of a child with more inattentive symptoms often do not feel that the diagnosis of ADHD applies to their child. In cases such as these, providing clarification and education about the subtypes of ADHD is often necessary. Joan also shows residual effects of dyslexia, which continue to affect her reading fluency and contribute to her difficulties in efficiently completing academic work.

Treatment

The treatment of ADHD has been reviewed elsewhere (DHHS, 1999); here, we summarize the main points of that review. The use of psychostimulant dopamine agonists, such as methylphenidate (Ritalin) and dextroamphetamine (Dexedrine) to treat ADHD is the most thoroughly researched application of psychopharmacology in child psychiatry. The efficacy and safety of these drugs in treating ADHD has now been well established. About 75–90% of children with ADHD show a favorable response to psychostimulant medication. More recently, a norepinephrine agonist, atomoxetine (strattera), has been shown to be an effective treatment for ADHD.

The side effects of psychostimulants are generally mild, especially compared to those of other psychopharmacological treatments, and usually abate with time and changes in dose. These side effects include decreased sleep and appetite, jitteriness, stomachaches, and headaches. Earlier concerns about growth retardation, precipitation of a tic disorder, psychostimulants as drugs of abuse, overdiagnosis of ADHD, or overprescription of psychostimulant drugs are not supported by research. There is nonetheless valid concern about the misdiagnosis of ADHD. Not all practitioners prescribing stimulant medication for ADHD have the time or the training to make this demanding differential diagnosis accurately.

Psychosocial treatments for ADHD mainly consist of behavioral intervention techniques for parents and teachers to help them better manage these children, who can be very disruptive in classrooms or families. Such treatments are particularly important for children who do not respond to medication or whose parents prefer not to use medication. In general, the efficacy of psychosocial treatments for improving ADHD symptoms is (1) less than that of psychostimulants (Pelham et al., 1998), and (2) greater for teachers than for parents.

The question naturally arises as to whether the combination of psychostimulant and behavioral interventions would be more efficacious than either alone. A large study funded by the National Institute of Mental Health addressed this question. This 3-year Multimodal Treatment of ADHD study

(MTA Group, 1998) compared four treatment conditions: medication alone, behavioral intervention alone, a combination of the two, and no treatment beyond what was already typically provided in the community. The behavioral intervention was intensive, involving parent training, school intervention, and summer treatment in a camp setting. The medication management was more intensive than what would typically be provided in a community setting. Subjects were randomly assigned to one of the four conditions, treated for 14 months, and followed for 22 months after that. There was a large main effect of medication treatment on ADHD symptoms, for which the addition of the behavioral intervention produced no added benefit. The behavioral intervention did improve outcome in some non-symptom-related areas.

Recently Klingberg et al. (2005) conducted a randomized, double-blind, placebo-controlled trial of computerized working memory training in children with ADHD. This training lasted more than 20 days and led to improvements in spatial and verbal working memory, response inhibition, complex reasoning, and parent ratings of ADHD symptoms. These improvements were still present 3 months after treatment ended. Hence this is a novel and promising treatment approach, but replication studies are needed.

There are also several unconventional therapies for ADHD, including the Feingold diet and EEG biofeedback, that have *not* been supported by careful treatment studies. These controversial therapies are discussed in more detail in Chapter 15.

In summary, psychostimulant treatment of ADHD is the gold standard. The criteria for establishing a particular treatment as empirically supported are reviewed in Chapter 14. According to these criteria, psychostimulant treatment qualifies as a Level I intervention. The empirical support for psychosocial treatments of ADHD is less strong, although these treatments may be helpful for cases in which a child does not respond to psychostimulants.

Table 9.4 summarizes clinical issues in ADHD.

TABLE 9.4. Clinical Summary Table: ADHD

Defining symptoms	• The critical symptoms described in DSM-IV-TR fall into two categories: inattention and hyperactivity–impulsivity. • Three subtypes of ADHD are defined, based on impairment in each of these two symptom dimensions: inattentive, hyperactive–impulsive, and combined.
Common comorbidities	• Over half of children who meet diagnostic criteria for ADHD qualify for a comorbid diagnosis. Common comorbidities include conduct disorder, depression, anxiety, Tourette syndrome, dyslexia, and bipolar disorder. • Children with ASD, schizophrenia, and ID often exhibit symptoms of ADHD, although DSM-IV-TR stipulates that these more serious primary diagnoses excludes an ADHD diagnosis.
Developmental history	• In infancy, symptoms may include a high activity level, less need for sleep, colic, frequent crying, and poor soothability. • In toddlerhood, characteristics include a low sense of danger, an unusual amount of energy, and a tendency to move from one activity to another very quickly. • During the early school years, children with ADHD are often referred because their behaviors are disruptive in the classroom. • In later school years, difficulties with organization may hinder school performance.
Diagnosis	• Diagnostic cutoffs on the inattentive and hyperactive–impulsive symptom dimensions require six of nine symptoms to be clinically significant in one or both dimensions. • Additional requirements for the diagnosis include that the symptoms (1) cause impairment; (2) are inconsistent with developmental level; (3) have been present for at least 6 months, with an onset before age 7; (4) are present in two or more settings; and (5) are not better accounted for by another mental disorder.
Prognosis	• ADHD is a chronic disorder across the lifespan. Many of the tasks of adult living require sustained effort, planning, and organization, which are areas of weakness for individuals with ADHD.
Treatment	• The use of psychostimulant drugs to treat ADHD is the most thoroughly researched application of psychopharmacology in child psychiatry. • About 75–90% of children with ADHD show a favorable response to psychostimulant medication. • Psychosocial treatments for ADHD mainly consist of behavioral intervention techniques for parents and teachers. In general, psychosocial treatments are less effective than psychostimulants for improving ADHD symptoms, although there are some promising new treatment approaches.

CHAPTER 10

Intellectual Disability

WITH LAUREN M. MCGRATH AND ROBIN L. PETERSON

HISTORY

Intellectual disability (ID), previously called mental retardation, has been recognized since antiquity, as witnessed by the distinction (expressed in pejorative terms) between those who had lost their reasoning ("lunatics") and those who had never developed it ("idiots"). However, in earlier times, those with ID were either neglected or placed in asylums. Efforts to train individuals with ID, to treat them humanely, and to understand their problems scientifically are much more recent and began with the Enlightenment in the 18th century, although much remains to be done to attain all three goals. Despite these efforts, stigma and abuse of those with ID (as well as those with other learning disorders) remain contemporary problems.

In France in 1799, Jean Itard found an abandoned boy with ID and possibly autism in a forest and attempted to train him, using instructional methods already in use with deaf persons (Achenbach, 1982). Itard's work with Victor, who became known as "the Wild Boy of Aveyron," is dramatized in François Truffaut's movie *L'Enfant Sauvage* (*The Wild Child*). Itard's efforts succeeded to some extent, showing that training could help those with ID—but Itard eventually abandoned Victor, who lived out his days in lonely custodial care. Edward Seguin (1812–1880) pursued more systematic efforts to train individuals with ID, both in France and in the United States (Achenbach, 1982). By the middle of the 19th century, several training schools for individuals with ID were established, and in 1876, the directors of these schools in the United States formed a society that later became the American Association on Mental Retardation (AAMR) (Hodapp & Dykens, 1996). The AAMR recently changed its name to the American Association on Intellectual and Developmental Disabilities (AAIDD). The AAIDD is the main professional organization in the field of ID; it publishes two journals and promotes research, intervention, and social policy efforts in this field.

Despite the good intentions of the founders of the present-day AAIDD, the training schools often devolved into custodial "warehouses." In addition, widespread acceptance of the "science" of eugenics at the end of the 19th century led to much more hostile attitudes toward those with ID. Eugenics conceived of familial ID as a threat to the gene pool; such a threat was dramatized by supposedly scientific accounts of extended families with limited intellectual functioning, such as *The Jukes* (Dugdale, 1877) and *The Kallikak Family* (Goddard, 1912). These concerns led to the reprehensible practice of enforced sterilization of those with ID. Since very little was actually known about the etiology of ID at the time, such a practice was not only ethically but also scientifically questionable.

The contemporary view of the treatment of ID is partly a humane reaction against this history of past abuses, and emphasizes the rights of those with ID. An important emphasis is on the concepts of "normalization" and "inclusion" or "mainstreaming." The basic idea behind these concepts is that, given appropriate accommodations, those with ID can and should be integrated as much as possible into normal life—in families, schools, and communities. We will return to the topic of treatment later in this chapter.

Scientific understanding of some of the causes of ID is actually quite recent; such causes include genetic syndromes, early neurological insults, polygenic inheritance, and environmental deprivation. Although Down's (1866) description of the syndrome that bears his name is over 140 years old, the genetic basis of Down syndrome (DS) was only discovered about 50 years ago (Lejeune, Gauthier, & Turpin, 1959). Our understanding of the molecular basis of FXS (discussed in connection with ASD in Chapter 8), another common genetic cause of ID, is much more recent still. The number of known genetic causes of ID is now more than 100 (Plomin et al., 1997), with more yet to be discovered. Other known genetic causes of ID include phenylketonuria, Lesch–Nyhan syndrome, neurofibromatosis, tuberous sclerosis, and Prader–Willi/Angelman syndrome, to name a few.

This chapter reviews general issues pertaining to ID and focuses on three genetic ID syndromes—DS, FXS, and Williams syndrome (WS)—that exemplify the progress made to date toward a neuroscientific understanding of ID. As we will see, each of these syndromes has a distinctive cognitive *and* social phenotype. The contrasting social phenotypes in these three disorders involve personality dimensions, such as gregariousness, empathy, and social anxiety, that are highly relevant for understanding other disorders. By tracing the complex developmental pathways that run from genetic alterations through brain development to these distinctive cognitive and social pheno-types, we are very likely to learn about the brain mechanisms underlying typical cognitive and social development, including brain mechanisms they share. In addition, ID syndromes present in a more extreme form dissociations that are also found in other disorders, and we discuss in more detail later, they provide a very important universality test for developmental theory.

DEFINITION

The definition of ID provides a good example of the issues involved in dimensional versus categorical conceptions of disorders, as well as the issues involved in etiological versus behavioral definitions. Part of what we call ID (especially mild ID) lies on a continuum—in this case, a continuum of intelligence and adaptive functioning, the two constructs used in definitions of ID. The IQ and adaptive behavior cutoffs for ID, as well as those for subtypes of ID, are inevitably somewhat arbitrary and have changed over the years. So ID defined in this way is not a syndrome, just as most of the learning disorders discussed in the earlier chapters are not syndromes (with the possible exception of ASD). On the other hand, there is clear bimodality in the lower tail of the IQ distribution, and many cases of moderate or more severe ID are part of a distinct distribution with distinct etiologies, as is discussed later. So there are many more known ID syndromes than is true for any other learning disorder described in this book. What makes them syndromes is that each has a distinct etiology that produces a distinctive physical and behavioral phenotype.

At first glance, it might appear that we should prefer etiological definitions of ID whenever they are available. But since those who share an etiology (such as trisomy 21, the cause of DS) nonetheless vary in their levels of cognitive and adaptive functioning, it is not at all clear that etiological definitions should replace behavioral ones, especially for most treatment purposes. Obviously, an individual with DS and mild ID needs different services from those needed by another individual with DS and moderate or severe ID. For any disorder, there is no doubt that etiological definitions will help focus medical interventions—but, short of a medical cure, we will also need behavioral definitions to guide treatments.

Most current definitions of ID (such as the one found in DSM-IV-TR) require three things: an IQ deficit, an adaptive behavior deficit, and onset before age 18 years. More specifically, the IQ must be at least 2 SDs below the mean on an individually administered IQ test (e.g., an IQ of 70 or lower on a Wechsler test). Earlier definitions had a higher IQ cutoff (1 SD below the mean), and did not require an adaptive behavior deficit. As a result, about 16% of the population met criteria for ID. Since many such individuals did not have significant social and occupational problems as adults, the validity of this diagnostic definition was questionable. The lower IQ cutoff of 2 SDs below the mean only identifies about 2% of the general population. Individuals with IQs that low are much more likely to have problems meeting the demands of everyday life, but even with a lower IQ cutoff, there will inevitably be some false positive diagnoses. This possibility is especially troublesome in ethnic and socioeconomic groups whose average IQ is below the population mean of 100, probably because of poorer health care, diets, and reduced educational opportunities.

To illustrate this problem, let us consider a hypothetical ethnic group with a mean IQ of 85, a normal distribution of IQ, and a SD similar in magnitude to that found in the general population (i.e., 15). In this particular case, about 16% of the subpopulation would fall below an IQ cutoff of 70, again raising questions about the validity of the definition. To eliminate the false-positive problem in some ethnic and socioeconomic groups, the adaptive behavior deficit criterion was added to the definition of ID in the 1970s. The combination of the two criteria—an IQ 2 SDs below the mean and equally extreme adaptive behavior deficit—is much more likely to identify individuals who are having significant problems in everyday life because of low intelligence.

The AAMR's controversial 1992 definition of ID essentially raised the IQ cutoff to 75. By changing the cutoff by just 0.33 SD, this definition *doubled* the number of those potentially eligible for the diagnosis. This change in cutoff has been controversial, and more recent definitions, such as that of DSM-IV-TR, have retained the lower cutoff (minus 2 SDs, or an IQ of 70).

In sum, the shifting IQ cutoffs in definitions of ID illustrate that imposing a cutoff on a continuum is somewhat arbitrary. Any cutoff will have a mix of costs and benefits in terms of research, external validity, clinical benefits to individuals, and social costs. Moreover, these different uses of the diagnosis will be unlikely to agree on the best cutoff. One can imagine that as the global economy increasingly demands technological sophistication from workers, arguments for raising the IQ cutoff for ID could become more common again.

Of the three diagnostic criteria for ID, the one that is least well defined is the adaptive behavior deficit. DSM-IV-TR requires that there must be a significant deficit in at least 2 (of 11) areas of adaptive functioning, such as self-care, communication, social skills, and occupational skills. Definitions of ID vary in how many areas of adaptive functioning they consider, and there is some controversy about which areas should count and how they should be measured. For instance, should a deficit in "leisure" (many academics and other professionals unfortunately have leisure impairments!)

count the same as a deficit in self-care? Some definitions distinguish as many as 10 or 11 areas of adaptive functioning, but factor-analytic studies of adaptive behavior inventories find a smaller number of underlying factors, with a single general factor accounting for most of the variance (reviewed in Hodapp & Dykens, 1996).

To illustrate some of these points, let us consider a commonly used measure of adaptive functioning, the Vineland Adaptive Behavior Scales (Sparrow, Balla, & Cicchetti, 1984; Sparrow, Cicchetti, & Balla, 2005). Both the original Vineland and its recent revision, the Vineland-II, have excellent psychometric characteristics in terms of reliability, construct validity, and discriminant validity. Each version clearly measures something besides IQ, because in normal children the correlation with IQ measures is about .30. The Vineland has three main scales, Communication, Daily Living Skills, and Socialization, whose internal validity is generally supported by factor analysis. Nonetheless, principal-components analyses of domain standard scores across eight age groups in the standardization sample for the original Vineland all found substantial general factors, which accounted for between 55% and 70% of the total variance. The Vineland is very likely psychometrically to be superior to clinical impressions of multiple domains of adaptive functioning recommended by the DSM-IV-TR. Moreover, these methods of assessing adaptive functioning may lead to conflicting and counterintuitive results with regard to whether a given child with an IQ under 70 has ID. A child may have a significant deficit on the Vineland Adaptive Behavior Composite, which best measures the general factor, but may not meet the DSM-IV-TR diagnostic criterion because only one of the three Vineland scale scores is below the cutoff. A second child, who if assessed on the Vineland may not be impaired on either the Adaptive Behavior Composite or any one of the three scales, may meet this criterion for an adaptive behavior deficit based on a clinical interview covering 11 areas of adaptive functioning. Obviously the first child will have a more significant overall adaptive behavior deficit than the second child, but only the second child will receive the diagnosis of ID.

In sum, diagnostic decisions about ID will vary as a function of which measure of adaptive behavior is used. This diagnostic uncertainty will be greater for individuals with milder deficits in IQ and adaptive behavior (i.e., those with IQs close to 70). Despite this uncertainty, the reliability of the diagnosis of ID is higher than that of many disorders because it requires the convergence of two separate behavioral criteria, IQ and adaptive behavior, each of which can be highly reliable.

The other continuum versus category issue in the definition of ID concerns severity subtypes of ID. These subtypes are clinically important, because they help predict both service needs and prognosis, but they are also somewhat arbitrary divisions of a continuum. Four subtypes are recognized in the DSM-IV-TR and ICD-10 taxonomies. These are defined by IQ ranges: "mild" (IQ = 50–55 to 70), "moderate" (IQ = 35–40 to 50–55), "severe" (IQ = 20–25 to 35–40), and "profound" (IQ < 20–25). In contrast, the 1992 AAMR definition eliminated these subtypes and replaced them with four levels of services required by an individual with ID: "intermittent," "limited," "extensive," and "pervasive." This change was motivated by the understanding that the kinds of services needed represent an interaction between the characteristics of an individual and his or her particular social context. This aspect of the 1992 AAMR definition has also been controversial, partly because the measurement of service needs is less precise and objective than the measurement of IQ. For instance, levels of funding available to service providers (such as schools, health maintenance organizations, and the Social Security Administration) could easily bias assessments of what services are needed.

EPIDEMIOLOGY

As the foregoing discussion makes clear, the prevalence of ID obviously depends on which cutoffs are used. Using the definition above (an IQ 2 SDs below the mean, an adaptive behavior deficit, and onset before age 18), the prevalence is between 1% and 3% (Hodapp & Dykens, 1996), with the majority having mild ID. The prevalence of the other three subtypes (moderate, severe, and profound) combined is 0.4%, or 4 per 1,000 (Hodapp & Dykens, 1996). Thus, depending on which overall prevalence estimate is used, between 60% and 87% of the total population with ID have mild ID.

ID is more common in males than in females; the male–femle ratio is about 1.5:1 (American Psychiatric Association, 2000). This male predominance is partly due to the large number of X-linked ID syndromes—the most common of which is FXS, which is discussed in more detail below. Because males have only one X chromosome, whereas females have two, they will manifest the phenotype caused by an abnormal gene on their X chromosome, whereas the phenotype in females with the same abnormal gene will be milder (or absent) because they have a normal copy of that gene on their second X chromosome. Comorbidity with other psychiatric diagnoses is a common aspect of ID; hence many individuals with ID have "dual diagnoses," and it is important that they receive appropriate treatment of both their ID and their comorbid disorder. Symptoms of ADHD are very common across most forms of ID.

Known genetic syndromes, such as DS or FXS, account for many cases of moderate or more severe ID. We now discuss the epidemiology of three of the best-known genetic ID syndromes, DS, FXS, and WS. Each represents a different type of genetic mechanism.

Down Syndrome

The most prevalent form of ID with a known genetic etiology is DS, which is found in 1 to 1.5 per thousand live births (Hodapp & Dykeus, 1996) and affects males and females equally. Although DS is genetic, most cases are not familial, as will be discussed later. Therefore, DS is not the most common *familial* form of ID with a known genetic etiology. Instead, FXS fits that description.

Fragile X Syndrome

Although FXS is familial, its transmission is not simply Mendelian, as will be discussed later. The prevalence of FXS varies somewhat across countries, probably because of founder effects; overall, it is found in about 1 in 4,000 males and about half as many females, so the population prevalence is about 0.019% (Sherman, 1996).

Williams Syndrome

Finally, WS is caused by a usually spontaneous, contiguous microdeletion of genes on chromosome 7. It affects both genders equally and occurs in about 1 in 25,000 births (.004%). About a quarter of individuals with Williams syndrome have moderate or worse ID.

Since the majority of individuals with DS and males with FXS have moderate or worse ID, together these two disorders come close to accounting for half of the total (0.4% of the population) of individuals with moderate or worse ID. WS accounts for less than 1% (0.25%) of this total. Although all three of these syndromes are genetic, only one (FXS) is familial, and the complexities of its transmission reduce familial risk. In addition, although males with FXS are technically fertile, they rarely reproduce because of their cognitive and behavioral problems. If most of the remaining causes of moderate or worse ID are likewise nonfamilial, we should expect little risk for cognitive delay in the relatives of probands with moderate or worse ID, contrary to what proponents of eugenics assumed a century ago.

ETIOLOGY[1]

Both genes and environment contribute to the etiology of ID. For instance, one of the most frequent environmental causes is fetal alcohol syndrome. In

[1] For a description of genetic technical terms, see Box 1.1 in Chapter 1.

this section, we first consider evidence that supports a difference in the etiology of mild versus moderate or worse ID, and then consider the etiology of the three ID syndromes discussed above (DS, FXS, and WS).

Mild versus Moderate or Worse ID

Both direct and indirect evidence supports the conclusion that the etiology of moderate or worse ID is substantially distinct from the etiology of mild ID. We have already seen that some of these etiologies of moderate or worse ID are nonfamilial (e.g., DS). Other nonfamilial organic etiologies, such as teratogens, perinatal complications, and postnatal neurological insults (e.g., meningitis and head injuries), are also much more common in moderate and worse ID (Hodapp & Dykens, 1996).

Moreover, as mentioned earlier, the lower tail of the IQ distribution is bimodal (Dingman & Tarjan, 1960), which also suggests distinct etiologies of ID for individuals in the second smaller distribution. Therefore, we should predict that siblings drawn from probands in this second smaller distribution should not be at risk for ID. Consistent with this prediction, the siblings of probands with moderate and worse ID have a mean IQ of 103 (Nichols, 1984). That is, they have regressed all the way back to the population mean, indicating that the etiology of the probands' extreme low IQ scores is nonfamilial; it cannot be due to either genes or environments shared by family members.

In contrast, mild ID is part of the lower tail of the IQ distribution and is clearly familial. In a classic family study of ID (Reed & Reed, 1965), 289 probands with mild ID and their relatives were examined. If mild ID is familial, the mean IQ of siblings of probands with mild ID should not regress all the way back to the population mean, unlike the case in moderate or worse ID. In the Reed and Reed (1965) study, the mean sibling IQ was about 1 SD below the population mean (i.e., about 85), thus supporting familiality. A second test of familiality involves transmission from parents to offspring. Reed and Reed (1965) found that if one parent had mild ID, the risk for ID in the children was 20%, whereas if both parents had mild ID, the offspring risk rose to 50%, again supporting familiality.

The distributional and etiological differences between mild and more severe ID have led to a distinction between "organic" and "cultural–familial" ID, which is called the "two-group" approach (Hodapp & Dykens, 1996). The implicit dualism involved in labeling some disorders "organic" and others not is discussed elsewhere (Pennington, 2002). In the current context, another problem with this distinction is that it might lead one to assume that the familial influences on mild ID are all environmental. Although we do not have a twin or adoption study of probands with mild ID per se, we

do know that the overall heritability of IQ is about 50%, and that twin studies of individuals with below-average IQs find a similar value (Plomin et al.,
1997). In a study of over 3,000 infant twin pairs, Eley et al. (1999) found
that the heritability of IQ in the lowest 5% was similar to that in the rest
of the sample. So the most parsimonious hypothesis is that IQ is similarly
heritable for those with mild ID and those with IQs over 70, which would
mean that mild ID is about 50% heritable. (As discussed earlier, moderate
ID and severe ID are less heritable.) Researchers using molecular methods
have recently begun to identify QTLs and candidate genes underlying the
heritability of IQ (see review in Posthuma & de Geus, 2006).

   However, it is also possible that environmental influences could be
stronger at the low end of the IQ distribution because children of parents
with low IQs would be exposed to a greater range of environmental adversities, including poorer health care, nutrition, and schools. These possibilities become even more salient when we consider minority groups who are
at greater risk for such adversities. Indeed, two twin studies have found
lower heritability of IQ in children of parents with lower education (Rowe,
Jacobson, & Van den Oord, 1999; Turkheimer, Haley, Waldron, D'Onofrio,
& Gottesman, 2003). These results demonstrate a G × E interaction in the
etiology of IQ. This kind of interaction, in which heritability is lower in
a higher-stress environment, is referred to as a "bioecological" interaction
(Bronfenbrenner & Ceci, 1994). The bioecological form of interaction contrasts with the more commonly encountered diathesis–stress G × E interaction, in which heritability is higher in high-stress environments. We next
consider the specific genetic mechanisms that operate in DS, FXS, and WS.

Down Syndrome

As discussed earlier, most (about 94%) cases of DS are not familial. Instead,
a parent with a normal chromosome number produces an offspring with an
extra copy of chromosome 21 (trisomy 21) through a process called "nondisjunction," which is failure of one of the paired chromosomes to separate
in meiosis. Nondisjunction is more likely in mothers (especially older ones)
than in fathers, because all of a mother's eggs are present in an immature
form before her birth, whereas new sperm are continually being produced
by fathers across their reproductive lifespan. In women of childbearing age,
each month one of these immature eggs goes through the final, reductive
division in meiosis, and becomes available for fertilization. Hence the older
the mother, the older the egg, and the older the egg, the greater risk for
nondisjunction, for reasons that are not completely understood. So, the risk
for DS is only 1 in 2,400 in mothers 15–19 years old, but rises to 1 in 40 in
mothers who are 45–49 years old.

Nondisjunction itself does appear to be familial. For instance, if a woman has already had one child with DS, her risk for a second child with DS is tripled (Rosenberg, 1986). The small remainder of cases of DS are caused by either translocation of an extra piece of the long arm of 21 to another chromosome or mosaicism, in which trisomy 21 occurs in some but not all cells. Both translocation and mosaic DS can be familial. A parent can be an apparently unaffected carrier, either because that parent has a benign translocation or because most of his or her mosaic cells are normal. These protective factors are not necessarily transmitted to the offspring.

Incidentally, nondisjunction is quite common across all the chromosomes, but most trisomies or monosomies are not viable, and lead to early, spontaneous abortions. More than half of all conceptions end early, and the majority of those are affected by nondisjunction. Thus viable "aneuploidies" (individuals with an abnormal chromosome number) can only involve a small number of extra or missing genes. This is the case if the aneuploid chromosome is small. Chromosome 21 actually has the fewest genes of any autosomal chromosome. The Y chromosome contributes to viable aneuploidies (e.g., 47,XYY); it has the fewest genes of any chromosome. The one exception is the X chromosome, which is large and gene-rich, but contributes to viable aneuploidies. However, all but one copy of the X chromosome is largely inactivated early in development (X inactivation is also called "Lyonization" in honor of Mary Lyon, who discovered it). Nonetheless, there is some cost to having the wrong number of inactive X chromosomes, since females without an inactive X (45,X) have Turner syndrome, and individuals with extra inactivated X's (such as 47,XXY males or 47,XXX females) have developmental disabilities.

So the genetic etiology of DS is due to an extra dose of the products of normal genes. Understanding this genetic etiology at the molecular level is a difficult task, because it requires that we (1) have identified all the genes on chromosome 21; (2) know which of these are overexpressed (other genes or epigenetic interactions may well produce dosage compensation for some of the genes on chromosome 21); and (3) know which of the overexpressed genes are expressed early enough in development to cause a congenital disorder. To understand the etiology of the neurobehavioral phenotype in DS, we need to add a fourth constraint—namely, that the gene is expressed in the brain, or at least affects brain development.

Earlier work with partial trisomies had established that only part of chromosome 21, on the long arm, is involved in the etiology of DS. But there are still many genes in that region. The physical map of chromosome 21 has been completed (Hattori et al., 2000), and it appears that the number of genes is only about 225, which is fewer than the size of the chromosome would predict (smaller chromosome 22 has about twice as many genes). A majority of these genes are in the DS region on 21q.

Work is now underway to determine which genes in this subset meet the other criteria listed above to qualify as correlates for the etiology of the neurobehavioral phenotype found in DS. Mouse models with trisomies of either single candidate genes or segments of the DS region have been constructed and are being tested for their neurological and neurobehavioral phenotypes; for a review, see Crnic and Pennington (2000). This review discusses some of the promising candidate genes that have already been identified. These candidates include the amyloid precursor protein gene (APP), which is also implicated in Alzheimer disease; a glutamate receptor subunit gene (CRIK1); the human minibrain homologue (MNB); and neuronal intracellular adhesion molecule (DSCAM).

In summary, DS has the most complicated genetic etiology of the three syndromes considered here, because it involves many more genes. Indeed, it is always possible that trisomy induces developmental instability in a general way, and that we will not be able to track specific phenotypic features of DS back to extra doses of specific genes (Reeves, Baxter, & Richtsmeier, 2001). Nonetheless, recent advances in mapping the human genome and constructing mouse models have accelerated progress toward understanding the genetic basis of the neurobehavioral phenotype in DS.

Fragile X Syndrome

FXS is a single-gene disorder in which the fragile X mental retardation 1 (FMR1) gene becomes inactivated (methylated), because it contains a large number (>200) of trinucleotide (i.e., cytosine–guanine–guanine [CGG]) repeats (Verkerk et al., 1991). Normal individuals have a small number (< 50) of repeats, but sometimes the number of repeats increases when gametes are produced, so that an FMR1 gene with a larger number (50–200) of repeats is transmitted to the offspring. A gene with this many repeats is called a "premutation," because it functions normally but increases the risk of an even larger number of repeats in the next (third) generation. If that number exceeds 200, the grandchild is considered to have the FXS mutation, because the FMR1 gene is very likely to be inactivated and will not produce the protein it codes for (FMR protein, or FMRP). The absence of this gene product in development is what causes FXS. A male grandchild with this mutation is very likely to have the full syndrome, including ID, because males only have one X chromosome. On the other hand, a female grandchild with this mutation on one of her X chromosomes will nevertheless have a normal FMR1 gene on her second X chromosome, so she can still produce some FMRP. How much FMRP she can produce partly depends on what proportion of her cells have this second X chromosome active, since the normal process of X inactivation leaves only one X chromosome active in each cell, as discussed earlier. This proportion is called the "X activation ratio," and it predicts the degree of phenotypic involvement in females with the fragile X mutation. So, because the FMR1 gene is on the X chromosome, FXS acts like a more typical X-linked disorder, and produces an excess of affected males with this syndrome. But unlike a typical Mendelian X-linked disorder (e.g., hemophilia), FXS also exhibits what is called "anticipation," which means that the severity increases and the age of onset decreases across generations. In contrast, in a Mendelian disorder, the phenotype stays the same across generations. Anticipation in FXS is explained by the expansion of repetitive sequences across generations; a similar phenomenon is found in Huntington disease, which also exhibits anticipation.

The degree of expansion across generations, and hence the degree of anticipation in both FXS and Huntington disease, depends on the gender of the transmitting parent, which is the second non-Mendelian aspect of these two disorders. In FXS, expansion is greater in a transmitting mother, whereas in Huntington disease, expansion is greater in a transmitting father. These are examples of a phenomenon called "imprinting." Imprinting is non-Mendelian, because it was classically assumed that gene expression did not vary as a function of which parent the gene came from.

In summary, the genetic transmission of FXS is complicated. In extended families with FXS, there will be (1) more cases in more recent generations (anticipation); (2) more males with FXS than females (X linkage); (3) more children with FXS born to mothers than to fathers with a premutation (imprinting); and (4) a wider range of phenotypic severity in females than in males with the mutation (partly because of variation in the X activation ratio in females). But understanding FXS at the gene level is a much simpler task than is the case for either DS or WS, because only a single gene (FMR1) is involved.

The role of FMR1 in brain development is now being elucidated (Garber, Smith, Reines, & Warren, 2006; Witt et al., 1995). The protein product of FMR1, FMRP, is an RNA-binding protein that is involved in the regulation of protein synthesis. In the brain, FMRP plays a role in synaptogenesis, dendritic spine maturation, and dendritic pruning (Galvez, Smith, & Greenough, 2005; Garber et al., 2006; Jacquemont, Hagerman, Hagerman, & Leehey, 2007), although the specific mechanisms remain to be elucidated (Veneri, Zalfa, & Bagni, 2004). The roles of FMRP in brain development are consistent with the observed brain and behavioral phenotype in FXS. For example, dendritic pruning is an important mechanism in brain development, which improves the efficiency of neural networks by eliminating excess synapses. A reduction in dendritic pruning would therefore help explain both an important aspect of the neurological phenotype (macrocephaly—abnormally large head circumference), as well as the ID in FXS.

Williams Syndrome

As mentioned earlier, WS is caused by a usually sporadic, contiguous dele-tion of genes on chromosome 7p11.23. This deletion is 1.5 megabases in length, is hemizygous (i.e., occurs only on one of the two copies of chromo-some 7), and involves at least 16 genes, 2 of which have been characterized (Mervis & Klein-Tasman, 2000). Recent molecular work has clarified what some of those genes are and how they influence the physical and cognitive phenotype. The physical phenotype includes characteristic facial features, cardiac abnormalities (particularly supravalvular aortic stenosis, or SVAS), and connective tissue features (see Mervis et al., 2000). Since there is an autosomal dominant form of SVAS, with some family members exhibiting other physical features of WS, researchers pursued the question of whether there might be a shared genetic etiology for WS and SVAS. Linkage studies of kindreds with familial SVAS eventually identified mutations in the elastin gene (ELN) on chromosome 7q as the cause of this familial disorder (Ewart, Jin, Atkinson, Morris, & Keating, 1994; Ewart et al., 1993a). Some of these families had microdeletions of portions of the ELN gene, raising the pos-sibility that an even larger deletion on 7q was the cause of WS. This hypoth-esis was confirmed by Ewart et al. (1993b) and in subsequent studies. ELN produces elastin protein, which is important in the heart and connective tis-sues; hence deletion of ELN could explain much of the physical phenotype in WS (Mervis et al., 2000).

But since ELN is minimally expressed in the brain, other genes must be involved in the cognitive and behavioral phenotype of WS. Subsequent studies identified a second gene in the WS deletion region on 7q11.23, LIM-kinase 1 (LIMK1), which was found to influence the deficit in spatial cog-nition found in WS (Frangiskakis et al., 1996). This deficit is not found in most individuals with familial SVAS.

In sum, research on the etiology of WS provides an example of a third genetic mechanism in the etiology of ID, microdeletions. As in DS, the genes involved are normal genes, but with abnormal expression. Whereas DS involves overexpression of some genes, WS involves underexpression. Theo-retically, 50% of the gene product is available in development because one of the two normal genes is missing. Work is currently proceeding to identify the remaining genes in WS deletion region and to trace their phenotypic effects. Because the size of the microdeletion in the WS region on 7q varies across individuals, it will be possible to evaluate how these new genes relate to different aspects of the WS phenotype.

There has been rapid progress in identifying genes involved in each of these three ID syndromes and relating them to aspects of the phenotype in each. This progress illustrates well the potential power of collaborations between molecular geneticists and cognitive neuroscientists for understanding the other disorders considered in this book.

BRAIN MECHANISMS[2]

In this section, the focus is on what is known about brain mechanisms in DS, FXS, and WS.

Down Syndrome

Nadel (1999) has reviewed what is known about brain development in DS. Broadly speaking, development appears normal at birth and is invariably abnormal by adulthood, since virtually all adults with DS have developed some of the neuropathological features of Alzheimer disease by about age 35. In addition, by adulthood, the brain is clearly microcephalic; differentially greater volume reduction occurs in the hippocampus, prefrontal cortex, and cerebellum (Kesslak, Nagata, Lott, & Nalcioglu, 1994; Logdberg & Brun, 1993; Raz et al., 1995; Weiss, 1991). Much less is known from the existing data about when these aspects of abnormal brain development first appear in individuals with DS.

A wide range of studies has found no differences at birth between brains of normal persons and brains of individuals with DS (e.g., Schmidt-Sidor, Wisniewski, Shepard, & Serson, 1990). Differences that appear in the first few months of life include delayed myelination, reduced growth of the frontal lobes, a narrowing of the superior temporal gyrus, diminished size of the brainstem and cerebellum, and a major reduction (20–50%) in the number of cortical granular neurons (Nadel, 1999). However, these differences in brain development are not invariant across all cases. So several features of the adult brain phenotype begin to emerge in the first years of life, including microcephaly (abnormally small head circumference) and reduced volumes of the cerebellum and frontal lobes. However, evidence for hippocampal volume reduction in the first years of life has not been reported.

Less is known about brain development in children and adolescents with DS. One structural MRI study of adolescents (Jernigan, Bellugi, Sowell, Doherty, & Hesselink, 1993) found a pattern of results similar to that found in adults–that is, microcephaly and relatively smaller volumes of frontal cortex, hippocampus, and cerebellum. These investigators compared a small sample ($n = 6$) with DS to both normal chronological-age-matched controls ($n = 21$) and adolescents with WS ($n = 9$). Both of the groups with ID had overall microcephaly, but only the group with DS had cerebellar volume

---

[2]For a description of neuroanatomical technical terms, see Box 1.2 in Chapter 1.

reduction relative to age controls. In the group with WS, despite microcephaly, the cerebellar volume was similar to that of age-matched controls. There were also contrasts between the groups with DS and WS in the proportions of grey matter for several other structures. The group with DS had a smaller proportion of anterior cortex and temporal limbic cortex, including the hippocampus, than either the group with WS or the chronological-age-matched control group had. In contrast, the posterior cortex, the lenticular nucleus, and the diencephalons were all proportionally larger in the group with DS than in the other two groups.

In summary, the adult brain phenotype in DS is characterized by both general (microcephaly) and specific (frontal lobes, hippocampus, and cerebellum) volume reductions, some of which may emerge earlier in development than others.

Fragile X Syndrome

Neuroanatomical abnormalities in FXS have included a decreased size of the posterior cerebellar vermis (Reiss, Aylward, Freund, Joshi, & Bryan, 1991), which may be related to abnormalities in sensory–motor integration, activity level, and social interactions. Mild ventricular enlargements have been demonstrated, which would be consistent with mild frontal or parietal atrophy, or hypersecretion of cerebrospinal fluid (Wisniewski, Segan, Miczejeski, Sersen, & Rudelli, 1991). Finally, there appears to be *enlargement* of some brain structures in FXS, since head circumferences are large. These findings are in contrast to the microcephaly found in DS and many other ID syndromes, and suggest a failure of neuronal pruning mechanisms in early brain development. As we have noted in Chapter 8, there is also evidence for macrocephaly in autism.

In summary, we do not yet know how the FMR1 mutation causes brain changes, or which brain changes cause the ID associated with FXS. However, the fact that this is a single-gene disorder in which the gene has been identified makes the elucidation of this causal pathway much easier than it will be for DS.

Williams Syndrome

In WS, structural studies have found a neurological phenotype that contrasts sharply with the one found in DS (Bellugi, Mills, Jernigan, Hickok, & Galaburda, 1999). Although there is microcephaly in both WS and DS, not all structures are equally reduced in size; nor are the same structures reduced in each syndrome. There is relative sparing of frontal, limbic, and cerebellar volumes in WS, whereas these volumes are reduced in DS (Bellugi et al., 1999). The affected limbic structures include the hippocampus, providing further evidence for a hippocampal deficit in DS. In contrast, there is sparing of the lenticular nuclei (part of the basal ganglia) in DS but not in WS. Posterior temporal cortex, including primary auditory cortex (Heschl's gyrus), is of normal size in WS, in contrast to DS (Bellugi et al., 1999). This difference could help explain both the hyperacusis (lower hearing thresholds) and the relatively preserved language development in WS. The neuroanatomical contrasts across these three ID syndromes are beginning to help us understand their contrasting neuropsychological phenotypes, which are discussed next.

NEUROPSYCHOLOGY

The neuropsychology of ID has been discussed in two earlier reviews (Pennington & Bennetto, 1998; Crnic & Pennington, 2000). The following discussion is based on those reviews. We know less about the neuropsychology of ID than we know about the neuropsychology of other learning disorders in this book, such as dyslexia and autism. Neuropsychologists have focused more on specific than on general developmental disorders. Nonetheless, the study of ID is relevant for fundamental issues concerning the nature of cognitive development (see Anderson, 2001). There are two fundamental facts about human cognitive development: (1) There are wide differences in diverse cognitive abilities both across age and between individuals at a given age; and (2) because differences are moderately correlated across wide content domains, there must be some general cognitive factors that partly explain individual and developmental differences in intelligence. The study of ID can help answer the following questions:

1. What are these general cognitive factors?
2. How do general cognitive factors underlying individual differences relate to those underlying developmental differences?
3. How do both relate to brain development?
4. How, despite these general influences, are there also differences in *specific* aspects of cognitive development?
5. How do these specific differences relate to brain development?
6. How universal are the hypothesized sequences of brain and behavioral development?

Some recent efforts to use a neuropsychological approach to study various ID syndromes have been much more concerned with which specific functions are relatively impaired or spared than with why there is an impairment in general intelligence. This approach tends to assume that the cognitive architecture consists of a set of relatively independent and isolable modules, and that the only difference between ID and other examples of brain damage or dysfunction is that more modules are dysfunctional in ID. In this view, we would study ID in much the same way we study more specific learning disorders, such as developmental dyslexia—by looking for the profile of specific strengths and weaknesses that characterizes a particular ID syndrome. However, as discussed earlier in the book, this approach to understanding developmental disorders has significant limitations (Oliver et al., 2000). Let us now place the six questions above in a historical context, and then consider what we have learned about them from the study of specific ID syndromes.

It is useful to view current work on the neuropsychology of ID in the context of issues that have been important in the history of psychological approaches to understanding ID (Hodapp, Burack, & Zigler, 1998). One key debate has been between those who espouse a developmental approach (Zigler, 1969) and those who espouse a specific-deficit approach, whether that deficit is thought to be in verbal mediation (Luria, 1961), stimulus traces (Ellis, 1963), attention (Zeaman & House, 1963), executive processes (Belmont & Butterfield, 1971), or some other cognitive process. The latter approach has attempted to account for all of ID, regardless of etiology, in terms of a single cognitive deficit. In contrast, the developmental approach has divided ID into organic and nonorganic types, and argued that for the nonorganic or cultural–familial type, there is a general slowing of development across all domains. Consequently, both the sequence of developmental acquisitions ("similar-sequence hypothesis") and the profile across domains ("similar-structure hypothesis") should be similar to what is found in typically developing children at the same mental age level. So the debate has centered on the relevance of specific versus general cognitive processes for understanding ID, as well as the relevance of etiology and, of course, development. These two positions have highlighted significant aspects of ID that any comprehensive neuroscientific account will have to explain, but each has committed significant errors.

In terms of aspects to explain, we have the fact that individuals with ID do develop; that they follow a typical sequence of developmental acquisitions much more often than not; and that performance on most, but not all, tasks is well predicted by mental age. In fact, development is even more robust in ID than some adherents of the developmental position expected, since these generalizations also apply to "organic" ID syndromes with known genetic causes, such as DS or FXS. So the hypotheses of similar sequence and structure have largely been supported. Both point to the potential importance of general cognitive processes in understanding ID, although a modularity theorist could conceivably argue that similarity in sequence and structure derives from independent modules, each slowed in its development to a similar extent. An important goal for the neuropsychological approach is to identify parameters of brain development that, when altered, would affect general cognitive processes and lead to this general slowing of development. Possible candidates include numbers of neurons, synaptic connections (either too few or too many), or neurotransmitter systems.

However, the specific-deficit approach is partly correct as well. There is now accumulating evidence of some degree of specificity in both developmental sequence and cognitive profile across ID syndromes. For instance, language development in WS contradicts an assumed universal sequence in two respects: Pointing does not precede referential labeling, and exhaustive sorting of objects does not co-occur with the vocabulary spurt (Mervis & Bertrand, 1997). In terms of profile, verbal short-term memory is above mental age level in WS and below it in DS, whereas the reverse is the case for visual–spatial skills (Klein & Mervis, 1999; Mervis, 1999; Wang & Bellugi, 1994). At the same time, this double dissociation across the two syndromes does not indicate independence of the two cognitive domains in ID, since there are moderate partial correlations (when age is controlled for) among these and other cognitive measures in WS (Mervis, 1999). In fact, greater correlations among various domains of cognition may be a general characteristic of ID (Detterman & Daniel, 1989). Moreover, development in the weak area can follow a typical developmental sequence (even though below mental age level), as has been shown in studies of the development of drawing skills in WS (Bertrand & Mervis, 1996; Bertrand, Mervis, & Eisenberg, 1997).

In summary, general developmental processes are robust in ID, even in so-called "organic" syndromes, but there is evidence of specificity as well. Both the general slowing of development and the different specific deficits that characterize different syndromes require a neuroscientific explanation. At the cognitive level, explanations have attempted to identify some fundamental process or processes that explain the general aspect of both developmental and individual differences in intelligence. One probably too simplistic position is that both developmental and individual differences can largely be reduced to differences in a single cognitive process, such as working memory (see Pennington, 1994). Another position, also probably too simplistic, is that a different fundamental cognitive process underlies each kind of difference. Hence Anderson's (2001) two-factor theory proposes that differences in speed of processing account for individual differences in intelligence, whereas working memory and inhibition account for developmental differences in intelligence. Research on ID syndromes allows us to test such theories.

The findings just reviewed also highlight that the developmental approach to understanding ID is a two-way street; not only does what we have learned about typical development help us understand ID, but research on ID syndromes also provides an important test of the generality of developmental theories. In fact, ID syndromes provide a particularly powerful test of putative universals in development, because (1) development proceeds more slowly in ID, allowing a more sensitive test of developmental sequences; (2) more dissociations are found both between (and within) cognitive and language development in ID; and (3) there are contrasting profiles of dissociations across ID syndromes.

In terms of errors, both approaches have been wrong in somewhat different ways about etiology. The specific-deficit approach has been wrong for ignoring etiology, and the developmental approach has been wrong for drawing too sharp a distinction between organic and nonorganic etiologies. All forms of ID must affect brain development in some way or another, and both genetic and environmental factors (and their interaction) are important in both syndromal and (currently) idiopathic mild ID (i.e., the cultural–familial subgroup discussed earlier). Recent research has found that as many as 30–50% of children with mild ID have a pathological etiology (Simonoff, Bolton, & Rutter, 1998). A medical geneticist would argue that some of the remaining cases are due to syndromes not yet recognized. But many cases of mild ID will be due to an accumulation of unfavorable genes and environmental risk factors. No one of these etiological factors will be pathological by itself.

Even when the etiology of mild ID is multifactorial in this way, the mechanisms of action of those alleles and environmental risk factors on brain and cognitive development will be important to understand and will probably reveal commonalities with mechanisms operating in so-called "pathological" cases. For instance, we have already explained that in DS and WS there are no pathological alleles, just extra or reduced doses of the products of normal alleles. Therefore, too sharp a line has been drawn between organic and nonorganic and between pathological and nonpathological; instead of a categorical distinction, we really have a continuum. From the perspective of developmental neuroscience, both typical and atypical development require an explanation in terms of genetic and environmental influences on brain development. Studying ID syndromes such as DS will identify what some of those influences are. We now turn to the neuropsychology of the three specific ID syndromes considered here: DS, FXS, and WS.

Down Syndrome

What is known about the brain phenotype in DS leads us to predict both overall neuropsychological dysfunction and somewhat more specific deficits on measures of prefrontal, hippocampal, and cerebellar functions. Because different aspects of the brain phenotype appear to emerge at different points in development, we would also predict different developmental trajectories for different domains of dysfunction. Specifically, we would predict that hippocampal dysfunction may appear later in development than dysfunction in other domains (Nadel, 1986). We now examine whether existing data support these hypotheses.

We begin with areas of cognitive development that have been thoroughly studied, including the level and trajectory of IQ, speech–language functions, short-term memory, and visual–constructive functions; we conclude with the few studies of hippocampal functions (i.e., allocentric spatial cognition and explicit long-term memory) in DS. To our knowledge, there are no previous studies of prefrontal functions in DS.

Level and Trajectory of IQ

DS does not specify a particular IQ, but instead exerts a powerful, downward main effect on IQ level. IQ in DS is also influenced by other genetic and environmental factors, just as it is in typically developing children. For instance, there is a positive relation between parental IQ and the IQ of individuals with DS, and part of this relation is very likely to be genetic, just as in children without ID.

In contrast to typically developing children, there is a progressive IQ decline in DS beginning in the first year of life. In other words, the ratio of mental age to chronological age is not constant (Hodapp & Zigler, 1990). By adulthood, IQ is usually in the range of moderate to severe ID (IQ = 25–55), with an upper limit on mental age of approximately 7–8 years (Gibson, 1978), though a few individuals with DS have IQs in the average range (Epstein, 1989). The trajectory of IQ in adulthood is also different in DS because of the increased risk of early onset Alzheimer disease; consequently, IQ declines much sooner in adulthood in DS than it would in typical aging (Epstein, 1989).

Little is known about the etiology of the virtually linear early decline in IQ across development in DS. Determining the brain bases of this trajectory DS could illuminate the relations between typical brain development and cognitive development. More specifically, dysfunction in either the prefrontal cortices, the hippocampus, or the cerebellum could conceivably reduce IQ in DS and affect its trajectory, but each in different ways. Each of these brain regions helps mediate general cognitive processes that operate across content domains. Hence dysfunction in each could be expected to have a general effect on cognitive development.

Speech, Language, and Verbal Short-Term Memory

Speech–language functions and verbal short-term memory have been extensively studied in DS and, other than IQ, are probably the best-documented aspects of its cognitive phenotype. They also decline early, thus contributing to the IQ decline, since IQ tests partly measure language development. The speech and language profile contrasts markedly with what is observed in autism, FXS, and WS—a finding that potentially limits the causal role for some speech and language processes in explaining ID across syndromes.

Several areas of speech and language development are delayed below mental age expectations in DS. Specifically, articulation (Fowler, Gelman, & Gleitman, 1994; Hulme & Mackenzie, 1992), phonology (Rondal, 1993), vocal imitation (Dunst, 1990), mean length of utterance, and expressive syntax (Fowler et al., 1994) are all below the expected mental age levels.

The development of verbal short-term memory also lags behind mental age in DS (Hulme & Mackenzie, 1992). This well-replicated deficit may help explain some of the speech and language difficulties found in DS, as a number of researchers have suggested for the syntactic deficit (Chapman, 1999; Fowler, 1998; Marcell & Weeks, 1988). The relation makes sense both theoretically and empirically. Theoretically, comprehending syntactic relations requires temporary memory storage of parts of a phrase. There are consistent moderate correlations between measures of verbal short-term memory and language in groups with developmental disabilities and those with typical development. Verbal short-term memory is a relative strength in WS, as is language, and the two are moderately correlated (r's = .47–.69) when chronological age is partialed out (Mervis, 1999).

Hulme and Mackenzie (1992) demonstrated that slower articulation is not responsible for the verbal short-term memory deficit in DS. They proposed that children with DS may not be rehearsing the to-be-remembered information in the articulatory loop. Consistent with the position we take here, they also suggested that deficits in verbal short-term memory may play an important causal role in ID.

Hence the verbal short-term memory deficit in DS probably helps explain the language deficit, which in turn contributes to the IQ deficit. Raitano-Lee (2006) tested whether the verbal short-term memory deficit in DS was due to decreased use of phonological or semantic codes (or both). She experimentally manipulated the phonological or semantic coding demands of verbal span tasks and found less use of phonological codes in children with DS than in mental-age-matched controls, but similar use of semantic codes. So the verbal short-term memory deficit in DS is due to a phonological deficit, similar to what is found in dyslexia, SSD, and LI. But we do not know the brain basis of the verbal short-term memory deficits in DS.

Visual–Constructive Functions

Certain spatial abilities are a strength relative to mental age in DS. For instance, Silverstein, Legutki, Friedman, and Takayama (1982) found that a group with DS outperformed a group with non-DS ID (individually matched for both chronological and mental age) on several drawing and other visual–constructive tasks from the Stanford–Binet test. This relative strength in DS contrasts with a relative weakness on similar tasks in WS (Wang & Bellugi, 1994; Wang, Doherty, Rourke, & Bellugi, 1995).

Long-Term Memory Functions

There are a few studies of long-term memory functions in individuals with DS across the lifespan, but most of this work has been done with adults. One exception is Mangan's (1992) study of preschool children (16–30 months old) with DS and chronological-age-matched controls on three spatial tasks, one of which (place learning and recall) tapped long-term memory functions. The group with DS performed worse than these controls on the learning portion of all three tasks, but was severely and selectively impaired on only the delayed-recall probes for the place-learning tasks. However, there was not a mental-age-matched control group in this study.

Carlesimo, Marrotta, and Vicar (1997) tested implicit (stem completion) and explicit verbal long-term memory (word list learning and prose recall), as well as explicit nonverbal long-term memory (the Rey–Osterrieth Complex Figure, Form B) in adolescents with DS ($n = 15$), non-DS ID ($n = 15$), and mental-age-matched controls ($n = 30$). They found similar verbal priming in all three groups for the stem completion tasks. For the two explicit tasks, the group with DS performed significantly worse than the other two groups in learning, but was not differentially impaired in delayed recall or recognition. In fact, the adolescents with DS improved on recognition trials, relative to their recall performance. These authors interpret their results as supporting a hippocampally mediated deficit in episodic memory in DS—one that particularly affects encoding. However, verbal memory tests are somewhat problematic in individuals with DS because of their well-documented language and verbal short-term memory deficits. Therefore, it would be valuable to see a test of nonverbal long-term memory in DS, using a task that does not depend on visual–motor skills.

Three studies of adults with DS have found particularly marked long-term memory deficits (Caltagirone, Nocentini, & Vicari, 1990; Devenny, Hill, Patxot, Silverman, & Wisniewski, 1992; Ellis, Woodley-Zanthos, & Dulaney, 1989). For example, Ellis et al. (1989) used pictures in a book to examine nonverbal long-term memory. Their group with DS was impaired at both recognizing pictures and remembering their locations—a result consistent with hippocampal dysfunction. However, a subset of this group performed very well on this task.

In summary, previous long-term memory research supports hippocampal dysfunction in DS. However, the only two studies in juvenile samples both have methodological shortcomings. So more work is needed to determine whether long-term memory dysfunction in DS occurs before adulthood and, if so, how early it occurs.

We (Pennington, Moon, Edgin, Stedron, & Nadel, 2003) conducted a study of long-term memory and executive functions in a sample of 28 individuals with DS (mean age = 14.7 years, *SD* = 2.7) compared to 28 typically developing children (mean age = 4.9 years, *SD* = 0.75) individually matched on mental age. Both neuropsychological domains were tested with multiple behavioral measures. "Benchmark" measures of verbal and spatial function demonstrated that this sample with DS was similar to others described in the literature.

The main finding was a significant group × domain interaction effect indicating differential long-term memory dysfunction in the group with DS. However, when chronological age was controlled for, there was a moderate partial correlation (*r* = .54) between long-term memory and executive function composite scores in the group with DS, and both composites contributed unique variance to the prediction of mental age and adaptive behavior in that group.

Overall, these results indicate a particular weakness in long-term memory functions in DS in the context of overall cognitive dysfunction. Interestingly, these results are similar to those found in a mouse model of DS. Such a model will make it easier to understand the neurobiological mechanisms that produce hippocampal dysfunction in DS.

Adaptive Behavior

The Pennington et al. (2003) study also provides evidence relevant to the theoretical issues discussed earlier. One domain of development—adaptive behavior—was *above* mental age level. So one determinant of adaptive behavior is chronological age, or time in the world. Nonetheless, adaptive behavior in DS is well below chronological age level and is correlated with IQ and mental age.

Executive Functions

Another domain of development examined in the Pennington et al. (2003) study—executive functions—was at mental age level. It may be that key aspects of psychometric intelligence (e.g., fluid intelligence) are closely related to executive functions (Pennington, 1994). Consequently, we would hypothesize that executive dysfunction is an important contributor to low IQ in all ID syndromes. Nonetheless, ID syndromes may vary in whether executive functions are at or below mental age level (as they are in FXS). No ID syndrome has yet been described in which these functions are above mental age level.

Three other domains of development—verbal short-term memory, structural language (such as lexical and syntactic skills), and long-term memory functions—are *below* mental age level in DS. As argued earlier, the verbal short-term memory deficit may help explain the structural language deficit. However, it seems very unlikely that the verbal short-term memory deficit can be explained by hippocampal dysfunction. In classical hippocampal amnesia, verbal short-term memory is spared (Shallice, 1988), as it is in children with early selective hippocampal damage (Vargha-Khadem et al., 1997), whose structural language development also appeared to be basically intact. Moreover, verbal short-term memory and hippocampally mediated long-term memory are doubly dissociable, since there are adults with a profound deficit in verbal short-term memory (Shallice, 1988) but intact explicit long-term memory.

Hippocampal dysfunction by itself is also unlikely as a sufficient explanation for the ID in DS, because the children with early selective hippocampal damage described by Vargha-Khadem et al. (1997) did not have ID.

So, as we return to the key issue of explaining the causes of both developmental and individual cognitive differences, the evidence from DS argues that *both* one- and two-factor theories are too simple. To explain the developmental profile in DS, we need at least four cognitive constructs: long-term memory, executive functions, verbal short-term memory, and another construct to explain the acquisition of adaptive behavioral skills that are above mental age level.

Fragile X Syndrome

Level and Trajectory of IQ

The average IQ of males with FXS declines with age, from a median value of 54 in younger males to about 44 in older males (Bennetto & Pennington, 2002). Longitudinal analyses of IQ in males with FXS have shown that this IQ decline is a real phenomenon and not an artifact of comparing different samples or using different IQ tests at different ages (Bennetto & Pennington, 1996, 2002).

In females with the fragile X mutation, the average IQ is higher, with a median value of 83 (Bennetto & Pennington, 2002), and there is not a decline with age. As explained earlier, this gender difference in IQ is explained by X-linked transmission. Approximately one-fourth of females with the full mutation have ID; most of the remainder exhibit learning problems (Hagerman et al., 1992; Staley et al., 1993).

Speech and Language Skills

Abnormalities in both speech production and language competence have consistently been noted in males with FXS, who often demonstrate delays in articulation and syntactic ability that are typically no different from those exhibited by typically developing children as they acquire language competence (Sudhalter, Scarborough, & Cohen, 1991). But males with FXS also show deviance in several areas of speech and language beyond that expected for their level of cognitive impairment. Their speech is often described as dysrhythmic, litany-like, and "cluttered." This latter term refers to a fast or fluctuating rate of talking, in which sounds or words are occasionally repeated or garbled (Hanson, Jackson, & Hagerman, 1986).

Males with FXS also show deviance in pragmatics and conversational skills. Their language is often described as perseverative and inappropriate or tangential in conversation style; furthermore, it is often marked by "pailalia" (direct self-repetition), echolalia (repetition of others), or frequent use of stereotypical statements. The deviant language pattern does not appear to be due to overall lower IQ: Males with FXS are more likely, for example, to perseverate on a topic, produce stereotyped vocalizations, and fail to read referential gestures in others than are males with DS (Sudhalter et al., 1990). Finally, women with FXS have also been shown to have less goal direction and organization in their thinking and speech than comparison women do (Sobesky, Hull, & Hagerman, 1994).

In contrast to their poor pragmatic skills, males with FXS who were administered on the Stanford–Binet Intelligence Scale: Fourth Edition showed strengths in vocabulary, verbal labeling, and verbal comprehension (Freund & Reiss, 1991). On achievement tests, such males have shown relative strengths in early reading skills and spelling ability (Hagerman, Kemper, & Hudson, 1985; Kemper, Hagerman, & Altshul-Stark, 1988).

Memory

On the memory subtests of the Stanford–Binet, males with FXS showed consistent weaknesses on short-term memory for sentences and bead memory (a visual memory task), but did relatively well on object memory (Freund & Reiss, 1991). The authors interpreted these results as suggesting that the memory deficit in FXS is dependent on the type of information to be remembered. Abstract visual information that is not easily labeled (e.g., bead memory) or information that requires sequencing or syntactic ability (e.g., sentence memory) may be difficult for males with FXS, because these tasks require organizational or analytic skill. Freund and Reiss found the same dissociation between abstract and meaningful visual memory in females with FXS. Other studies of females with FXS have found a consistent pattern of relative weakness on subtests that require visual–spatial, quantitative, and auditory short-term memory skills (e.g., Brainard, Schreiner, & Hagerman, 1991; Kemper, Hagerman, Ahmad, & Mariner, 1986). However, long-term memory for meaningful verbal information is a significant strength for females with FXS, and they often perform above mental age level in this area (Bennetto & Pennington, 2002).

Spatial Abilities

Both males and females with FXS have demonstrated an apparent deficit in spatial ability. Visual–spatial tasks, such as Block Design on the Wechsler tests, are typically among the lowest-scoring IQ subtests in profiles of individuals with FXS (see Kemper et al., 1986; Theobold, Hay, & Judge, 1987). Kemper et al. (1986) found a deficit in spatial short-term memory in a group of males. Mazzocco, Hagerman, Cronister-Silverman, and Pennington (1992) found a pattern of weaker figural than verbal memory in a sample of females with FXS. Individuals with FXS also typically show deficits in arithmetic (Dykens, Hodapp, & Leckman, 1987; Kemper et al., 1986).

Executive Functions

There is clear evidence of a specific deficit in executive functions in women with FXS (Bennetto, Pennington, Porter, Taylor, & Hagerman, 2001; Mazzocco et al., 1992; Mazzocco, Pennington, & Hagerman, 1993). Moreover, X activation ratio in such women predicts the degree of executive dysfunction (Bennetto et al., 2001). Furthermore, in these studies, the deficits in executive function remained after the authors covaried out the effects of IQ. There is preliminary evidence of executive deficits in males with FXS as well (Bennetto & Pennington, 2002).

In addition to impairment on standard tests of executive functions, individuals with FXS tend to show a pattern of deficits on other tasks that is consistent with impaired executive functioning. Boys with FXS obtained lower Sequential Processing scores than Simultaneous Processing scores on the original Kaufman Assessment Battery for Children (Dykens et al., 1987; Kemper et al., 1988). Tasks of sequential processing, such as imitating sequential hand movements, often rely on an individual's ability to hold a sequence of actions on line in working memory and formulate a motor plan to execute a response. Other tasks of motor sequencing have been shown to be sensitive to frontal lobe deficits (Kolb & Whishaw, 1990). This dissociation between performance on sequential and simultaneous tasks provides further neurocognitive differentiation between individuals with FXS and DS. In contrast to boys with FXS, individuals with DS showed no differences between levels of simultaneous and sequential processing (Hodapp et al., 1992; Pueschel, Gallagher, Zartler, & Pezzullo, 1987).

Social and Behavioral Phenotype

The social and behavioral phenotype in FXS has also been studied. Some of this has already been described in Chapter 8, since males with FXS have some of the symptoms of autism. One striking symptom is marked avoidance of eye contact, as well as social anxiety and shyness. Nonetheless, they have more interest in social interactions than individuals with autism do. Females with FXS exhibit shyness, social anxiety, and mood problems (Hagerman, 1999).

The constellation of behavioral problems often observed in individuals with FXS is also consistent with a deficit in executive functioning. These include difficulty with attentional control, distractibility, impulsivity, and difficulty with transitions or shifting from one cognitive set to another (Hagerman, 1987). A deficit in executive functioning would also help to explain a number of the deviant speech and language areas. For example, perseverative thinking, difficulty with topic maintenance, and tangential conversational style are all consistent with such a deficit. Evidence consistent with this hypothesis was found in an experimental study of discourse processing in females with FXS (Simon, Keenan, Pennington, Taylor, & Hagerman, 2001). The discourse deficit in this sample correlated with both X activation ratio and a measure of verbal working memory.

Williams Syndrome

The neuropsychology of WS provides an interesting contrast to what is found in both DS and FXS. The following summary of the neuropsychological phenotype in WS is based on three reviews (Bellugi et al., 1999; Mervis, 1999; Mervis & Klein-Tasman, 2000).

Level and Trajectory of IQ

The average IQ in WS is somewhat higher than that found in DS and FXS, and falls in the mild range of ID, with a mean IQ of about 60. For instance, in a sample of 100 individuals with WS, the mean IQ was 60, with a range from 40 to 100 (Bellugi et al., 1999). In another sample of 38 children and adolescents with WS, the mean IQ was 59.3 ($SD = 10.7$), with a range from 38 to 84 (Mervis, 1999). Roughly 25% of individuals with WS will have IQs and adaptive behavior scores above the cutoff for ID; roughly half will fall in the mild range of ID; and the remaining 25% will have moderate or worse ID (Mervis & Klein-Tasman, 2000). Also in contrast to both DS and FXS, there is not evidence for a decline in IQ in WS. Raw scores on both language and spatial IQ measures show a moderate positive correlation with age (r's = .55–59) across childhood, whereas standard scores are not significantly correlated with age (Mervis, 1999). If there was an IQ decline, the correlation of raw scores with age would be smaller, and there would also be a significant *negative* correlation between standard scores and age.

Speech and Language Skills

Another notable contrast is in speech and language skills. Groups with WS have been found to have both verbal short-term memory (i.e., digit span) and receptive vocabulary are above mental age level, and grammatical understanding at mental age level (Bellugi et al., 1999; Mervis, 1999). In contrast, groups with DS are *below* mental age level on these aspects of language development. In both DS and WS, there are moderate correlations between verbal short-term memory and language skills; these, together with research on verbal short-term memory and language in typical development, suggest that verbal short-term memory plays an important role in both typical and atypical language development. In the other two ID syndromes considered here, DS and FXS, and in autism, we have seen dissociations between structural language competence (phonological, lexical, and syntactic development) and pragmatic competence. Pragmatic language is a relative strength in groups with DS, despite their deficit in structural language, whereas it is a deficit in both autism and FXS, despite relatively preserved structural language. In WS, it appears that at least some aspects of pragmatic language are a "super" strength. Individuals with WS are chatty and seek social contact; indeed, their narratives exhibit "hyperaffectivity," a greater than normal use of affective prosody to convey meaning (Bellugi et al., 1999).

Spatial Cognition

WS is also distinct from these other syndromes in terms of spatial cognition, which is consistently *below* mental age expectations in this disorder, whereas it is a relative strength in autism and DS. For instance, subjects with WS are very poor at drawing and block design tasks, as well as on spatial tasks that do not require production of a spatial pattern (i.e., judgment of line orientation; see Bellugi et al., 1999). Their performance on block design is very consistently poor, both in absolute terms and relative to their other abilities. Thus an operational definition of this profile on the original Differential Ability Scales (an IQ test with a spatial component) showed excellent sensitivity and specificity (both above .90) in discriminating individuals with WS from those with other developmental disabilities (Mervis, 1999); the sensitivity and specificity of this profile are holding up in new samples (Mervis & Klein-Tasman, 2000). Despite this pronounced deficit in spatial cognition, individuals with WS are relatively unimpaired in recognizing faces (Bellugi et al., 1999) and perform similarly to other groups in processing global aspects of spatial stimuli (Mervis, 1999). In fact, reducing the salience of the global pattern on a block design model by leaving spaces between blocks improved the performance of individuals with WS, just as it does for individuals with other developmental disabilities or for younger typically developing children (Mervis, 1999).

Although there is a marked dissociation between verbal and spatial cognition in the cognitive profile in WS, these dissociated domains nonetheless tap some common processes. For instance, the partial correlations (controlled for age) between a block design measure and three verbal measures—backwards digit span (arguably a measure of verbal working memory), receptive vocabulary, and receptive syntax—ranged from .50 to .52 (Mervis, 1999). This result argues for the importance of considering general as well as specific cognitive processes in this ID syndrome (an issue that has been discussed earlier).

Executive Functions

There is less research on executive functions in WS than in the other syndromes considered here. One study found that children with WS performed similarly on two executive tasks to a group of children with Prader–Willi syndrome; the two groups were also similar in both mental and chronological age (Tager-Flusberg, Sullivan, & Boshart, 1997). This one result suggests that executive functions are not spared in WS. Other comparisons are needed to determine whether executive functions are below mental age level in persons with WS, as they are in those with FXS and in older individuals with autism.

Social and Behavioral Phenotype

WS also has a distinctive social and behavioral profile—one that contrasts interestingly with some of the other ID syndromes considered here. Both clinical observations and formal temperament and personality measures document "high gregariousness, strong orientation toward other people, high empathy, high sensitivity to criticism, and high anxiety" (Mervis & Klein-Tasman, 2000, p. 157). Strong social drive appears early in the development of children with WS; at early ages, they stare very intently at a new person (Mervis & Klein-Tasman, 2000). This intensity of eye contact is the direct opposite of what is observed in FXS. Theory-of-mind performance in WS sheds light on potential dissociations within the domain of social cognition. Despite their empathy and hyperaffectivity, individuals with WS consistently perform at or below MA level on false-belief tasks (Tager-Flusberg, Boshart, & Baron-Cohen, 1998; Tager-Flusberg & Sullivan, 2000; Tager-Flusberg et al., 1997). Since social behavior in WS is the *opposite* of that in autism in many ways, it is striking that there is nonetheless a deficit on theory-of-mind tasks in WS. This result further questions whether a deficit in representational or cognitive theory of mind could be the primary deficit in autism. How could such a primary deficit be associated with opposite profiles of social behavior? Instead, other aspects of intersubjectivity—perhaps those related to social orientation, emotion, and empathy—may be more important in accounting for the opposite social phenotypes found in WS and autism. Tager-Flusberg and Sullivan (2000) have distinguished social-cognitive aspects (i.e., representational theory of mind) and social-perceptual aspects (e.g., emotion perception and empathy) of social knowledge. They argue that children with WS are impaired at the former but not the latter. Deficits in social-cognitive knowledge could interfere with maintaining friendships, which is a problem for individuals with WS despite their high social drive (Mervis & Klein-Tasman, 2000). Friendships usually require communication skills that depend on taking another's knowledge into account. Being chatty and empathic, but nonetheless talking about topics that are irrelevant for the listener, could alienate potential friends.

In summary, across these three ID syndromes and autism, we have evidence for associations and dissociations that have implications for developmental theory. In terms of associations, problems with executive functions and attention are found in all four syndromes; problems with false-belief tasks are widespread as well. We also have evidence for three double dissociations: (1) spatial cognition versus structural language (DS vs. WS), (2) structural language versus pragmatic language (DS vs. autism and FXS), and (3) pragmatic language versus spatial cognition (autism vs. WS). These double dissociations provide evidence that these different cognitive domains can develop somewhat independently of each other. But we would not want to argue for total independence, because even the areas of strength in each ID syndrome are still below age level, and because dissociated domains are nonetheless correlated, as illustrated above. So various ID syndromes appear to share a general cognitive deficit that affects all domains of cognitive development to some extent, whereas they may differ in their profiles of strengths and weaknesses in specific cognitive domains. Therefore, the challenges for a neuroscientific account of ID are to specify cognitively what this general deficit is, and to identify which aspects of altered brain development produce this general cognitive deficit and which lead to the specific cognitive profiles.

There has been considerable progress toward an integrated neuroscientific understanding of these three ID syndromes—indeed, *more* progress than for many of the disorders considered in this book. What we learn about pathways running from genes to brain to behavior in these ID syndromes is likely to provide useful hypotheses for studying other disorders.

Table 10.1 summarizes research on ID.

DIAGNOSIS AND TREATMENT

As described in this chapter, many genetically based ID syndromes have unique features in their behavioral presentation within the context of gen-

TABLE 10.1. Research Summary Table: ID

Definition	• Most current definitions of ID require (1) an IQ deficit (at least 2 SDs below the mean on an individually administered IQ test), (2) an adaptive behavior deficit, and (3) onset before age 18 years. • Four subtypes of ID are defined by IQ ranges: mild (IQ = 50–55 to 70), moderate (IQ = 35–40 to 50–55), severe (IQ = 20–25 to 35–40), and profound (IQ < 20–25).
Epidemiology	• Prevalence is between 1% and 3%, with the majority having mild ID. • ID is more common in males than females; the male–female ratio is about 1.5:1. The male predominance is partly due to the large number of X-linked ID syndromes. • Known genetic syndromes account for many of the cases of moderate or more severe ID, especially fragile X syndrome (FXS) in males and Down syndrome (DS). • DS is the most prevalent form of ID with a known genetic etiology (0.17%) and affects males and females equally. Most cases are not familial. • FXS is the most prevalent familial form of ID with a known genetic etiology (0.019%). It affects more males than females. • Williams syndrome (WS) affects both genders equally, and its prevalence is about 0.004%.
Etiology	• Nonfamilial etiologies are much more common in moderate and more severe ID, whereas familial etiologies are much more common in mild ID. • The overall heritability of IQ is about 50%, so mild ID can be estimated to be about 50% heritable. Moderate and severe ID are less heritable. • DS results from an extra copy of chromosome 21 (trisomy 21). • FXS is a single-gene disorder in which the fragile X mental retardation 1 (FMR1) gene on the X chromosome becomes inactivated. • The genetics of FXS is complicated and involves X linkage, anticipation, and imprinting. • WS is caused by a usually sporadic, contiguous deletion of genes on chromosome 7p11.23.
Brain bases	• DS: Although brain development appears normal at birth, by adulthood, the brain shows neuropathological features of Alzheimer disease and is microcephalic, with differentially greater volume reduction in the hippocampus, prefrontal cortex, and cerebellum. • FXS: Neuroanatomical abnormalities have included a decreased size of the posterior cerebellar vermis, mild ventricular enlargements, and enlargement of some brain structures (consistent with the large head circumferences). • WS: Microcephaly, with relative sparing of frontal, limbic, and cerebellar volumes (the opposite pattern from DS).

(continued)

TABLE 10.1. (continued)

Neuropsychology	• A neuropsychological explanation of ID must explain both the general slowing of development and the different specific deficits that characterize different ID syndromes.
	• DS:
	  • Progressive IQ decline beginning in first year of life. By adulthood, IQ is usually in the moderate to severe ID range.
	  • Relative strengths include adaptive behavior and visual–spatial abilities. Executive functions are consistent with mental age. Relative weaknesses include long-term memory, speech, language, and verbal short-term memory.
	• FXS:
	  • The average IQ of males declines with age from a median value of 54 in younger males to about 44 in older males.
	  • In females with the fragile X mutation, the average IQ is higher, with a median value of 83, and there is not a decline with age.
	  • Relative strengths include vocabulary, verbal labeling, verbal comprehension, reading, and spelling. Relative weaknesses include pragmatics, conversational skills, short-term memory, visual–spatial skills, arithmetic, executive functions, social skills, attention, and impulsivity.
	• WS:
	  • The average IQ falls in the mild range of ID, with a mean IQ of about 60. No evidence for a decline.
	  • Relative strengths include verbal short-term memory, receptive vocabulary, pragmatics, and social drive. Children show a notable weakness in visual–spatial skills.

eral similarities resulting from ID. This section focuses on the similarities in presenting symptoms, history, and behavioral observations that can be expected for a child with ID, regardless of the etiology.

Presenting Symptoms

The early presenting symptoms in children with ID are often related to speech–language delays, because language skill is one of the most easily observable aspects of early cognitive development, whereas nonverbal reasoning is more difficult to assess. These children are often identified and treated for speech–language delays before they receive the broader diagnosis of ID. When a child has entered grade school, parents may identify learning delays and note that their child is struggling with grade-level work, seems to be learning more slowly than peers, and/or has difficulty mastering new concepts. Parents often ask whether their child has a learning disability or has a particular learning style. At feedback, psychoeducation about the similarities and differences between a more specific learning disorder and ID is sometimes helpful for parents to optimally support their child's learning.

The primary presentation of a child with ID may also appear emotional or behavioral in nature. The child may be susceptible to intense outbursts and tantrums, perhaps even exhibiting aggressive behavior. Attentional difficulties are also common. Socioemotional immaturity and other social difficulties that affect peer relationships may also be concerns for parents.

History

Children with ID often present with general developmental delays starting in infancy. One of the first developmental tasks of infancy is feeding, which requires coordinated motor movements, and so children with ID often have trouble nursing. Motor and language milestones are also often delayed. These delayed milestones are often the first triggers for parents to seek out an evaluation and/or therapeutic services. During the toddler years and beyond, a child may exhibit delayed emotion regulation skills and be prone to intense outbursts and temper tantrums, as noted above. Play behavior during the toddler years will be simpler and more concrete than that of a typically developing child. In addition, adaptive behavior may begin to show delays during this period; the child may have difficulty moving toward independence in such tasks as toileting, eating, dressing, and bathing.

When the child enters kindergarten and the grade school years, school difficulties may become more evident. As observed above, concerns may be raised about the child's maturity and progress with academic skills. The child is likely to have particular difficulty with academic tasks requiring abstract reasoning. Parents and teachers may observe that the child needs lots of repetition in order to learn new information. And, once the information is learned in one context, the child may have difficulty generalizing it to other contexts. Parents and teachers often express frustration that the child is able to do certain problems on one day but cannot do the same problems on the following day. These difficulties with retention and generalization are characteristic of a child with ID. Thus, although a child with ID will be able to learn new material, it will take many repetitions, which may frustrate the child. In this context, it is not surprising that attention difficulties are common in ID, although this issue is not likely to account completely for the attention problems in ID. Consistent failure in the school setting may also be an important trigger for the development of comorbid psychopathology, such as anxiety and depression.

It is also important to note that children with ID often develop compensation strategies in the classroom that can mask their difficulties with comprehension. For example, a teacher may check in with a child to see whether he or she understands, and the child may respond enthusiastically, "Yes, that is interesting!" Unfortunately, these compensation strategies may result in the child's being assigned work that is far above his or her academic skills.

Social difficulties often become evident once a child enters the school context. These social difficulties are often secondary to the child's cognitive limitations because the child is often interested in other children and interactive. However, because the other children are at different developmental levels, the maintenance of true friendships can be challenging. The child's language-based difficulties can also have an impact on social relationships. For example, difficulties with language comprehension and expression can make conversations difficult. The child may have trouble following a conversation and say things that seem irrelevant or tangential. In addition, group-based activities may be particularly problematic because the child will have difficulty following the quick verbal banter of the other children and understanding the evolving structure/rules of games, making the group setting particularly overwhelming.

Behavioral Observations

When working with a child with suspected ID, it is important to look for evidence of facial dysmorphology that is consistent with known genetic ID syndromes.

During testing, the child may show inordinate difficulty on tasks requiring abstract reasoning and problem solving (e.g., WISC-IV Matrix Reasoning), but may perform better on more concrete tasks (single-word reading, spelling, simple math computations). This concrete style may also be evident in the child's interpretations of figurative language (e.g., "Hold your horses"), which may be very literal. On the WISC-IV Similarities task, the child may have difficulty abstracting similarities and revert to the more concrete strategy of telling what is different about the items.

During conversations, the child's language may be characterized by short, simple utterances. The child may also show a delay in internalization of self-talk, so that he or she talks out loud during tasks to regulate behavior. The clinician may need to slow down his or her own language, simplify instructions, and repeat instructions in response to behavioral cues from the child that the information is confusing, overwhelming, or too fast-paced. The child may also show delays in metacognition (e.g., not asking for clarification when he or she does not understand instructions).

Case Presentations

Case Presentation 9

Background. Tori is an 8-year-old girl who will be entering second grade in a few weeks. She is old for her grade because she repeated kindergarten, due to her parents' and teacher's concerns that she was "immature" and not making expected progress. She has already received special education services for "speech–language disability," and in first grade she received extra help for literacy and math as well. Her parents have requested this evaluation to get more information about "what is in the way of Tori's learning and how we can help her."

Tori was the result of an uncomplicated pregnancy and birth. Her Apgar scores were good. Tori had some trouble nursing in the perinatal period, and though her mother had planned on breastfeeding exclusively, Tori's diet had to be supplemented with formula so that she would grow adequately. Parents described her as a happy, easygoing baby, but noted that she reached all developmental milestones more slowly than her older brother. Tori sat unassisted at 9 months, never crawled, and walked unassisted at 17 months. Her language development was quite delayed: Her parents report that she had only about 10 words just before she turned 3, used two- to three-word phrases at 3, and did not speak in sentences until 4 years of age. Because of these delays, she was evaluated by the state early intervention program at age 2½ and diagnosed with a mixed expressive–receptive language disorder, for which she received regular speech–language therapy.

Tori's parents have identified a number of concerns in addition to her language development and academic progress. Her father describes her as "uncoordinated"; he notes that she cannot ride a two-wheeled bike and that she struggles to learn routines in her ballet class. Her mother volunteered in Tori's first-grade class once a week and is concerned about her social development. By her mother's description, "Tori thinks everybody is her friend and doesn't know when the other kids are being mean to her." Outside of school, Tori enjoys watching Disney movies and then reenacting scenes from them. She also likes listening to music and playing with her stuffed animals.

Tori's parents report no history of learning or academic problems themselves. Her mother completed an associate's degree and works as a dental assistant. Her father completed a 4-year college degree and works as a banker. Tori has an 11-year-old brother without difficulties.

Tori's diagnostic testing is summarized in Table 10.2.

Discussion. Although Tori's striking language delays could be consistent with a specific diagnosis of LI, her history makes it clear that her cognitive limitations extend into the nonverbal realm, and that ID is likely to be the appropriate diagnosis. Tori's language remains poor for her age, and she certainly will continue to benefit from interventions and support in this area, but her LI is not *specific* in the sense that her language skill is not discrepant from other intellectual abilities.

From her earliest days, Tori did not quite meet developmental expectations. As a newborn she had difficulty with nursing. A general develop-

TABLE 10.2. Test Summary, Case 9 (Tori)

Construct	Standard score/ cutoff
General intelligence	
WISC-IV Full Scale IQ	60
Crystallized intelligence[a]	
WISC-IV Verbal Comprehension Index	69
Similarities	3
Vocabulary	5
Comprehension	6
Fluid intelligence	
WISC-IV Perceptual Reasoning Index	65
Block Design	6
Picture Concepts	4
Matrix Reasoning	3
WISC-IV Working Memory Index[b]	68
Digit Span	5
Letter–Number Sequencing	3
WISC-IV Processing Speed Index[c]	70
Coding	3
Symbol Search	6
Adaptive behavior	
SIB-R	62
Academic	
Reading	
History	
Learning and Behavior Quest. Reading History items	<55
Word recognition	
WJ III Letter Word ID	82
TOWRE Sight Word Efficiency	76
Phonological coding	
WJ III Word Attack	73
TOWRE Phonemic Decoding Efficiency	71
Paragraph fluency	
GORT-4 Fluency	70
Reading comprehension	
GORT-4 Comprehension	70
Math	
WJ III Math Fluency	79
WJ III Calculation	74
WJ III Applied Problems	66

(continued)

TABLE 10.2. *(continued)*

Construct	Standard score/ cutoff
Spelling	
WJ III Spelling	81
Oral language	
General	
CELF-4 Core Language	74
Semantics	
PPVT-4	85
Phonological awareness[d]	
CTOPP Elision	70
CTOPP Phoneme Reversal	65
Verbal Memory	
WRAML Sentence Memory	65
WRAML Story Memory	75
CTOPP Nonword Repetition	75
Verbal processing speed	
CTOPP Rapid Naming Composite	75
Problem solving/nonverbal reasoning	
Children's Category Test	58
Attention and hyperactivity–impulsivity	
ADHD Rating Scale–Inattention	
Parent	4/9
Teacher	5/9
ADHD Rating Scale–Hyperactivity–impulsivity	
Parent	3/9
Teacher	4/9
Visual–spatial	
Rey–Osterrieth Complex Figure Test (Copy)	65
Beery–Buktenica Test of Visual–Motor Integration	61

Note. WISC-IV, Wechsler Intelligence Scale for Children—Fourth Edition; SIB-R, Scales of Independent Behavior—Revised; WJ III, Woodcock–Johnson III Tests of Achievement; TOWRE, Test of Word Reading Efficiency; GORT-4: Gray Oral Reading Test—Fourth Edition; PPVT-4, Peabody Picture Vocabulary Test, Fourth Edition; CELF-4, Clinical Evaluation of Language Fundamentals—Fourth Edition; CTOPP, Comprehensive Test of Phonological Processing; WRAML, Wide-Range Assessment of Memory and Learning.
[a]See also Oral language—Semantics.
[b]See also Oral language—Verbal memory.
[c]See also Oral language—Verbal processing speed, and Academics—Math—WJ III Math Fluency.
[d]See also Verbal memory—CTOPP Nonword Repetition for another test of phonological awareness.

mental delay was further evident in the ages at which she met motor and language milestones. In contrast, her early social development represented an area of relative strength. By her parents' report, Tori was interested in others and interactive from an early age. Her current social difficulties are probably secondary to her cognitive limitations. Because her typically developing same-age peers are at different levels of cognitive development from hers, it will be difficult for her to develop true friendships with them. If she remains in a regular classroom, her parents and teachers should explore ways for Tori to be exposed to other children functioning at her mental level (e.g., Special Olympics or other special activities).

The most striking aspect of Tori's test scores is the pervasiveness of her difficulties; she has performed in the impaired range on nearly every test given her. Her WISC-IV Full Scale IQ, together with a measure of her adaptive functioning, qualifies her for a diagnosis of mild ID. Like most children with ID, Tori struggles greatly with tasks requiring abstract reasoning or problem solving. This difficulty is evident in her very poor scores on such tests as the Similarities and Matrices subtests of the WISC-IV, as well as the Children's Category Test. On the Similarities subtest, Tori's responses were very concrete, even for an 8-year-old. For example, when asked how a shirt and a shoe are alike, she looked at her outfit and said, "They both have yellow on them." In contrast, Tori has performed somewhat better on rote tasks, such as single-word reading and spelling and solving simple math problems. Her highest score is on the PPVT-4, which falls in the low-average range. This test often represents a relative strength in children who have received a good deal of environmental language support (e.g., speech–language therapy, enriched home environment).

Many children with ID have very poor attention. In the supportive, one-on-one testing environment, Tori's attention was adequate. However, parent and teacher ratings indicate that she does have at least some difficulty in this area. It may be that she has difficulty attending primarily because much of the information she encounters is confusing or otherwise overwhelming to her. However, children with ID can sometimes benefit from both medical and behavioral interventions used for children with ADHD, so Tori's parents and teachers should monitor this issue carefully.

The etiology of Tori's difficulties is unclear. Her physical appearance is normal (i.e., not dysmorphic). There is no obvious environmental cause for her delay, such as anoxia or another brain injury, and there is no relevant family history. Her parents' occupations and educational levels indicate that Tori's IQ is probably well below theirs. We recommend referring all children with ID of unknown etiology for a genetics evaluation. Sometimes such an evaluation will identify an underlying genetic syndrome, and this information can be useful to the family from a genetic counseling point of view. In addition, some genetic syndromes associated with ID are correlated with specific medical problems, for which the child can then be followed. Rarely, a genetics evaluation will identify an underlying disorder for which there is a known medical treatment (as in the case of some metabolic disorders).

Case Presentation 10

Background. Will is a 7-year-old boy who is currently in second grade. Will has been referred for an evaluation because of learning delays, hyperactivity, anxiety, and poor social skills.

Will's family history is unremarkable. His mother describes her pregnancy and delivery as uncomplicated. However, Will's developmental milestones were delayed, especially his speech–language milestones. He began to walk at 15 months, and he was very clumsy. It was not until Will was 3 years old that he began to say several words. His medical history includes recurrent otitis media with effusion, which was treated with the placement of ear tubes when he was 2 years old. During Will's toddler years, his parents became increasingly concerned about the fact that he became very anxious in new surroundings and with new people. He would scream and have tantrums in these novel settings, and he was difficult to soothe. Will entered preschool when he was 3 years old. At that time, his teachers noted some unusual repetitive behaviors, such as hand flapping and sniffing. The teachers also described Will as overactive, distractible, and susceptible to tantrums and angry outbursts when he was overstimulated. According to Will's parents, he struggled to connect with other children. Although he was interested in other children and would approach them, it seemed that he did not know how to act when he approached. He had particular difficulty with making eye contact.

These behavioral and social concerns have continued as Will has progressed into grade school. He continues to struggle with peer relationships and remains very anxious and shy, particularly in social situations. His teachers describe him as hyperactive with a very short attention span. This year, Will began taking methylphenidate to improve his distractibility and hyperactivity. Will's parents and teachers report that they have seen improvement in these symptoms with the medication. Despite these improvements, his parents are very concerned that Will is struggling with grade-level work and seems to be learning more slowly than his peers. He currently receives special education pull-out services to support his learning in academic subjects.

Will's diagnostic testing is summarized in Table 10.3.

Discussion. One of the recommendations from this evaluation was for Will to have genetic testing, because his behavioral phenotype and physical characteristics are characteristic of FXS. The characteristic behavioral

TABLE 10.3. Test Summary, Case 10 (Will)

Construct	Standard score/ cutoff
General intelligence	
WISC-IV Full Scale IQ	62
Crystallized intelligence[a]	
WISC-IV Verbal Comprehension Index	73
Similarities	5
Vocabulary	9
Comprehension	2
Fluid intelligence	
WISC-IV Perceptual Reasoning Index	75
Block Design	4
Picture Concepts	8
Matrix Reasoning	6
WISC-IV Working Memory Index[b]	65
Digit Span	5
Letter–Number Sequencing	3
WISC-IV Processing Speed Index[c]	62
Coding	2
Symbol Search	4
Adaptive behavior	
SIB-R	68
Academic	
Reading	
History	
Learning and Behavior Quest. Reading History items	70
Word recognition	
WJ III Letter Word ID	85
TOWRE Sight Word Efficiency	74
Phonological coding	
WJ III Word Attack	80
TOWRE Phonemic Decoding Efficiency	72
Paragraph fluency	
GORT-4 Fluency	65
Reading comprehension	
GORT-4 Comprehension	75
Math	
WJ III Math Fluency	58
WJ III Calculation	65
WJ III Applied Problems	68

(continued)

TABLE 10.3. *(continued)*

Construct	Standard score/ cutoff
Spelling	
WJ III Spelling	75
Oral language	
General	
CELF-4 Core Language	69
Semantics	
PPVT-4	80
Phonological awareness[d]	
CTOPP Elision	80
Verbal memory	
WRAML Sentence Memory	65
CTOPP Nonword Repetition	60
WRAML Story Memory	85
Verbal processing speed	
CTOPP Rapid Naming Composite	65
Executive functions	
Inhibition	
Gordon commission errors	60
Set shifting	
WCST	59
Attention and hyperactivity–impulsivity	
Gordon omission errors	65
ADHD Rating Scale–IV Inattention	
Parent	7/9
Teacher	6/9
ADHD Rating Scale–IV Hyperactivity–impulsivity	
Parent	8/9
Teacher	8/9
Visual–spatial	
Beery–Buktenica Test of Visual–Motor Integration	58
Social communication	
SCQ	10/40 (cutoff = 15)

Note. WCST, Wisconsin Card Sorting Test; SCQ, Social Communication Questionnaire. For other abbreviations, see Table 10.2.
[a]See also Oral language—Semantics.
[b]See also Oral language—Verbal memory.
[c]See also Oral language—Verbal processing speed, and Academics—Math—WJ III Math Fluency.
[d]See also Verbal memory—CTOPP Nonword Repetition for another test of phonological awareness.

phenotype involves language delays, hyperactivity, inattentiveness, autistic features (e.g., poor eye contact, hand stereotypies, repetitive behaviors), shyness and social anxiety, and hyperarousal by stimuli. As described, Will's history includes many of these features. Will also shows physical features consistent with FXS, including a long face, prominent ears, prominent chin, and hyperextensible finger joints. Genetic testing has confirmed a diagnosis of FXS. Will shows a mosaic pattern, with some of his cells having a pre-mutation and the rest of his cells having a full mutation; hence a proportion of his cells are able to produce FMRP. As a result, Will is not as severely affected as a typical male with a full mutation. The mean IQ in this most affected group is typically in the moderate range of ID, whereas the mean IQ in males with mosaicism typically falls in the mild range of ID.

An important rule-out for this case presentation is ASD, since Will shows difficulties with social-communicative skills. Although Will shows some autistic features, his score on the SCQ is below the autism screening threshold. This result is consistent with his parents' report that he does show some difficulties relating to other children and making eye contact, but he is interested in other children and seems motivated to interact with them.

Will's WISC-IV Full Scale IQ score and his adaptive behavior score are consistent with mild ID. On the WISC-IV, Will's lowest scores are on the Working Memory Index and Processing Speed Index, indicating that short-term memory and cognitive efficiency are areas of relative weakness for him. Will's scores on the Verbal Comprehension Index and Perceptual Reasoning Index are relatively stronger, although he shows quite a bit of scatter on the subtests of these. Within the Verbal Comprehension Index, Will shows a particular weakness on the Comprehension subtest, which is a test of real-world social knowledge and reasoning. Will's lower score on this subtest is consistent with his weaknesses in social development. Within the Perceptual Reasoning Index, Will shows a particular weakness on the Block Design subtest. Children with FXS often score poorly on this subtest because of visual–spatial deficits that are characteristic of this syndrome's neuropsychological profile. This weakness is also evident in Will's score on the Beery–Buktenica Test of Visual–Motor Integration.

Will's academic skills are generally consistent with his cognitive abili-ties, although the pattern of scores shows some strengths and weaknesses. Children with FXS frequently have trouble with math, and this pattern is evident in Will's scores. In contrast, Will shows relative strengths in single-word reading and spelling.

Will has a history of speech–language delay, and he continues to show weaknesses in use and understanding of language on the CELF-4. Behavioral observations also indicate that Will shows weaknesses in the pragmatics of language. He perseverates on words, phrases, and topics, and shows poor topic maintenance. Consistent with the typical FXS neuropsychological profile, Will shows weaknesses in short-term auditory memory (e.g., WISC-IV Working Memory Index, CTOPP Nonword Repetition, WRAML Sentence Memory), relative to his memory for more meaningful information (e.g., WRAML Story Memory). Will also shows a relative strength on a test of single-word receptive vocabulary, the PPVT-4.

Children with FXS often show executive function deficits consistent with some of the behavioral problems that are characteristic of the syndrome, such as inattention, hyperactivity, impulsivity, and difficulty with transitions. These behavioral characteristics overlap considerably with the symptoms of ADHD, and so it is not surprising that Will's parents' and teacher's ratings on ADHD questionnaires meet symptom thresholds for an ADHD diagnosis. In fact, Will has begun taking ADHD medication with beneficial effect. Will's performance on executive function tests indicates weaknesses on tests of inhibition (Gordon Diagnostic System commissions) and set shifting (the WCST).

In summary, Will is a child with FXS who has mild ID. He is not as severely affected as some males with FXS, because he shows a mosaic genetic pattern. He shows several behavioral, physical, and neuropsychological features that are characteristic of this syndrome.

Treatment

Treatments for ID generally do not remediate the core underlying intellectual deficits, but aim to improve quality of life by reducing associated problems and improving adaptive functioning (Hartley, Horrell, & Maclean, 2007). A key early finding was the failure of institutionalization as a treatment for ID. Compared to individuals with ID raised in their own homes, institutionalized individuals showed a wide range of poor outcomes, including shorter life expectancy (Centerwall & Centerwall, 1960; Dupont, Vaeth, & Videbech, 1986; Shotwell & Shipe, 1964). These findings led to a gradual change in practices, so that people with ID are now likely to live in private homes or in community-based group homes. Although most of these community-based group homes provide dramatically better environments than large institutions, there is little evidence that group living is preferable to semi-independent living. For example, one study found few outcome differences for adults with ID living semi-independently versus those living in group homes; any differences favored semi-independent living, even after preexisting differences in ability were controlled for (Stancliffe & Keane, 2000). Such findings have substantial public policy implications because of the higher cost of group homes.

By federal mandate, early intervention services are available to children with ID during the first 5 years of life. Once children are identified, they can receive services in their homes (at no cost to their families) until age 3, and then through their public school district until age 5. Children receive a range of services tailored to their needs, including physical, occupational, and speech–language therapies. Early intervention is generally associated with positive outcomes, though results have seldom been as dramatic or long-lasting as providers and parents would hope. Evidence for early intervention as an effective treatment is strongest for children at risk for ID due to environmental factors, such as poverty or prematurity (Ramey, Ramey, & Lanzi, 2007). Even among children with genetic ID syndromes, early intervention can have positive effects, but these are more likely to relate to academic outcomes or broader family function than to long-lasting changes in intelligence (Hines & Bennett, 1996).

ID is associated with a wide range of treatable emotional and behavioral problems. Applied behavioral analysis, a highly structured behavioral treatment, is an empirically supported intervention for problem behaviors in ID. Common problem behaviors include aggression, self-injurious behavior, or difficulty with basic self-care (e.g., feeding, toileting). Individuals with ID are also at increased risk for psychopathology, including internalizing disorders such as anxiety or depression. Attentional difficulties are also extremely common in ID. Although prevalence estimates vary widely, children with ID are probably four to five times more likely to have a psychiatric disorder than are children with typical-range intellectual abilities (Matson & Laud, 2007). It is important that individuals with ID be assessed and treated for these dual diagnoses. There are few well-controlled treatment studies of psychopathology that occurs specifically in ID, but some common behavioral interventions (e.g., cognitive-behavioral therapy for depression) will need to be tailored for developmental level. In addition, depending on the specific brain pathology underlying the ID, established psychopharmacological interventions may not work as they would in individuals without neurological conditions (Matson & Laud, 2007).

Prevention

Depending on etiology, some forms of ID are preventable. One of the most impressive prevention studies is the Abecedarian Project, a randomized controlled trial of intensive early intervention services that began in 1972. Newborns were enrolled in the study based on a number of environmental risk factors, including poverty and low parental education, but none of the children had genetic ID syndromes or known neurological disorders. The treatment group received high-quality, coordinated services, including early education, pediatric care, and family social support. The comparison group received nutritional supplements, social services, and low-cost pediatric care. Children in the treatment group showed significantly higher IQ scores, beginning at age 18 months and continuing at least until age 21 years. The size of the IQ difference was nearly 1 *SD*, meaning that substantially fewer children in the treatment group fell below the ID cutoff. Thus high-quality early intervention can prevent some cases of ID of predominantly environmental etiology (see Ramey et al., 2007).

A few genetically based forms of ID, most notably metabolic disorders, can be prevented with appropriate medical treatment. Perhaps the best example is phenylketonuria. Children with the gene for this disorder lack the enzyme to metabolize phenylalanine. If they follow a typical diet, the resulting brain damage inevitably leads to ID. However, when babies are identified early and fed a restricted diet, IQ can be normal. Currently, all newborns born in this country are screened for phenylketonuria, and it is estimated that thousands of cases of ID have been prevented (National Institutes of Health, 2000).

Prenatal screening and diagnosis provide the possibility of another form of prevention. It is now standard practice that all pregnant women, regardless of maternal age, be offered prenatal screening for DS and other chromosomal disorders. Such screening is essentially risk-free and can be completed as early as late in the first trimester. Women who are at high risk because of maternal age, family history, or a positive early screen are additionally offered more invasive diagnostic procedures (chorionic villus sampling or amniocentesis) and may choose to terminate pregnancy with an affected fetus. Of course, not all families will find this form of prevention ethically acceptable.

The guidelines for establishing a particular treatment as effective are discussed in Chapter 14. The degree to which ID treatments can be considered "well established" or even "probably efficacious" varies with both the treatment goals and the etiology of ID. In general, medical treatment for metabolic forms of ID, and prevention of ID of primarily environmental etiology, have more rigorous research support than do behavioral interventions for genetic ID syndromes. For example, many early intervention studies do not use randomized assignment or appropriate control groups, which reduces the strength of the conclusions that can be drawn from them. It is particularly difficult to use the strongest research designs for evaluation of ID treatments, since parents and clinicians are eager to offer all forms of possible help to a child with such substantial developmental problems.

Table 10.4 summarizes clinical issues in ID.

TABLE 10.4 Clinical Summary Table: ID

Defining symptoms	• General learning and developmental delays. • Speech–language delays. • Attention problems. • Social difficulties.
Common comorbidities	• Comorbidity with other psychiatric diagnoses is a common aspect of ID. • Attentional difficulties are very common across most forms of ID.

Developmental history	• Motor and language milestone delays.
	• Toddler years:
	  • Outbursts and temper tantrums stemming from delayed emotion regulation skills.
	  • Simple, concrete play behavior.
	  • Adaptive behavior delays.
	• School-age years:
	  • Difficulty with academic tasks, especially those requiring abstract reasoning.
	  • Difficulty with retention and generalization of information.
	  • Social difficulties stemming from cognitive and language limitations.

Diagnosis	• Most current definitions of ID require (1) an IQ deficit (at least 2 *SD*s below the mean on an individually administered IQ test), (2) an adaptive behavior deficit, and (3) onset before age 18 years. • The adaptive behavior deficit is the least well defined.
Prognosis	• Although there are no effective treatments for remediating the core cognitive deficit in ID, there are treatments that are successful at improving quality of life.
Treatment	• Institutionalization is not an effective treatment for ID and generally leads to poorer outcomes. • By federal mandate, early intervention services are available to children with ID during the first 5 years of life. • Early intervention is generally associated with positive outcomes, though results have seldom been as dramatic or long-lasting as providers and parents would hope. • Applied behavioral analysis, a highly structured behavioral treatment, is an empirically supported intervention for problem behaviors in ID. • Treatments for dual diagnoses need to be tailored to developmental level.
Prevention	• High-quality early intervention can prevent some cases of ID of predominantly environmental etiology. • A few genetically based forms of ID, most notably metabolic disorders, can be prevented with appropriate medical treatment. • Advances in prenatal screening and diagnosis have provided the possibility of another form of prevention, although these issues clearly intersect with the ethics of the family.

CHAPTER 11

Developmental Coordination Disorder

HISTORY

Developmental coordination disorder (DCD) has been recognized for at least 100 years under different labels, including "congenital maladroitness," "motoric deficiency," "minimal brain dysfunction," "clumsy child syndrome," and "developmental dyspraxia" (Tupper & Sondell, 2004). The symptoms of DCD are more subtle than those found in cerebral palsy (CP), muscular dystrophy, or Tourette syndrome, so it is not surprising that those disorders attracted clinical attention first. All three were first described in the 19th century (Tupper & Sondell, 2004). In contrast to these three disorders, most research on DCD has appeared in the last 20 years, and much remains to be done to understand it.

DEFINITION

The DSM-IV-TR definition of DCD (American Psychiatric Association, 2000) requires substantial motor delays or deficiencies in everyday activities. The person's motor deficits must be age- and IQ-discrepant, and must be associated with functional impairment. They must also be idiopathic—that is, not due to a medical condition such as acquired brain damage (as is found in CP) or a peripheral disorder (like muscular dystrophy), or to a PDD such as autism. If DCD is associated with ID, the motor difficulties must be worse than the child's level of ID would predict. In contrast, the ICD-10 (World Health Organization, 1992) definition of this disorder excludes ID.

227

Children with DCD are slower to acquire early motor milestones, and by definition, their problems in balance and in gross and fine motor coordination interfere with everyday activities (e.g., dressing, eating, riding a bicycle, playing sports) and with academic skills, particularly handwriting (Zoia, Barnett, Wilson, & Hill, 2006). Many children with DCD have associated visual–spatial deficits, even on tasks without a motor component, and their processing speed is slow (Dewey & Bottos, 2006). The combination of fine motor and visual–spatial deficits is reminiscent of NVLD, which is discussed in Chapter 13. In regard to developmental course, there is evidence that motor difficulties in DCD persist into adolescence and adulthood (Dewey & Bottos, 2004).

EPIDEMIOLOGY AND COMORBIDITIES

The estimated prevalence of DCD is roughly 5–10% of the population (American Psychiatric Association, 2000; Henderson & Hall, 1982). There is disagreement in the literature as to whether there is an unequal gender ratio for DCD. Some researchers report a male–female ratio of 3:1 (Zoia et al., 2006), while others find that equal numbers of each gender are affected (Hoare & Larkin, 1991). As explained for dyslexia in Chapter 6, gender ratios can be affected by selection artifacts, with referred samples often being more likely to have a male preponderance than population samples. In a recent large volunteer twin sample in Australia, the prevalence of DCD was 8%, and the male–female ratio was nearly equal (1.31:1) (Martin, Piek, & Hay, 2006).

DSM-IV-TR cites SSD and LI as common comorbidities of DCD, in addition to ID, and says that DCD is generally evident early in development because of failure to achieve motor milestones at typical ages. Another frequent comorbidity of DCD is ADHD. From 30% to 50% of children with ADHD also meet diagnostic criteria for DCD (Kadesjo & Gillberg, 1998; Kaplan, Dewey, Crawford, & Fisher, 1998; Pitcher, Piek, & Hay, 2003).

ETIOLOGY[1]

Although birth injuries and other neurological insults can certainly produce the symptoms of DCD, the DSM-IV-TR definition of DCD requires it to be idiopathic. We were able to find only one genetic study of DCD, a large volunteer twin study (Martin et al., 2006). This study used parent report measures of ADHD and DCD in a sample of 1,285 school-age twin pairs.

[1] For a description of genetic technical terms, see Box 1.1 in Chapter 1.

The researchers replicated substantial heritabilities for the three ADHD sub-types (.74–.98), and they also found substantial heritabilities for each of the four scales of their DCD questionnaire (.64–.85). Bivariate heritability between ADHD and DCD was most pronounced for the inattentive subtype of ADHD and varied across the scales of the DCD questionnaire, being most robust for the fine motor/handwriting scale (shared additive genetic component of .25–.66) and less consistent or negligible for the other three scales. This finding makes sense, given the high prevalence of handwriting problems in ADHD.

So this study provides evidence that DCD is heritable on its own. Despite the methodological confound of possible rater bias, which would artificially increase evidence for shared genetic influence, perhaps the most striking result from this study is the evidence that DCD is substantially genetically distinct from ADHD. This result argues for its validity as a distinct disorder, despite its high comorbidity (up to 50%) with ADHD. Obviously, much more work is needed on the etiology of DCD.

BRAIN MECHANISMS[2]

The brain mechanisms of more severe acquired or syndromal motor disorders are fairly well understood and thus provide a theoretical basis for possible brain mechanisms in DCD. These more severe motor disorders include CP, Huntington disease, Parkinson disease, and acquired apraxia.

The neural systems underlying skilled motor performance can be broadly divided into the pyramidal and extrapyramidal systems. The pyramidal system includes the primary and secondary motor areas in the frontal cortex (including the supplementary motor area and the frontal eyefields), and the corticospinal tract, which projects to the spinal motor neurons. So the planning and initiation of a voluntary skilled movement is mediated by these frontal motor areas, and a motor act itself occurs when spinal motor neurons activate particular muscle groups. The pyramidal system is required for rapid and precise control of voluntary skilled movements—serving a tennis ball, playing the piano, painting a picture, and so on. Damage to the pyramidal system on one side produces hemiparesis and hemiplegia.

The extrapyramidal system consists of several structures that modify and coordinate movements initiated by the pyramidal systems. Structures included in the extrapyramidal system include the basal ganglia, cerebellum, and portions of the brainstem (e.g., the substantia nigra). Well-known extrapyramidal motor syndromes include Parkinson disease and Huntington disease.

---

[2]For a description of neuroanatomical technical terms, see Box 1.2 in Chapter 1.

One of the best-understood motor disorders in children is CP, which can affect either the pyramidal or extrapyramidal system, or both. CP is a disorder of movement and posture caused by an acquired brain lesion that occurs early in life—usually prenatally or perinatally, but sometimes in the early postnatal period (Blondis, 2004). There are several symptomatic subtypes of CP, each correlated with different lesion locations in the motor systems. The most common form of CP is spastic CP; "spastic" in this context means that increased muscle tone and reflexes impair mobility. Spastic CP accounts for roughly 75% of all CP cases. Spastic CP is due to hypoxic–ischemic lesions in the pyramidal motor system, usually in the periventricular white matter underlying cortical motor areas (Blondis, 2004). Spastic CP is divided into subtypes, based on which limbs are affected and whether dysfunction is lateralized. "Diplegia" means that both legs are affected; "quadriplegia" means that all four limbs are affected; and "hemiplegia" means that dysfunction is lateralized because of a unilateral pyramidal lesion. The next most common subtype of CP is extrapyramidal or dyskinetic CP, which is characterized by abnormal movement patterns and postures (called "choreathetosis" and "dystonia"). The usual lesion site is in the basal ganglia. Extrapyramidal CP accounts for roughly 14% of CP cases (Blondis, 2004). The remaining two rarer types of CP, hypotonic CP (characterized by a generalized decrease in muscle tone) and ataxic CP (characterized by wide-spaced stance and unsteady gait), are associated with cerebellar dysfunction (Blondis, 2004).

Modern neuroimaging studies of CP (reviewed in Dewey & Bottos, 2004) have greatly advanced our understanding of the underlying neuropathology of this disorder. Ultrasonography, CT, and structural MRI have all been used to understand CP and have contributed to the clinical–anatomical correlations that define CP subtypes.

Because of what we know about the neurology of CP and other neurological disorders that affect motor function, it is plausible to look for the neural correlates of DCD in motor areas of the brain, including the frontal cortex, the basal ganglia, and the cerebellum (Dewey & Bottos, 2004). Neuroimaging studies (reviewed earlier) have examined these structures in disorders comorbid with DCD, such as dyslexia and ADHD; however, no neuroimaging studies of children with DCD seem to have been performed to date, so these neural hypotheses remain to be tested.

NEUROPSYCHOLOGY

It is well known in adult neurology and neuropsychology that the motor system is very sensitive to neurological disease, so it should not be too surprising that the developing brain can readily be perturbed in a variety of ways to produce motor dysfunction. Certainly, the example of CP illustrates that this is true.

However, other structures in the brain besides the motor systems discussed earlier are needed to produce a skilled movement. Action must be coupled with perception of the ever-changing environment and actions must serve adaptive goals of organisms. On the perceptual side, the dorsal visual system in the superior parietal lobe (sometimes called the "where" or "how" system) coordinates bodily space with extrapersonal space in the coordination of movements. On the planning side, the prefrontal cortex is important in selecting goals to pursue and strategies to meet them, whereas the secondary and primary motor areas convert these abstract strategies into motor plans that can be executed. So it should be clear that our tendency to dismiss symptoms as "just motor" and therefore to split thought from action is mistaken. Voluntary motor acts, and even involuntary ones, are exquisitely cognitive, requiring very precise coordination of representations in very different metrics and modalities.

This wider view of what is required for motor control has informed research on the neuropsychology of DCD. For instance, the frequent finding of visual–spatial deficits in DCD (Dewey & Bottos, 2004) is consistent with the role of the superior parietal lobe in skilled movement. Researchers have also found intact procedural learning (Wilson, Maruff, & Lum, 2003), but impairments in motor imagery (Katschmarsky, Cairney, Maruff, Wilson, & Currie, 2001; Maruff, Purcell, Tyler, Pantelis, & Currie, 1999; Wilson, Maruff, Ives, & Currie, 2001), anticipatory postural adjustments (Jucaite, Fernell, Forssberg, & Hadders-Algra, 2003), and working memory (Alloway, 2007), as well as reduced inhibition (on the Simon task—Mandich, Buckolz, & Polatajko, 2002). These findings make it clear that more than low-level, output processes are implicated in DCD; instead, it appears to involve several aspects of higher-level motor control. But whether there are valid neuropsychological subtypes of DCD remains to be determined.

The field, however, generally agrees that developmental dyspraxia, a deficit in skilled voluntary sequenced movement, is distinct from DCD in general. The motor problems in DCD also seem to be partly distinct from those found in ASD. Dewey, Cantell, and Crawford (2007) found that children with ASD had gestural deficits (both to command and to imitate) that were not accounted for by their motor coordination problems, which they shared with children with DCD and DCD + ADHD. Since failure to perform gestures to command is a defining feature of developmental dyspraxia, these results suggest that the motor phenotype of ASD includes developmental dyspraxia, whereas typical DCD or the DCD + ADHD combination does not.

DIAGNOSIS

As noted earlier, the DSM-IV-TR diagnosis of DCD requires documenting age- and IQ-discrepant motor performance that is associated with functional impairment, as well as excluding confounding conditions. To document a motor deficit, clinicians use a standardized motor test, such as the appropriate portions of the Bayley Scales of Infant and Toddler Development, Third Edition (Bayley, 2005) or the Griffiths Mental Development Scales (Griffiths, 1967) in infants and toddlers, or the Movement Assessment Battery for Children (Henderson & Sugden, 1992) or the Bruininks–Oseretsky Test of Motor Proficiency (Bruininks, 1978) for children ages 4–14 years. Functional impairment in everyday activities can be documented by history or by a motor scale on an adaptive behavior measure like the Vineland-II (Sparrow et al., 2005). Just as with any developmental disorder, diagnosis of DCD should not proceed in a vacuum, but should consider whether disorders that frequently co-occur with DCD are present (such as ADHD, ASD, RD, or LI).

TREATMENT

The treatment of DCD and other motor disorders of childhood is reviewed by Michaud (2004) and in Polatajko, Rodger, Dhillon, and Hirji (2004). Polatajko et al. (2004) divide motor treatments into two broad groups of approaches: "process-focused" approaches, which are aimed at remediating postulated underlying causes (e.g., neurodevelopmental treatment and sensory integration therapy), and "performance-focused" approaches, which concentrate on skill acquisition, task modification, and environmental accommodation. Performance-based approaches include cognitive-behavioral treatment, conductive education, compensation, and exercise.

Polatajko et al. (2004) performed a meta-analysis of 106 studies concerned with treatment of childhood motor disorders, including CP, DCD, spina bifida, Tourette syndrome, muscular dystrophy, and acquired brain injury. Only 30 of these articles involved actual research evaluations of treatments, but some of these articles were meta-analyses. The remaining articles were classified as descriptive or as expressing an opinion about treatment.

The results of the Polatojko et al. (2004) meta-analysis were as follows. There was no evidence of efficacy for neurodevelopmental treatment for CP (e.g., Brown & Burns, 2001; Pless & Carlsson, 2000) or of sensory integration therapy (SIT) for DCD (see review in Chapter 15; Michaud, 2004). The review by Michaud (2004) reached the same conclusion about the effectiveness of SIT for motor disabilities in children. So neither process-focused approach was supported as effective. Among the performance-focused approaches, there was some positive evidence for a cognitive-behavioral approach—namely, cognitive orientation to daily occupational performance (CO-OP). CO-OP is a client-centered approach in which the child selects goals for everyday motor activities, and the therapist analyzes performance breakdowns that interfere with skill acquisition and helps the child develop strategies to overcome these performance breakdowns. There was insufficient evidence to support the efficacy of other performance-focused approaches, although some support was found for exercise as a treatment for CP and muscular dystrophy. Another treatment for motor disorders, called patterning, also lacks empirical support (see review in Chapter 15).

In sum, there is one empirically validated best practice for particular motor disorders in childhood (CO-OP), and there are some treatments that should be avoided because research has failed to find that they are efficacious. These treatments include patterning, neurodevelopmental treatment, SIT, and conductive education. Clearly, more research is needed on effective treatments for DCD and other motor disorders of childhood.

CHAPTER 12

Mathematics Disorder

HISTORY

In 1925, Henschen coined the term "acalculia" to describe acquired deficits in arithmetic. Later, other behavioral neurologists distinguished subtypes of acalculia associated with different lesion locations. These included an "aphasic" subtype associated with left perisylvian lesions, a "spatial" subtype associated with right-hemisphere lesions, and a "planning and perseveration" subtype associated with frontal lesions (Badian, 1983; Berger, 1926; Hecaen, Angelergues, & Houillier, 1961, 1979; Luria, 1966). These three subtypes could be thought of as secondary acalculias, in which deficits in arithmetic are caused by a broader cognitive deficit that would produce other symptoms. In contrast, the fourth subtype, called "semantic dyscalculia" or "primary anarithmia," is considered to be a primary acalculia. It is characterized by a pure deficit in the understanding of numerical quantity and is associated with lesions of the left inferior parietal sulcus, which is immediately posterior to the angular gyrus (Dehaene, 2003). The conclusion that it is primary and specific is based on performance dissociations across patients with acquired lesions, and on neuroimaging data of typical individuals performing mathematical tasks (Dehaene, 2003).

This list of acquired subtypes of acalculia makes it clear that there are multiple cognitive components of arithmetic operations. Since mathematics includes a great deal more than arithmetic, there are quite likely to be different kinds of mathematics disorders beyond arithmetic disorders, but most research on acquired acalculia and on developmental mathematics disorder (MD) has focused on problems with arithmetic. Even when MD is restricted to problems with arithmetic, analyzing it is inevitably much more complicated than analyzing a disorder like dyslexia, where the impaired skill (recognition of printed words) is much narrower.

As is true for dyslexia, LI, and DCD, initial work on developmental problems with arithmetic was heavily based on earlier work with acquired disorders. So the initial name for MD was "developmental dyscalculia." This term was introduced by Kosc (1974), who did the first systematic study of children with arithmetic problems. Since then, considerable research has been done on MD, which is reviewed in the following sections.

DEFINITION

DSM-IV-TR (American Psychiatric Association, 2000) defines MD as a substantial discrepancy between a child's performance on individually administered tests of math skills and what is expected in children of similar age, intelligence, and education. In addition, this skill deficit must be associated with functional impairment. If a sensory disorder is present, the math problems must exceed what might be expected from the sensory disorder alone.

This definition, like that of DCD, requires both age and IQ discrepancy, but adds the requirement of education discrepancy. The logic of this third discrepancy is that math, like reading, depends on instruction, and that failure in math because of inadequate instruction is not a disorder. As is the case with many other DSM diagnoses, the degree of discrepancy is not operationally defined. And as with most other learning disorders considered in this book, the diagnostic cutoff is somewhat arbitrary, because the relevant skills are normally distributed. In studies of MD (reviewed in Butterworth, 2005), typical cutoffs have ranged from the 25th to the 35th percentile, usually with an IQ cutoff (e.g., 80).

EPIDEMIOLOGY AND COMORBIDITIES

Using definitions of this sort, several population studies have found prevalences of 3–6.5% for MD (Shalev & Gross-Tsur, 2001). In Gross-Tsur, Manor, and Shalev's (1996) study of an Israeli population, a two-stage procedure was used. First, a citywide screening of over 3,000 children ages 10–11 identified those scoring in the bottom 20% on a group-administered arithmetic achievement test. This group of roughly 600 children were then given individual IQ and math assessments. Those obtaining an IQ greater than or equal to 80, and scoring at or below the mean of children two grades younger, were classified as having developmental dyscalculia (MD). There were 140 such children (4.6% of the original 3,000), with a nearly equal male–female ratio (1.1:1).

So the prevalence of MD in this and other studies (6.3% in Badian, 1983; 3.6% in Lewis, Hitch, & Walker, 1994) is higher than the 1% figure cited in DSM-IV-TR, which is based on clinic samples. The explanation for this discrepancy could be that children with isolated MD are less likely to be referred. In my clinical experience, it is much rarer for our clinic to see a child with specific MD than with specific RD.

Comorbidities

From the subtypes of acquired acalculia discussed earlier, one would expect cases of MD to be comorbid with language, spatial (e.g., NVLD), or attention problems. Indeed, there are elevated rates of comorbidity between MD and LI, RD, and ADHD in epidemiological studies, and studies of MD without RD find associated spatial problems (as reviewed in Chapter 13 on NVLD). Manor, Shalev, Joseph, and Gross-Tsur (2001) found that 26% of children with LI were later diagnosed with MD. In the Gross-Tsur et al. (1996) study, 17% of the children with MD also had RD, and 26% also had ADHD, leaving 57% with MD without RD or ADHD. Badian (1983) found that 43% of her sample of children with MD also had RD, and that 52% of her sample of children with RD also had MD. Badian's (1983) study did not address comorbid ADHD. Lewis et al. (1994) found that 64% of their sample with MD also had RD, and that 37% of their sample with RD also had MD. Although the estimates vary across these studies from different countries, they all agree on the comorbidity of MD and RD, and on the existence of a substantial number of children with MD but without RD. So specific and possibly primary MD appears to exist and thus requires a neuropsychological explanation.

ETIOLOGY[1]

There is evidence that MD is familial and heritable, but there is much less research on its etiology than on most of the other learning disorders covered in this book. Shalev, Manor, and Kerem (2001) found a sibling relative risk (lambda) of 5–10, which is in the range found for most learning disorders.

Using a twin design, we (Alarcon, DeFries, Light, & Pennington, 1997) found that MD was heritable. This study used the DeFries–Fulker regression method to examine the heritability of the group deficit in probands selected for either MD only or MD + RD. Of all probands who met the criteria for MD, 58% also met criteria for RD, which is a rate of comorbidity similar to that found in other English-speaking samples (Badian, 1983; Lewis et

---

[1]For a description of genetic technical terms, see Box 1.1 in Chapter 1.

al., 1994). The heritability value for MD overall was significant (.38 ± .18). When the sample was divided by proband subtype (MD + RD vs. MD only), the resulting heritability values were .41 ± .21 and .32 ± .37, respectively, indicating a somewhat greater heritability for MD + RD. In a separate study, Light and DeFries (1995) found significant bivariate heritability for RD and MD in the same twin sample. Subsequent studies have replicated this finding of heritability of MD (e.g., Haworth, Kovas, Petrill, & Plomin, 2007). In sum, there is evidence that MD is familial and heritable, and that some of the genetic influences on MD are shared with genetic influences on RD. In addition, there are also two genetic syndromes that produce MD as part of their phenotype, Turner syndrome and FXS in females; these are discussed in Chapter 13.

This evidence for genetic influences on MD converges with several studies (Haworth et al., 2007; Knopik & DeFries, 1999; Thompson, Detterman, & Plomin, 1991; Wadsworth, DeFries, Fulker, & Plomin, 1995) that have found heritability for typical individual differences in mathematics (e.g., .62–.75 in Haworth et al., 2007, and .67 in Knopik & DeFries, 1999). Likewise, there is also evidence for shared genetic influences on typical individual differences in mathematics and reading skills (Knopik & DeFries, 1999; Light, DeFries, & Olson, 1998), similar to what Light and DeFries (1995) found for low mathematics and reading scores. Knopik and DeFries (1999) found that 58% of the covariation between reading and math composite scores was due to genetic influences shared by reading and math. The study by Light et al., (1998) examined which cognitive factors accounted for the covariation between reading and math scores. They found that verbal IQ and nonword-reading ability accounted for most of this covariation, and that this relation was genetically mediated in both probands with RD and controls.

So both MD and individual differences in math across the entire distribution are moderately heritable and share genetic influences with reading and language measures. It would be valuable to examine whether there is distinct genetic covariation between MD and spatial or executive skills. A positive finding would provide some additional external validity for these hypothesized subtypes of MD.

In sum, MD has several identified genetic influences, including polygenic influences on low math scores (Alarcon et al., 1997) and two genetic syndromes, Turner syndrome and FXS in females. The association between RD and MD seems to be largely genetically mediated and acts through both phonological and broader language skills. Taken together, the genetic research reviewed here provides some validity for three subtypes of MD—a language-related form comorbid with RD, a spatial subtype found in Turner syndrome, and an attentional/executive subtype found in females with FXS—but more work is needed to validate these subtypes.

BRAIN MECHANISMS[2]

What we know about brain mechanisms in MD is limited by the scarcity of neuroimaging studies of MD itself. On the other hand, we do know a fair amount about the brain mechanisms that mediate skill in mathematics in adults, and this research is reviewed by Dehaene (2003) and Shalev and Gross-Tsur (2001). The adult research includes dissociations found among patients with acquired brain lesions, neuroimaging studies of nondisabled subjects, and neuroimaging studies of patients with dyscalculia (including females with Turner syndrome). Because mathematics can be selectively spared or impaired when a lesion impairs reading, language, or semantics for nonmathematical content, dyscalculia researchers argue for some specificity to the neural structures mediating mathematical performance in adults. Of course, there are alternative explanations for seeming content-based dissociations (Farah, 2003; Van Orden, Pennington, & Stone, 2001). So these dissociations may not actually localize modules for mathematics in general or for component mathematical operations.

According to Dehaene (2003), these results indicate that a distributed bilateral cortical network involving portions of the parietal and frontal lobes supports mathematical operations, such that different localized lesions in this network are associated with impaired performance on different mathematical tasks. As mentioned earlier, one key brain region in this network appears to be the left inferior parietal region posterior to the angular gyrus. As reviewed by Dehaene (2003), this region is activated in typical adults performing arithmetic calculations or comprehending the magnitude of a number, regardless of input or output modality, or even awareness of a numerical stimulus. Moreover, activity is proportional to difficulty, whether indexed by number of calculations, size of numbers involved, or numerical distance between them (in a comparison task). Patients with acquired lesions to this left inferior parietal region have severe deficits in even simple calculations or numerical comparisons, and are said to have "pure semantic acalculia," which is also called "primary anarithmia." The one patient with developmental dyscalculia or MD who has been studied with neuroimaging (magnetic resonance spectroscopy) had a localized abnormal signal overlapping this inferior parietal region in the left hemisphere (Levy, Levy, & Grafman, 1999). On the basis of all these data, Dehaene (2003) argues that this bilateral inferior parietal region supports the semantic representation and manipulation of numerical quantity, which he labels "numerical intuition" or a "mental number line."

The importance of bilateral parietal structures for arithmetic is also supported by neuroimaging studies of females with Turner syndrome. These

---

[2]For a description of neuroanatomical technical terms, see Box 1.2 in Chapter 1.

studies have found abnormalities in bilateral parietooccipital areas, both with structural (Murphy, DeCarli, & Daly, 1993; Reiss et al., 1993; Reiss, Mazzocco, Greenlaw, Freund, & Ross, 1995) and with functional (Clark, Klonoff, & Hadyen, 1990) scans.

Although this convergence of evidence is impressive, we still need a computational model of how this inferior parietal region accomplishes these functions and what its inputs and outputs are. In addition, there may be portions of adjacent parietal cortex or other parts of the brain that are also sensitive to numerical quantity, so the "mental number line" may not be as localized as Dehaene (2003) argues.

The other brain region identified by Dehaene (2003) is the inferior frontal cortex on both sides. It is more activated by larger exact language-dependent calculations, such as multiplication, whereas the inferior parietal site is more important for approximation.

NEUROPSYCHOLOGY

Like studies of RD, studies of MD have benefited from a mature developmental and cognitive science—in this case, a science of mathematical skill. Interest in the development of mathematical concepts was stimulated by the seminal studies of Piaget (1952). More recent research (e.g., Geary, 1994; Gelman & Gallistel, 1986; Wynn, 1998) has given us a clearer understanding of the roots of mathematical knowledge in infancy and its development through the acquisition of counting skills and calculation strategies.

This normative developmental framework has been used to analyze the performance of children with MD (Butterworth, 2005; Geary, Hoard, Byrd-Craven, & DeSoto, 2004). Although children with MD have often learned number names and some aspects of counting procedures, there is evidence that their core understanding of numerosity or cardinality is impaired, which is reminiscent of the deficit found in semantic acalculia (Dehaene, 2003) discussed earlier. This evidence includes (1) a study by Koontz and Berch (1996), which found that children with MD have a decreased ability to "subitize" (i.e., automatically recognize the numerosity of small sets of three or fewer items without counting them); (2) a study by Landerl, Bevan, and Butterworth (2004), which found slower reaction times on tests of dot counting and number magnitude comparison in children with MD than in either children with dyslexia or typical controls; and (3) a study by Geary, Hanson, and Hoard (2000), which found small decreases in the accuracy of number magnitude comparisons in first graders with MD.

This impairment in the core understanding of numerosity would be expected to undermine later development of counting and calculation strategies, and the evidence is consistent with that view. Gelman and Gallistel

(1986) have described the five implicit principles of counting that typical children learn. These principles are one-to-one correspondence (also called "itemizing"), stable order of counting names, "cardinality" (the fact that the last-counted number is the cardinal magnitude of the set), "abstraction" (the fact that any set of items can be counted), and "order irrelevance" (the fact that the same cardinal number is achieved, regardless of the order of the count). The abstraction and order irrelevance principles are not necessary for practical success at counting, and young children sometimes deduce two nonessential counting principles that contradict order irrelevance—namely, a "standard direction" principle (e.g., counts have to start at the left side of a set) and an "adjacency" principle (i.e., counts must proceed from one contiguous item to the next).

As reviewed by Geary et al. (2004), first- and second-grade children with MD + RD or with MD only were able to identify violations of the first three counting principles (one-to-one correspondence, stable order, cardinality) but were more likely than their typical agemates to endorse the nonessential adjacency principle, and in first grade were less likely to detect double counts of the first item. Importantly, children with RD (but not MD) did not differ from typical controls, which means that these counting problems were not secondary to RD.

Clearly, problems with an understanding of numerosity and counting principles may lead to problems with arithmetic. Typical children initially solve simple sums by counting all the items in both addends, then learn to count up from the larger addend, and then start to solve harder sums by reducing them to simpler ones (e.g., 6 + 5 = 5 + 5 + 1). This sequence reflects an increasing understanding of the relations among number facts, as well as increased use of memory-based strategies for remembering. Eventually, typical children master all their number facts and do not have to rely on counting.

As reviewed by Geary et al. (2004), it has been found in several countries that children with MD + RD or with MD only make more counting errors in simple calculations and persist in simpler counting strategies (e.g., counting all) longer than controls do. Most dramatically, both children with MD + RD and those with MD only are much worse than typical controls at learning their math facts and applying them automatically—a deficit that is still present at the end of elementary school. Although both groups with MD perform worse on these skills than a group with RD only, the group with MD + RD is more impaired than the group with MD only. So while RD does not appear to cause MD in the comorbid group, it may exacerbate it. It is well known that many children with RD are poor at memorizing math facts, presumably due to their poor phonological memory. It would be useful for future research to test whether some children with MD have problems with memorizing math facts that cannot be accounted for by problems in phonological memory.

At the level of number, counting, and arithmetic skills, there is considerable empirical support for the typical and atypical developmental trajectories just presented. However, because the data come from different studies at different ages, we do not have strong evidence that early numerosity problems cause inefficient counting or that both of these undermine mastery of math facts. But these are certainly plausible hypotheses that need to be tested.

Where there is less agreement in the field of MD is whether MD is primary—namely, a core deficit in numerosity per se (e.g., Butterworth, 2005)—or secondary to a more general deficit in verbal working memory or spatial cognition (Geary et al., 2004). So we do not know whether the neuropsychological explanation of MD lies within the domain of number itself or whether it is secondary to a more general cognitive problem. Similarly, it is uncertain whether there are valid neuropsychological subtypes of MD, such as the traditional subtypes of acquired dyscalculia discussed earlier, although there is some initial evidence supporting such subtypes.

DIAGNOSIS AND TREATMENT

The DSM-IV-TR diagnosis of MD requires an IQ test and an individually administered mathematics achievement test (e.g., the Woodcock–Johnson III). The achievement test must contain math subtests that assess both knowledge and automaticity of math facts and math problem solving. Given the research discussed earlier, careful observation of the process by which a child solves problems, including the child's use of counting strategies and the automaticity of his or her math facts, should be helpful.

Since MD is frequently comorbid with LI, RD, and ADHD, these disorders should be ruled in or out in a child suspected of having MD, since they may modify the severity, nature, and treatment of MD. Shalev and Gross-Tsur (2001) also advise screening for medical illnesses (e.g., epilepsy) and genetic syndromes (e.g., Turner syndrome or FXS in females).

In regard to treatment, there has been very little research. One pilot study (Kaufmann, Handl, & Thony, 2003) found that a treatment program focused on basic understanding of the numerical concepts discussed earlier benefited the calculation skills of children with MD.

CHAPTER 13

Nonverbal Learning Disability

HISTORY AND DEFINITION

The field of learning disabilities has long recognized that a small number of children present with what is called "right-hemisphere learning disability" or "nonverbal learning disability" (NVLD) (Denckla, 1979, 1983; Rourke, 1989; Rourke & Finlayson, 1978; Rourke & Strang, 1978; Semrud-Clikeman & Hynd, 1990; Tranel, Hall, Olson, & Tranel, 1987; Weintraub & Mesulam, 1983). In these accounts, problems with math, handwriting, and social cognition are all viewed as part of the same right-hemisphere syndrome. But math and handwriting deficits are already covered by other diagnoses (see Chapters 11 and 12), and social-cognitive deficits are covered by ASD (see Chapter 8). So a key issue is whether NVLD is a distinct disorder. In other words, NVLD is less well-validated than all the other disorders in Part II, but we include it here because it is better validated than the two disorders in Chapter 4, CAPD and SMD.

Moreover, although the co-occurrence of these symptoms in some patients is indisputable, it is nevertheless conceptually clearer to consider deficits in either math or handwriting separately from deficits in social cognition. In our clinical experience, there are certainly children who present with specific deficits in math and/or handwriting without deficits in social cognition. Conversely, there are patients with clearer social-cognitive deficits who do not have math or handwriting problems. Moreover, adult studies in both nondisordered individuals and patients with acquired brain lesions support the dissociability of spatial and social cognition (Bryden & Ley, 1983; Etcoff, 1984).

Another name for the hypothesized learning disorder discussed here is "developmental Gerstmann syndrome" (Benson & Geschwind, 1970;

Kinsbourne & Warrington, 1963); this is named by analogy with "acquired Gerstmann syndrome," in which there are deficits in calculation, spelling, finger position knowledge, and right–left discrimination. This constellation of symptoms has been considered a left parietal lobe syndrome, but, as discussed in Chapter 5, Benton (1961, 1977, 1992) found that these four symptoms did not co-occur with any greater frequency than they did with other symptoms of left parietal lobe damage. NVLD may have the same problem, namely that its defining symptoms do not co-occur distinctly enough to justify calling NVLD a syndrome. Moreover, the construct of Gerstmann syndrome suggests a left hemisphere locus for the symptoms of NVLD, whereas more recent evidence suggests that specific developmental problems in math and handwriting (but not reading) are more likely to result from right-hemisphere dysfunction.

Another definitional issue concerns what kind of specific math or handwriting disorders characterize NVLD. In Chapter 6, my colleagues and I discuss the frequent co-occurrence of math and handwriting problems with developmental dyslexia. Although the reasons for handwriting problems in dyslexia are not well understood, it does not appear to reflect a spatial processing problem, but rather a linguistic or motor sequencing problem. The math problems found in children with dyslexia are of a different sort from those found in children without reading and spelling problems (Rourke, 1989; Strang & Rourke, 1985b). Briefly, children with dyslexia have trouble memorizing math facts and understanding "word" problems because of their reading problem. Sometimes they missequence numbers they write, but they usually do not have basic conceptual problems with mathematical understanding. In contrast, nondyslexic children with poor math performance appear to have fundamental conceptual problems in understanding mathematics. In some of these children, these conceptual problems appear to be secondary to a deficit in right-hemisphere spatial cognition. This distinction is also supported by the adult clinical literature, in which math and handwriting deficits are frequent concomitants of acquired aphasia, but can occur as a consequence of lesions in non-language-related areas that do not produce aphasia (Hecaen & Albert, 1978; Luria, 1966). With these definitional points clearly in mind, let us examine what is known about NVLD or right-hemisphere learning disability.

EPIDEMIOLOGY

Rourke (1989) estimated the prevalence of NVLD within a learning disability clinic sample to be only 5–10%; this is considerably less than the prevalence of either dyslexia or ADHD, which together would account for the large majority of such clinic samples. Denckla (1979) found a somewhat lower prevalence: 1% of patients in a learning disability clinic sample of 484 cases. So NVLD is a rare disorder.

ETIOLOGY[1]

Aside from an association with two specific genetic syndromes, Turner syndrome and FXS (see Chapters 8 and 10) in females, little is known about possible genetic or environmental causes of NVLD. There are no family, twin, adoption, segregation, or linkage studies of NVLD.

Both math and handwriting problems are found in girls with Turner syndrome, who do not have reading problems (Money, 1973; Pennington, Bender, Puck, Salbenblatt, & Robinson, 1982). Turner syndrome is caused by nondisjunction during meiosis of the paired X chromosomes, resulting in a gamete with no X chromosome. If such a gamete is involved in a successful conception and birth, a phenotypically female individual with only one X chromosome (45,X) is the result.

In terms of cognitive phenotype, individuals with Turner syndrome tend to have depressed nonverbal IQs and problems with a variety of visual–spatial tasks (Alexander & Money, 1966; Cohen, 1966; Garron, 1977; Shaffer, 1962). Although their pattern of deficits is often interpreted as due to selective right-hemisphere dysfunction (Christensen & Nielsen, 1981; Silbert, Wolff, & Lilienthal, 1977), several neuropsychological studies have found deficits on a wider range of tasks (McGlone, 1985; Pennington et al., 1985; Waber, 1979). These latter studies support the interpretation that the brain dysfunction in Turner syndrome is better described either as diffuse or as predominantly (but not exclusively) nonverbal, rather than as involving focal right-hemisphere dysfunction. The same caveat should be borne in mind when other examples of "right-hemisphere learning disability" are considered.

Interestingly, problems in affective discrimination and psychosocial adjustment have been found in girls with Turner syndrome (McCauley, Kay, Ito, & Treder, 1987), and these were not simply attributable to the girls' short stature. So it is possible that Turner syndrome is one cause of NVLD.

The other genetic syndrome with a phenotype similar to NVLD also involves the X chromosome: FXS in females. Briefly, the similarities to NVLD are deficits in executive functions, worse problems in math than in reading and spelling, intact structural language but impaired pragmatic language, and social anxiety and shyness. In summary, both Turner syndrome and FXS in females appear to be possible genetic causes of what is called NVLD.

---

[1] For a description of genetic technical terms, see Box 1.1 in Chapter 1.

In regard to environmental causes, there are also few data. Weintraub and Mesulam (1983) discussed etiology in their 14 cases; they found evidence for an acquired insult in 9 of these (e.g., infantile hemiplegia, perinatal complication, or early-onset nonfamilial seizure disorders). Such acquired insults were only present in 1 of the 11 cases reported by Tranel et al. (1987). Rourke (1989) lists several other possible etiologies of NVLD, including moderate to severe closed head injury (presumably early in development), unsuccessfully treated hydrocephalus, cranial radiation, and congenital absence of the corpus callosum. Only the last etiology is developmental. So it appears that acquired brain damage may produce NVLD, as well as two known genetic syndromes. But the evidence for idiopathic NVLD apart from ASD (see Chapter 8) or MD (see Chapter 13) is virtually nil.

BRAIN MECHANISMS[2]

There are very few data in the area of brain mechanisms for NVLD as well, so more direct validation of the right-hemisphere hypothesis regarding NVLD is needed. Voeller's (1986) study addressed the issue of brain mechanisms most directly. She selected 15 children with right-hemisphere findings on neurological exam and/or computed tomography (CT) scan from a clinic population of 600 children referred for a pediatric neurological exam. Thus her sample, unlike others in this area, began with patients identified according to a neurological criterion and then studied their behavioral and neuropsychological characteristics, which turned out to be similar to those reported in other studies of right-hemisphere learning disability. These results provide partial validation of the right-hemisphere hypothesis—"partial" because her sample was not an unbiased sample of children in the general population with right-hemisphere neurological findings. Quite conceivably, there could be such children with right-hemisphere neurological findings who have not come to clinical attention and do not have the social and behavioral difficulties characteristic of this syndrome. Neurological tests were also reported for the Weintraub and Mesulam (1983) and Tranel et al. (1987) samples. In the former, these were motor signs on the left, especially asymmetrical left-arm posturing during complex gait, found in 12 of 14 patients. In Tranel et al. (1987), only 2 of 11 patients had asymmetrical motor findings, and none had any abnormalities on CT scan. Five of seven EEGs in this study had mild diffuse abnormalities—a finding that does not differentiate these patients from groups with ADHD or other learning disorders. Modern neuroimaging techniques would be interesting to pursue in patients with

---

[2]For a description of neuroanatomical technical terms, see Box 1.2 in Chapter 1.

these disorders, and would provide a better test of the hypothesized right-hemisphere localization.

NEUROPSYCHOLOGY

The neuropsychological hallmark of NVLD is a significant verbal IQ > non-verbal IQ discrepancy. As discussed above, these children show weaknesses in visual–spatial skills and social cognition. They show strengths in verbal tasks; indeed, children with the NVLD profile are often good readers. However, their reading strengths tend to be in word decoding, whereas they may show weaknesses in reading comprehension.

For the symptoms of NVLD to make sense, there needs to be a connection between deficient visual–spatial skills and social deficits. Rourke (1989) argues that the same underlying right-hemisphere neuropsychological disorder leads to both the cognitive and social deficits in NVLD. In Rourke's (1989) model, the disruption of right-hemisphere functioning is caused by early damage or dysfunction in white matter connections, especially long white matter connections important for intermodal integration, for which the right hemisphere is specialized. In contrast, left-hemisphere functional development is hypothesized to be less vulnerable to white matter dysfunction, and thus more likely to be spared.

But, the social deficits found in NVLD could be correlated symptoms that are not related in a causal way to the deficient visual–spatial skills. Arguing for this possibility are data indicating that the processing mechanisms in the right hemisphere that mediate spatial cognition are dissociable from those that mediate social cognition. Developmental insults to the right hemisphere may frequently impair both sets of mechanisms, producing the observed correlation between deficits in each area that are found in the studies just reviewed. In at least two of these studies, subjects were selected in part because they exhibited this pattern of correlated deficits, so we really do not know in an objective way what the extent of the correlation is. In our clinical experience, there are certainly children with specific math and handwriting problems who do not have deficits in social cognition.

DEVELOPMENTAL COURSE

There has been only one small ($N = 8$) adult follow-up study of children with NVLD (Rourke, Young, Strang, & Russell, 1986). In that study, the outcomes were poor: All of the subjects exhibited continuing emotional and social difficulties and were working in jobs below their educational level. Some had been diagnosed with schizophrenia as adults. These results are consistent with the kinds of problems found in the adult patients described by Tranel et al. (1987) and Weintraub and Mesulam (1983). Rourke (1989) reports that although children with NVLD may present with characteristics of ADHD in the early school years, their clinical symptoms switch to internalizing ones later, including a higher rate of suicidal behavior in adolescence.

Because the subjects in all these studies were ascertained clinically, we really do not know what proportion of children with visual–spatial deficits have (and do not have) concomitant social and emotional problems, and what proportion of each of these groups has social and emotional problems as adults. We do know that the adult outcome of patients with Turner syndrome, who have visual–spatial deficits, is quite like that of typical individuals in many cases, so the same dissociation is likely to hold in idiopathic cases of NVLD.

In terms of early development, the only data available are from retrospective case histories. Strang and Rourke (1985a) summarized these data; they reported greater delays in motor than in language milestones; decreased exploratory activity; hypoactivity, echolalia, and other pragmatic deficiencies in language usage; hyperlexia in some cases; poor peer relations; and overdependency on parents. This type of early history is reminiscent of that seen in children with higher-functioning autism or Asperger syndrome. Once again, we are faced with the issue of the degree of overlap between NVLD and ASD. Rourke (1989) believes that what he calls NVLD and Asperger syndrome overlap considerably, whereas he views autism as distinct because of the greater language pathology in most autistic children.

In a later study, Rourke and colleagues (Klin, Volkmar, Sparrow, Cicchetti, & Rourke, 1995) applied Rourke's diagnostic criteria for NVLD to a series of cases previously diagnosed by clinical experts as having Asperger syndrome. They found a very high rate of NVLD in the sample of individuals with Asperger syndrome. This suggests that Rourke's syndrome of NVLD may be equivalent to Asperger syndrome, in which case we do not need both categories. Clinicians attempting to make a differential diagnosis between NVLD and Asperger syndrome or high-functioning autism (M. T. Stein, Klin, & Miller, 2004) may be faced with an impossible task.

SUMMARY OF VALIDITY OF NVLD

So it appears that the NVLD profile can be found in many children with Asperger syndrome or high-functioning autism, although it has yet to be determined whether the overlap between ASD and NVLD is so large that NVLD is a redundant diagnostic category. Children with developmental problems in spatial cognition and relatively normal social cognition, such as girls with Turner syndrome, would need to be placed in a different diagnostic category, such as MD. A different diagnosis from NVLD for girls with Turner syndrome is justified by their distinct developmental trajectory. The early development of children with Turner syndrome (Berch & Bender, 1990; Robinson, Lubs, & Bergson, 1979) is different from the early developmental profile of children with NVLD just presented. These girls do not have motor milestone delays, echolalia or other obvious pragmatic deficiencies, or the kinds of social problems exhibited by children with NVLD.

To conclude, much more needs to be known about the developmental course of children with visual–spatial deficits, the academic difficulties they have, and the degree to which they are at risk for social deficits and poor adult outcome. To answer these questions, prospective studies of unselected samples of children with visual–spatial problems are needed.

It needs to be emphasized that a child with a large verbal IQ > nonverbal IQ disparity does not necessarily have a disorder, even if his or her spatial skills are significantly below the mean. There is wide variation in spatial skills in the typical population, and not all apparent spatial deficits cause functional impairment. So, unless a child's spatial deficit is associated with functional impairment in academic or social skills, no disorder is present.

In sum, we do not yet have sufficient evidence to accept NVLD as a valid learning disorder apart from either ASD, MD, or DCD all of which are covered in the DSM-IV-TR (ASD in the category of PDDs).

PART III

IMPLICATIONS FOR PRACTICE AND POLICY

This last section of the book considers what needs to be done to translate the emerging science of learning disorders into practice. In the chapters on specific disorders, my collaborators and I have already identified the gaps in existing knowledge that future research needs to fill, and I am cautiously optimistic that future research *will* fill these gaps. But I think that concerted new efforts need to be mobilized to translate the existing science of learning disorders into practice and policy.

Chapter 14 first considers general issues that have impeded this translation, and then discusses how the spread of evidence-based practice (EBP) is transforming practice and policy. Chapter 15 demonstrates how research can be fruitfully applied to practice by critiquing controversial therapies. The discussion of less well-validated learning disorders in Chapter 4 is also relevant to the issue of EBP. In addition, both Chapters 14 and 15 touch on public policy issues as they emerge in this discussion.

CHAPTER 14

Evidence-Based Practice
Barriers and Benefits

This chapter first considers barriers to applying science to practice and policy in the field of learning disorders. It then describes what evidence-based practice (EBP) is and how it can transform practice and policy in the field of learning disorders. The first barrier is essentially human gullibility.

SCIENCE VERSUS DOGMA

Humans, including clinicians, are notoriously susceptible to questionable or even false beliefs and practices, which can easily become fads or dogmas. Once a questionable belief or practice is advocated by an authority, it is quickly imitated by followers and transmitted to others. We humans are a uniquely successful species because of the benefits of cultural transmission, but cultural transmission can also be a liability. The ease of accepting the "argument from authority," compared to the effort involved in testing beliefs, means that we are quite likely to be susceptible to false claims. This is all the more true when we are faced with threats to our well-being, such as the threats posed by disease and disability.

A number of excellent books have been written about our susceptibility to mistaken beliefs, including Carl Sagan's (1995) *The Demon-Haunted World* and Michael Shermer's (1997) *Why People Believe Weird Things: Pseudoscience, Superstition, and Other Confusions of Our Time*. Because every human shares this susceptibility, the first steps in scientific training are skepticism about and critical analysis of beliefs, especially our own pet theories. What we think we have seen with our own eyes can easily turn out to be wrong. As Karl Popper (1959) pointed out, the proper goal of science is to falsify hypotheses, not to confirm them. Those hypotheses that cannot be falsified are tentatively held to be true. Because every individual observer is fallible, we only count as true those observations that can be replicated across multiple observers.

Consequently, the history of science is filled with disproven beliefs: The earth is flat; the sun revolves around the earth; the speed of a falling object varies with its weight; life spontaneously generates from mud; vapors spread disease; and so on. Similarly, the history of science is filled with discarded constructs, such as phlogiston (the hypothesized substance underlying combustion), ether (the medium for the transmission of light), and absolute simultaneity (which depends on absolute as opposed to relative time). Each of these beliefs and constructs embody theories about how the world works, and each was firmly held to be true or real by some or all of the best minds of the day. It took careful logical analysis and rigorous experiments to show that these beliefs were false and that these constructs were not real.

Similarly, most of the history of medicine is prescientific and is filled with disproven beliefs and erroneous practices. Everyone has heard of the use of leeches and other methods to bleed patients, but they may not realize how drastic this practice was. Some early distinguished physicians, like Benjamin Rush, attempted to drain 80% of the body's blood, often killing the patient (Vyse, 2005).

Two of the greatest scientists in the history of medicine, William Harvey (1578–1657) and Thomas Willis (1621–1675), were also general practitioners. They pioneered the use of empirical methods to learn how the heart circulates blood (Harvey) and to describe the anatomy of the brain (Willis). But as clinicians, they used treatments from the time of Galen (who lived in the 2nd century C.E.) in their clinical work (Zimmer, 2004). Faced with a patient with what we now know as tuberculosis, Willis bled him with leeches and prescribed the following: a roasted apple stuffed with frankincense and candy, the milk of an ass mixed with rose water, and a bowl of turtle soup (Zimmer, 2004, p. 104). This prescription is an early example of polypharmacy. If the prescription actually worked, how would Willis have known which component (or components) made the difference? Willis also provided the first clinical case description of a patient with psychosis associated with bipolar disorder, but his medical treatment of her now seems barbaric. To control her mania, he bound her with chains and ropes; bled her; gave her enemas; and had her drink a concoction of laudanum, barley, poppy flowers, and cardiac syrup. She died within days (Zimmer, 2004, p. 105). Thus, even as these two great English scientists helped lay the foundations of modern medicine during the 17th century, their clinical therapies were at least 1,500 years old.

The fourth example is much more recent. The famous biologist Lewis Thomas (1974) recalled in *Lives of a Cell: Notes of a Biology Watcher* that in his boyhood one could identify a doctor's house because of the presence of large stone balls in the front yard. In the early 20th century, a common treatment for abdominal pain was to place a heated stone sphere on the patient's stomach. When this treatment practice fell out of favor, physicians put these stone balls outside as garden decorations.

So these stories highlight several pertinent facts about the history of medical treatments: (1) They have been prescientific or unsubstantiated until very recently; (2) there is a long time lag between scientific discovery and its impact on practice; (3) even brilliant physicians have been susceptible to customary practices and treatment fads; and (4) faced with a suffering patient, there is considerable pressure on a clinician to do something, even something that harms the patient.

Although there have been many dramatic advances in the scientific understanding of medical diseases in the last 100 years or so, the lag or gap between science and practice remains. For most of the 20th century, physicians were trained in anatomy and physiology, but received little research training per se and relied mainly on observations from clinical experience to refine their diagnostic and treatment decisions. While clinical practice certainly refines certain skills, such as surgical ones, it is well known that such unsystematic observations can lead to biased beliefs about diagnosis and treatments (Dawes, 1994; Groopman, 2007). So we can still find unreliable diagnostic tests, mistaken diagnoses, and unsubstantiated treatments in the practice of modern medicine. As discussed later, the emphasis on evidence-based medicine in training physicians is actually quite recent, emerging only in the last few decades. One factor driving this new emphasis is economics: Medical care is less expensive and more effective if best practices are followed. So those institutions that pay for medical care, including health insurance companies and government agencies, now insist on empirically supported procedures to help contain medical costs. The same is true in the United Kingdom and Canada, where medical care is provided by a national health service.

But an even more important factor for the emergence of evidence-based medicine is the rapid accumulation of scientific research on diagnostic procedures and treatments. To be a competent modern physician, a practitioner must be able to critically evaluate these new research findings and incorporate them into practice (Evidence-Based Medicine Working Group, 1992).

So, if human susceptibility to mistaken beliefs has characterized much of the history of medicine, it is not too surprising to find mistaken beliefs and controversial therapies in the much younger field of learning disorders. Chapter 15 provides many examples of these. What is encouraging is that we already have much of the knowledge base and methods necessary to close this gap between science and practice in the field of learning disorders. Changes in training and policy that could accomplish this goal are discussed later.

But now let us consider a second impediment to applying science to practice in the field of learning disorders—namely, how worthwhile values can lead to dubious treatments.

HOW VALUES CAN MISLEAD PRACTICE

One of the founders of empirical science, Francis Bacon, distinguished facts from values, making it clear that science is only about facts. In other words, science describes what is, but practice and policy are concerned with what ought to be. Deciding what ought to be inevitably requires decisions about values.

How society cares for those with disabilities depends on its values and the resources it has to implement those values. A nomadic tribe with limited resources may not be able to care for disabled relatives, and some such societies have left these relatives to die. In any society, the most vulnerable members are susceptible to mistreatment and exploitation, even when prevailing values support humane treatment for all. So an alternative measure of a society's level of development is the degree to which it protects the rights of its weakest members. Although the United States has the largest gross domestic product of any country in the world, it scores lower on these alternative indices of development, such as promoting child health or caring for disabled persons. Therefore, an important value in the field of learning disorders in the United States (as elsewhere) is protecting the rights of those with disabilities.

Important progress was made in recognizing and legislating these rights in the 1970s in the United States, Canada, and Western Europe (Mazurek & Winzer, 1994). These advances grew out of the United Nations' endorsement of universal human rights in 1948 (due largely to the efforts of Eleanor Roosevelt) and to the civil rights movement of the 1950s and 1960s. The civil rights movement led to laws that protected ethnic minorities from discrimination, including such practices as segregated schooling. Subsequent laws in the 1970s did the same for people with disabilities, including reducing the segregation in their schooling. Before these laws were passed, children with certain disabilities (e.g., vision and hearing impairment, significant intellectual disability [ID], and cerebral palsy [CP]) did not attend public schools; instead, they were educated in special schools for those with each type of disability

In 1975, the Education for All Handicapped Children Act—the first version of the Individuals with Disabilities Education Act (IDEA)—became federal law in the United States. This landmark law involved several key changes in special education policy. These changes mandated the identification and evaluation of children with disabilities, and guaranteed an appropriate free public education and placement in the least restrictive environment. This legislation also stipulated the process by which a child suspected of having a disability would be evaluated to qualify for an individualized education program, and the rights and roles of the child's parents in this process (Hallenbeck & Kauffman, 1994). IDEA ended the segregated schooling of children with certain disabilities, and was an important step forward in the struggle for universal human rights.

A second key piece of legislation was the Americans with Disabilities Act (ADA), which was passed in 1990. ADA protects people with disabilities from discrimination in employment, accommodations, transportation, and telecommunications. Together, IDEA and ADA gave people with disabilities the same access to education, employment, and the wider world as people without disabilities. These laws led to an emphasis on the integration of people with disabilities into society through the provision of various accommodations.

Within special education, these developments have led to a doctrine of integration or "full inclusion." For instance, progress across countries in special education can be measured first by whether there is any special education, and second by the degree of integration in special education (Mazurek & Winzer, 1994). Some countries have very limited special education (e.g., South Africa and New Guinea); some have segregated special education (e.g., Japan, Russia, and Taiwan); and some have integrated special education (e.g., the Scandinavian countries, the United Kingdom, New Zealand, and the United States).

One can endorse the values embodied in these laws and international changes in the treatment of people with disabilities, but still question whether rigid adherence to the principle of full inclusion always leads to the best educational outcomes for children with disabilities. Full inclusion, at least at times, provides an example of how a noble value has become a dogma that impedes best practice.

Unfortunately, this and other dogmas have been buttressed by adaptation of a postmodern philosophy in schools of education. Howard and Silvestri (2005, p. 205), in a critique, summarize this philosophy as holding that "science is an antiquated and mechanistic approach" and that "quantitative methods that rely on logical positivism should be replaced with the qualitative methodologies of deconstruction and discourse." When applied to special education, this postmodern philosophy views disabilities as just socially constructed phenomena. On this view, what children with disabilities need most is social acceptance, and so accommodation and inclusion become more important than treatment. I hope that the data reviewed in the earlier chapters make it clear how ludicrous this postmodern conception of disabilities is. Disabilities are the results of real, physical brain differences, and these brain differences need scientifically based treatment just as any other physical illness does.

Consequently, debates about inclusion are some of the most divisive in the history of special education (Hallenbeck & Kauffman, 1994). Some advocates of full inclusion argue for an elimination of special education altogether, because any distinctions are discriminatory. But critics of this approach say that it mistakenly makes the place where education occurs the only relevant criterion, without considering its content or efficacy (Mock & Kauffman, 2005). Surveys of regular education teachers generally find that these teachers are uncomfortable with full inclusion, mainly because they have not been trained as special educators; research is also discouraging about whether it provides beneficial outcomes for children with disabilities (Mazurek & Winzer, 2005).

One of the problems with full-inclusion logic is that physical presence in a setting does not guarantee meaningful inclusion or participation. A child with autism may lack the very social and communicative skills necessary to participate in the interactions in a regular classroom. A child with ID may lack the language and/or cognitive skills to participate in these interactions. Their physical presence may provide a superficial measure of conformity to a worthwhile moral principle, while at the same time depriving them of the very interventions they need to be capable of genuine inclusion. So full inclusion is a good example of unintended consequences: An admirable value (of human rights for people with disabilities) has led to an educational dogma with potentially harmful results.

Some other examples of educational practices based more on dogmatic values than on empirical research are the repudiation of labeling and the whole-language approach to reading instruction. Giving labels to people with disabilities is mistrusted because it may lead to stereotyping and discrimination, but without accurate diagnoses it is hard to plan appropriate interventions, as previous chapters have explained. The whole-language approach embraces the admirable value that the goal of reading is learning about the world, not just decoding printed words. But, as discussed in Chapter 6, children need to learn decoding skills before they can read to learn.

EVIDENCE-BASED PRACTICE

So how can the field of learning disorders overcome these barriers to effective practice? I think that the example of EBP provides a very useful model. Although modern science has transformed our understanding of medical disorders, it has taken the more recent movement of evidence-based medicine to translate that science into practice. So this section briefly reviews the history of, and criteria for, EBP in both medicine and clinical psychology.

History of EBP

As reviewed by Spring (2007), the movement toward EBP began in the United States in the early 1900s with a survey by Abraham Flexner of all 155 American medical schools. This survey was initiated by the American Medical Association and sponsored by the Carnegie Foundation in order to standardize medical education and ensure quality in medical practice. After visiting all 155 schools, Flexner recommended in 1910 that the vast majority (124) be closed because they provided inadequate training. By the mid-1930s, more than half had actually shut down. Later reformers in American medicine have kept the focus on the persisting gap between science and practice, and have contributed to the emergence of EBP.

In the United Kingdom, Archibald Cochrane promoted important reforms in the National Health Service by implementing the use of randomized controlled trials to guide practice decisions. He reasoned that because health care funds are limited, they should only be spent to provide therapies whose efficacy has been proven in high-quality trials of this type. Doing otherwise would increase inequities in care, because money wasted on ineffective treatments for some would deprive other patients from receiving effective treatments. There is now an international voluntary organization named in his honor (The Cochrane Collaboration), dedicated to conducting and disseminating systematic reviews of randomized controlled trials (*www. cochrane.org*).

A third contributor to the EBP movement was David Sackett, a clinical epidemiologist in Canada. He and his colleagues developed a process by which medical practitioners could conduct EBP in real time. To make this process possible, innovations were needed in both medical training and access to the relevant research literature.

As reviewed by Spring (2007), the EBP model described by Sackett, Rosenberg, Gray, Haynes, and Richardson (1996) consists of three components: the best available research evidence bearing on the patient's problem; the clinical expertise of the health care provider; and the patient's individual characteristics, values, and preferences. The first component is paramount and provides the range of best practices that the provider can both recommend to the patient and help him or her understand and consider. So EBP is not equivalent to empirically supported therapies (ESTs); rather, data on ESTs constitute part of the first component of the clinical decision-making process in EBP. This EBP model has now been adapted by the fields of nursing, social work, and clinical psychology (see, e.g., American Psychological

Association, 2005). To understand the critical first component of EBP, it is important to understand how treatments are validated.

How Treatments Are Validated

There are well-established research designs for evaluating the efficacy of a treatment. One key requirement is a control group. Since people with disorders are by definition at the extremes of symptom dimensions, over time their symptoms may become less extreme, partly because of regression to the mean. Even though learning disorders are chronic conditions, children with learning disorders still develop. So, over time, their skills will improve and problematic behaviors may lessen. Consequently, without a control group, one cannot know whether changes in the treated group are due to the treatment or would have occurred anyway. A second key requirement is that participants must be randomly assigned to the treatment and control groups, and that random assignment must actually lead to equivalent groups. Without random assignment, treatment may be confounded with uncontrolled group characteristics. An important third requirement is to control for the expectations of both the experimenter and the participants. In a drug study, this is accomplished with double-blind trials of a treatment versus a placebo. To control for expectations in a behavioral treatment study, an experimental treatment must be contrasted with an alternative treatment of similar duration and intensity, but lacking the key "ingredient" of the experimental treatment. Otherwise, participants in the experimental treatment condition may outperform untreated controls because of a placebo effect and not because of the treatment itself. Those who implement the treatments should be monitored for the fidelity of implementation, and they should be unaware of the study's hypotheses. Moreover, participants should not know which is the experimental treatment. For some behavioral treatments, a crossover design can be used. In the second part of the study, the experimental group now gets the alternative treatment and the control group gets the experimental treatment. If the experimental treatment consistently outperforms the alternative treatment in a crossover design, that provides strong evidence of its efficacy.

Both beneficial and adverse treatment effects must be tested for statistical significance, and the treatment effect must be large enough to be clinically meaningful. Finally, and very importantly, the efficacy of the treatment must be replicated by other independent investigators besides the originator(s) of the treatment. If a new treatment is consistently replicated, and if the balance of beneficial versus adverse effects is acceptable, it is considered validated.

So it takes at least several years of rigorous scientific work to validate a new treatment, and validation goes through several stages. Therapies differ in their degree of empirical validation, but we do not accept them as completely validated until all the criteria discussed above are met.

Levels of Empirical Support

Nonetheless, it is useful to lay out the levels of empirical support that professional groups consider when evaluating a therapy. One such grading system (Table 14.1) has been proposed by the Agency for Healthcare Research and Quality of the U.S. Department of Health and Human Services (2000; West et al., 2002).

The empirical criteria outlined in the preceding section correspond to Level I evidence in this scheme. A therapy that has been adequately tested has either consistent negative or positive evidence from well-designed experimental treatment studies. For instance, the recommendations that certain hospitalized older patients take one baby aspirin a day to prevent heart attacks, and that older people receive the pneumonia vaccine, are based on positive Level I evidence; the noneffectiveness of taking vitamin C to prevent the common cold is supported by negative Level I evidence—a consistent lack of a treatment effect in well-designed studies.

If a treatment only has Level II evidence, more research is needed before it is either validated or invalidated. *So a treatment supported by Level II evidence is still experimental and not ready for clinical dissemination.* Most of the controversial therapies for learning disorders described in the next chapter do not even have Level II evidence in their favor; their support comes

TABLE 14.1. Scheme for Grading Strength of Evidence in Medical Research

Grade	Criteria
I	Evidence from studies of strong design; results are both clinically important and consistent, with minor exceptions at most; results are free from serious doubts about generalizability, bias, and flaws in research design. Studies with negative results have sufficiently large samples to have adequate statistical power.
II	Evidence from studies of strong design but there is some uncertainty due to inconsistencies or concern about generalizability, bias, research design flaws, or adequate sample size. Or, evidence consistent from studies using weaker designs.
III	Evidence from a limited number of studies of weaker design. Studies with strong design either have not been done or are inconclusive.
IV	Support solely from informed medical commentators based on clinical experience without substantiation from the published literature.

Note. From West et al. (2002, p. 71).

from either uncontrolled studies (Level III) or just clinical experience (Level IV).

Division 12 of the American Psychological Association (Chambless et al., 1998) proposed a similar set of criteria for empirically supported psychological interventions (Table 14.2), usually referred to as ESTs (see above). These criteria are virtually identical to the ones discussed earlier, but they specifically include well-replicated-single case designs, which are often utilized by scientists trained in applied behavioral analysis. As long as the single cases have been sampled adequately, criterion II (below) is scientifically justified.

TABLE 14.2. Criteria for Empirically Supported Psychological Interventions

Well-established treatments

  I. At least two good between-group design experiments demonstrating efficacy in one or more of the following ways:

    A. Superior (statistically significantly so) to pill or psychological placebo or to another treatment.

    B. Equivalent to an already established treatment in experiments with adequate sample sizes.

OR

  II. A large series of single-case design experiments ($N > 9$) demonstrating efficacy. These experiments must have:

    A. Used experimental designs and

    B. Compared the intervention to another treatment as above.

Further criteria for both I and II

  III. Experiments must be conducted with treatment manuals.

  IV. Characteristics of the client samples must be clearly specified.

  V. Effects must have been demonstrated by at least two different investigators or investigating teams.

Probably efficacious treatments

  I. Two experiments showing the treatment is superior (statistically significantly so) to a waiting-list control group.

OR

  II. One or more experiments meeting the well-established treatment criteria IA or IB, III, and IV, but not V.

OR

  III. A small series of single-case design experiments ($N \geq 3$) otherwise meeting the well-established treatment criteria.

Note. From Chambless et al. (1998, p. 4). Copyright 1998 by Division 12, American Psychological Association. Reprinted by permission.

How to Bring EBP to the Field of Learning Disorders

Because of the emergence of EBP in several health care fields (Spring, 2007), including medicine and clinical psychology, it will be easier to bring EBP to the treatment of learning disorders by all professionals. In what follows, I recommend changes in training and policy to accomplish this goal.

Training

In the fields of medicine and clinical psychology, future practitioners are being trained in the research skills necessary to evaluate new assessments and therapies. But the scientist-practitioner model has had much less impact in the fields of education, speech–language pathology (Koenig & Gunter, 2005), and occupational therapy, with the result that these fields are more susceptible to fad diagnoses and treatments.

A stronger emphasis on scientific training in both initial graduate education and continuing education could eventually address this problem. The accrediting bodies in these fields should require higher standards for scientific training in graduate and continuing education in these fields. This recommendation is particularly important for those in leadership positions in these fields. Decisions about educational and therapeutic intervention programs in schools and clinics should be made by policy makers with the relevant scientific training, sometimes in consultation with outside experts.

A "Food and Drug Administration" for Behavioral Assessments and Treatments?

Public money for education and health care funds much of the clinical work that is done with children with learning disorders. For many of these disorders, scarce public money does not begin to meet all the real clinical needs these children have. What is disturbing is that some of this scarce public money is wasted on controversial therapies. If there were greater accountability for how existing resources are spent, this public money could be used more effectively.

So it seems reasonable to demand greater accountability for public money spent on educational and clinical interventions for children with learning disorders. One way to accomplish this would be to set up a national agency that would evaluate behavioral assessments and treatments. Since some of the websites in Appendix B provide readily accessible research evaluations of treatments, including treatments of learning disorders, this accountability might be achieved by building on these existing resources.

A new medical treatment must be carefully evaluated by the U.S. Food and Drug Administration (FDA) before it is deemed safe and effective for clinical application. Health insurers, both private and public (e.g., Medicare, Medicaid, and the Child Health Insurance Program), do not ordinarily reimburse for treatments that have not been approved by the FDA. More generally, health insurers have rigorous and specific standards for what constitutes "reasonable and customary care" for various medical illnesses. Recently, Medicare and Medicaid have gone a step further and based reimbursement levels on performance, including whether doctors and hospitals are actually implementing proven therapies (e.g., administration of the pneumonia vaccine for hospitalized older patients).

There is nothing approaching this level of accountability in the diagnosis, treatment, and education of children with learning disorders. This was possibly justifiable in the past, when there was much less research on these topics, but it is not justifiable today. If an FDA-style national agency or some other clearinghouse were established to set science-based standards for the diagnosis, treatment, and education of children with learning disorders, then there would be much clearer guidance for how public dollars should be spent.

INTEGRATING THE SYSTEMS THAT SERVE CHILDREN WITH LEARNING DISORDERS

Learning disorders pose a considerable public health burden, because they are prevalent and chronic disorders, but public health policy for dealing with them is uneven and at times poorly integrated. There ought to be a seamless integration of the efforts of health care providers and educators to promote early identification and empirically validated treatment of learning disorders. Achieving this goal will require the previously discussed changes in training of professionals, and the regulation of behavioral assessments and treatments just discussed. It will also require implementation of better early screening for these disorders and better early intervention. Given the current educational and health care systems in the United States, these kinds of changes in public health policy sound hopelessly unrealistic and perhaps unattainably expensive. But such practices are already in place in other developed countries. Moreover, one of the lessons of other changes in public health policy (such as conducting early screening for phenylketonuria, putting fluoride in the drinking water, or vaccinating children for polio) is that they not only greatly reduce human suffering; they also save enormous amounts of money.

Health economists evaluate the impact of various disorders by estimating their "burden"—how much they reduce the productivity of affected individuals. A disorder's burden on society in terms of lost productivity is a function of the prevalence, severity, and chronicity of the disorder. One commonly used measure of burden is "disability-adjusted life years," which is the years of productive life lost to premature death or disability, adjusted for the severity and duration of the disorder. A wider notion of burden would include the costs of caring for individuals affected with that disorder.

The World Health Organization now issues regular reports on the global burden of disease. In some underdeveloped countries, malaria would have the highest disease burden in terms of disability-adjusted life years, because of the prevalence and chronicity of that disease in those countries. In contrast, Murray and Lopez (1996) found that in established market economies, where malaria and other infectious illnesses are less prevalent, cardiovascular conditions topped the list, accounting for 18.6% of the total burden. But mental illness ranked second, accounting for 15.4% of the total burden.

Murray and Lopez (1996) studied disease burden in adults and so did not consider the burden posed by learning disorders. Because of their prevalence, severity, chronicity, and cost of care, it is clear that learning disorders pose a considerable burden. For instance, epidemiologists have estimated the lifetime costs to society for a person with autism to be $4 million in 1998 dollars (Newschaffer & Curran, 2003). Even with a very conservative estimate of the prevalence of autism (say, 1 per 1,000), there would be about 300,000 affected individuals in the United States, with a total lifetime cost of over $1 trillion. Improvements in public health and educational policy could reduce this burden and be cost-effective. What would these improvements look like?

Currently the front line for identifying learning disorders consists of primary care pediatricians and school systems. Schools have procedures in place (i.e., early intervention, child find) for the early identification of more severe learning disorders, such as ID, CP, speech–language problems, and autism, but not for dyslexia or ADHD. Primary care pediatricians also screen for these and other disorders (e.g., CP, hearing loss, vision impairment), but they are often not extensively trained about other developmental disabilities or learning disorders. So one recommendation would be to increase the training of pediatricians in these areas. Another would be for schools to implement early screening for all learning disorders.

CHAPTER 15

Controversial Therapies

This chapter illustrates the principles of EBP (outlined in Chapter 14) by reviewing controversial therapies for learning disorders. This review is based partly on a very useful book, *Controversial Therapies for Developmental Disabilities* (Jacobson, Foxx, & Mulick, 2005a) and an earlier review of controversial therapies for learning disorders by Silver (1995).

In previous chapters, I have discussed the empirical support for most mainstream interventions for the learning disorders covered in this book. As the reader has probably noticed, not all treatments have reached Level I validation, suggesting that more research would be very beneficial. Nevertheless, these mainstream treatments have received better validation than the controversial therapies discussed further below.

There are many labels to describe treatments that promise more than they deliver, including "prescientific," "pseudoscientific," "unsubstantiated," "alternative," "quick fixes," "fads," "quackery," and even "snake oil." A somewhat more neutral term is "controversial therapies," which is the term used in this chapter. The essential characteristic of a controversial therapy is either that its efficacy has not been demonstrated in rigorous treatment studies, or that it has been tested scientifically and found not to work.

Although there are controversial therapies for every human disorder, the field of learning disorders has more than its share (Jacobson et al., 2005a), and new ones seem to appear every day. While there is an emerging science of learning disorders, it has not yet influenced some areas of practice very much at all. It seems ironic that controversial therapies for these well-validated learning disorders are perhaps even more prevalent than they were 20 years ago. Why should the field of learning disorders be particularly susceptible to controversial therapies?

Some of these reasons are reviewed by Vyse (2005). Although learning disorders are chronic neurodevelopmental conditions for which no cures are available, parents and sometimes practitioners hope for cures. So if available ESTs (as defined in Chapter 14) do not offer a cure, or at least as much improvement as parents and practitioners hope for, it is tempting to turn to a treatment that promises a cure or dramatic improvement. A second reason is that the best available treatment may be time-consuming and expensive, while some alternatives are quicker and cheaper.

A third important reason for the persistence of controversial therapies is the nature of the therapy "market" for behavioral interventions. First of all, a lot of public and private money is spent on the treatment of learning disorders, which affect roughly 20% of all children. So in hard-nosed economic terms, this is a lucrative market. Second, there is a tremendous disparity between the research and development costs for a validated therapy and those for an unvalidated one. Although the same disparity exists for medications, the medication market is regulated (by the FDA). Alternative medicines still abound, but their claims to efficacy are monitored by the FDA. Behavioral therapies are much less regulated, and thus there is no penalty for making false claims about efficacy. So a pseudoscientific behavioral therapy can be developed quickly with little initial investment of time or money and then marketed. As Mark Twain once said, "a lie has gotten halfway around the world by the time the truth gets its boots on." The World Wide Web has made advertising such therapies much easier and has probably contributed to their proliferation. As described later, some of these controversial therapies have been used with very large numbers of children at considerable public expense. One clear policy implication is that there should be more careful regulation of behavioral and educational interventions.

Yet another reason for the proliferation of controversial therapies for learning disorders is that they are sometimes supported by a proprietary professional group, as sensory integration therapy (SIT; see below) is supported by occupational therapists. Or a therapy may be advocated by an authority the parent respects, such as a teacher or clinician. Sometimes the claim that the treatment is grounded in neuroscience research makes it more convincing. The public has become aware of the dramatic advances in neuroscience. Just adding neuroscience terminology to an explanation otherwise judged to be vacuous increases its plausibility significantly (Weisberg, Keil, Goodstein, Rawson, & Gray, 2008). Finally, such a therapy may be more consonant with a parent's own ideology, such as a preference for "natural cures" over medications. Since controversial therapies for learning disorders are prevalent and appealing, it is important to teach clinicians and parents how to recognize such therapies before wasting valuable time and money on them.

HOW TO RECOGNIZE A CONTROVERSIAL THERAPY

Smith (2005) has reviewed characteristics of controversial treatments, and these are summarized here. One thing that makes a therapy controversial is that its theoretical basis does not fit with our scientific understanding of the disorder it is supposed to treat. For instance, it does not make sense to use vestibular stimulation to treat dyslexia, because as far as we know, the vestibular system is not involved in the cause of dyslexia (see the "Cerebellar–Vestibular Treatment" section for a fuller discussion). So theoretical plausibility is one criterion for evaluating therapies. Other warning signs besides theoretical implausibility are making unrealistic promises (e.g., that a therapy will "cure" a learning disorder), making vague claims that cannot be studied, or claiming to be beneficial for many different disorders. If the different disorders have different underlying causes, it is very improbable that the same treatment will be effective for all of them. Still other warning signs include (1) the use of sophisticated technology in applications that have not yet been validated; (2) criticisms of validated treatments, or promises of much greater benefits than such treatments provide; (3) support by subjective evidence, such as anecdotes, case histories, testimonials, or surveys; and (4) appeals to the popularity or longevity of the treatment. Just as is the case in the investment market, if something looks too good to be true, it probably is.

But the most important criterion is whether the treatment has been empirically validated in rigorous treatment studies, as described in Chapter 14. If the treatment has not been empirically validated, it is by definition experimental and not ready for dissemination to the public. Treatments whose efficacy is supported only by clinical observations, uncontrolled studies, or anecdotes are not empirically validated, and one could argue that it is unprofessional and unethical to disseminate them.

WHY CONTROVERSIAL BEHAVIORAL TREATMENTS ARE HARMFUL

In mainstream medicine, drugs are not approved for clinical use until they have been rigorously investigated for efficacy in double-blind, randomized controlled trials, which also evaluate their potential side effects. Almost all laypersons recognize the potential harm of taking an untested drug, and so would be reluctant to agree to such a treatment for themselves or their loved ones. They would also regard a practitioner who prescribed untested drugs as unethical and guilty of malpractice. Yet when laypersons turn to behavioral or educational treatments, especially for children, their standards often become much more lenient. They may tend to think that such treatments can do no harm, and that the professionals advocating them are caring people who want to help children with problems (which they often are). But good intentions are not sufficient for ethical practice.

This uncritical way of thinking about behavioral or educational treatments for children is mistaken in several ways. First, because children generally do not decide what treatments they receive, those who care for them—parents, clinicians, and educators—have an even higher ethical obligation than those who care for adults. Second, ineffective behavioral and educational treatments *do* cause harm, because they waste valuable resources (both time and money) that could be devoted to proven treatments. This is all the more urgent when the optimum time in a child's development for intervention is being wasted on ineffective treatments. For most of the learning disorders in this book, early intervention is more effective than later intervention. Third, seemingly innocuous behavioral and educational interventions can cause harm more directly by stigmatizing children or leading them to make inaccurate attributions about the nature of their symptoms.

Therefore, parents, educators, and health care professionals need to be especially vigilant to make sure that treatments that are applied to children are ESTs. In a time when dollars for health care and education are harder and harder to come by, we could free up considerable financial resources by stopping ineffective treatments. So it is incumbent on parents of a child with a learning disorder to educate themselves about effective treatments so they can be good advocates for their child. An even greater obligation falls on the shoulders of clinicians who diagnose and treat children with learning disorders. They should be knowledgeable about best practices and avoid controversial therapies.

The remainder of this chapter reviews specific controversial therapies for the disorders covered in this book. Similar to the "process focused" approaches for treating DCD discussed in Chapter 11, the logic of nearly all the controversial therapies reviewed here is (1) that a disorder in some higher aspect of cognition, such as reading, language, attention, or social cognition, is caused by a lower-level deficit in one modality of perception (e.g., auditory, tactile, or visual), or in some aspect of motor skill; (2) that the lower-level deficit can be remediated with practice (because of brain plasticity); *and* (3) that fixing the lower-level deficit will improve the deficit in higher cognition. Accordingly, these three assumptions need to be tested empirically for each therapy.

In other words, it needs to be demonstrated (1) that the particular lower-level deficit is actually present in children with the particular learning disorder that the treatment targets; (2) that the treatment can ameliorate this particular deficit; and, most crucially; (3) that ameliorating this deficit also remediates the learning disorder itself. We would also like to know whether it does so more effectively than other available treatments, especially if they cost less in terms of time and money. Since training of a particular skill rarely transfers to other skills, it is particularly important that research on these treatments meet this third empirical criterion of differential effectiveness in treating the actual clinical symptoms that define the disorder.

In contrast, a "performance-based" therapy that more directly targets the deficient area of higher cognition has fewer underlying assumptions and so has greater face validity. For example, a child with reading disorder (RD) should be given practice in component reading skills; a child with language impairment (LI) should receive practice in component language skills; and so on. We still need to test which components to target, and which intervention methods actually work.

So, in evaluating each of these controversial therapies, we will want to see whether these three empirical criteria have been met, and whether the controversial therapy works better than a more conventional "performance-based" therapy that more directly targets the deficient area of higher cognition.

These controversial therapies are organized into the following broad categories: (1) auditory treatments, (2) visual treatments, (3) motor–vestibular treatments, and (4) other therapies.

AUDITORY TREATMENTS

Controversial therapies in the auditory category include auditory integration training (AIT), the Tomatis method, and Fast ForWord (FFW). All three share the view that altered auditory processing lies at the root of various learning disorders, and that modified auditory input can reorganize the auditory system to improve auditory processing *and* thus improve deficits in higher-level cognition.

Auditory Integration Training

AIT has been reviewed by the American Speech–Language–Hearing Association (ASHA, 2004), the American Academy of Pediatrics (AAP, 1998), Silver (1995), and Gravel (1994); what follows is based on those reviews. This approach was developed by a French physician, Guy Berard, and is based on the theory that some individuals have overly sensitive or undersensitive hearing at specific frequencies. These deviations in peripheral hearing are postulated to contribute to a wide range of disorders—not only autism spectrum disorder (ASD) and other learning disorders, but also depression, migraine headaches, and epilepsy. The theory underlying AIT shares with the theory of sensory integration dysfunction or sensory modulation disorder—SMD (see Chapter 4 and the discussion of SIT below) the idea that some children have altered sensitivities to sensory stimuli that cause distress, and that these altered sensitivities can be treated with modified sensory input.

A special device, an AudioKinetron, is used to diagnose hyper- and hypoacusis and the frequencies at which these altered sensitivities occur. Treatment consists of listening to computer-modified music that is tailored to the individual patient's profile of altered sensitivities, so that some frequencies are amplified (to increase sensitivity) and others are filtered out (to reduce hyperacusis). The altered auditory input is hypothesized to reorganize the auditory cortex so that the peripheral hearing profile is brought within a typical range, thus leading somehow to alleviation of the symptoms of the patient's learning or other disorders.

This therapy is considered controversial because our current scientific understanding of the disorders for which AIT is prescribed does not include problems in peripheral hearing as a cause. More to the point, current scientific understanding does not recognize any processing problem that is shared by all these various disorders. As discussed earlier, a claim that a treatment will cure multiple disorders should make us skeptical, because distinct disorders have different causes and so require different treatments. But the most important problem with AIT is the lack of peer-reviewed empirical research addressing the three criteria listed above: that this particular auditory problem is present in all these patient groups, that AIT reverses this deficit, and that AIT also reverses the symptoms of these various disorders. Both Gravel (1994) and the AAP (1998) caution against its use as a treatment for ASD.

Tomatis Method

The Tomatis method was also developed by a French physician, Alfred Tomatis. It too postulates peripheral hearing differences, including abnormal ear dominance, that can be reversed through controlled auditory stimulation. The Tomatis website (*www.tomatis.com*) claims that this treatment has helped individuals with ASD, dyslexia, ADHD, Down syndrome, and SMD.

Once again, we have a claim that the therapy benefits multiple disorders with distinct causes, and we do not have peer-reviewed, published research addressing the three criteria listed above. Nonetheless, the Tomatis website lists over 20 Tomatis treatment centers in North America and over 50 in Europe, suggesting that this treatment is widely utilized.

Fast ForWord

FFW was developed by Paula Tallal, PhD, and her colleagues at Scientific Learning Corporation (*www.scilearn.com*). Because Tallal's previous research had documented auditory temporal processing deficits in children with acquired LI, children with developmental LI, and some children with RD, she and her colleagues sought to develop a treatment that would remediate this auditory deficit and help affected children improve their language and literacy skills. So, unlike the developers of AIT and the Tomatis method, Tallal had done careful research to meet the first criterion discussed above— namely, that the postulated deficit is present in the disorders targeted by the treatment.

The FFW treatment consists of seven computer games, three of which are aimed at improving the discrimination and memory of speech sounds (phonemes and syllables) and four of which target higher-level language skills, including vocabulary, syntax, and morphology (e.g., plural and past-tense forms of words). Each game requires a child to make judgments about auditory presentations of either speech sounds, words, or sentences that have accompanying visual displays. The initial auditory presentations are acoustically modified so that the duration of rapid speech cues (such as for-mant transitions in stop consonants) is gradually increased. As the child's accuracy increases, the degree of acoustic modification decreases until the child is being trained with natural speech. Treatment is intensive, lasting 100 minutes a day, 5 days a week for up to 6 weeks.

FFW represents a much more subtle case of a controversial therapy than AIT or the Tomatis method. It was developed by serious scientists; it is based on an apparently plausible and extensively studied hypothesis about the cause of language problems; and the initial validation studies appeared in *Science*, one of the most prestigious scientific journals in the world (Mer-zenich et al., 1996; Tallal et al., 1996). So FFW appears to have much more scientific validity than AIT or the Tomatis method. Partly because of this scientific appeal, many more children have been treated with FFW, and it has achieved much more acceptance among speech and language patholo-gists and other professionals than has either AIT or the Tomatis method. In sum, FFW represents a particularly important case study of a controversial therapy.

So what makes FFW controversial? First, despite apparent theoretical plausibility and some empirical support, the hypothesis of auditory tem-poral processing deficits as a cause for LI or RD has not fared that well, as discussed in Chapters 6 and 7. Although auditory temporal processing defi-cits are sometimes found by other researchers to be present in these groups, that is not always the case, and there are alternative explanations for why they are present. Moreover, the development of speech and language is not as dependent on brief cues in the speech stream as Tallal's theory assumes (Marshall, Snowling, & Bailey, 2001; Mody, Studdert-Kennedy, & Brady, 1997; Nittrouer, 1999; Rosen, 2003), and auditory temporal deficits, though present in some children with LI and RD, are less robust than deficits in phoneme awareness or phonological memory (Bishop, Adams, Lehtonen, & Rosen, 2005; Ramus et al., 2003).

Second, and more importantly, the evidence in favor of this treatment is only Level III evidence, whereas rigorous Level I studies find no treatment effect. Most of the evidence for treatment efficacy comes from studies by the originators of FFW themselves (e.g., Merzenich et al., 1996; Tallal et al., 1996), and these studies are hard to interpret because the experimental group received other treatments besides acoustically modified speech. So, even though the experimental group performed better than the controls, the effect of acoustically modified speech was not isolated in the design. A study by Habib et al. (2002) did just that by examining natural speech versus acoustically modified speech within FFW. Across a range of language and reading measures, the researchers did not find an advantage for acoustically modified speech. In addition, most of the results presented by Merzenich et al. (1996) and Tallal et al. (1996) are pretest–posttest difference scores for the FFW group and not differences relative to an untreated control group. So we do not know whether these pre–post differences in the FFW group would have occurred anyway because of regular school instruction, development, or just regression to the mean. Independent studies that appear to provide support for the efficacy of FFW (e.g., Temple et al., 2003) also lacked an untreated control group (see review in Olson & Wise, 2006).

Third, and most importantly, independent Level I treatment studies that included untreated control groups have found much weaker treatment effects on trained skills and no effects on spontaneous speech and language or reading—the key targets of FFW (see reviews in Koenig & Gunter, 2005; Olson & Wise, 2006). Hook, Macaruso, and Jones (2001) and Pokorni, Worthington, and Maison (2004) compared FFW to two other commonly used reading interventions: the Orton–Gillingham program and the Lindamood Phoneme Sequencing Program (Lindamood & Lindamood, 1998). FFW produced gains on phoneme awareness and speaking and syntax measures similar to the trained stimuli used in FFW, but not significant gains in reading or broader language skills (see review in Olson & Wise, 2006); that is, the training did not generalize.

Two recent, large randomized controlled trials tested FFW as a reading intervention in economically disadvantaged urban school districts (Borman, Benson, & Overman, submitted; Rouse & Krueger, 2004). Rouse and Krueger (2004) conducted a carefully designed treatment study of a large group ($N = 512$) of elementary-school-age children who were administered extensive pre- and posttreatment measures of reading and language skills. Children were randomly assigned to FFW or to a no-treatment control condition, and were well matched on background variables. The study found no effect of FFW on reading or broader language skills. Similar results were found in the second treatment study, conducted in the Baltimore public schools (Borman et al., submitted).

Finally, there have been two recent randomized controlled trials comparing FFW to other treatments for LI, including computerized ones (Cohen et al., 2005; Gillam et al., 2008). Neither study found a treatment advantage for FFW on either language skills or auditory temporal processing measures.

In sum, the weight of evidence means that instead of calling FFW a controversial therapy because it has not been tested empirically (as is true for most of the therapies reviewed in this chapter), we should call it a disproven therapy because it has been tested and has not met the empirical criteria discussed earlier. Some but not all studies find that children with LI and RD have auditory temporal processing deficits (criterion 1), and treatment studies have shown that FFW improves these deficits (criterion 2). However, in the large randomized controlled trial by Gillam et al. (2008), which was funded by the National Institutes of Health, all three other treatments improved such auditory deficits as much as FFW did. So, contrary to what the theory behind FFW predicts, acoustically modified speech is not necessary for improving auditory deficits. Perhaps each treatment actually remediated these deficits in different ways, or perhaps children in each group just improved because of practice, development, and regression to the mean. In any case, FFW did not show differential efficacy in improving auditory deficits. Most importantly, criterion 3 was not met across independent Level I studies of FFW. In these studies, there was generally no transfer from FFW training to the clinical symptoms.

FFW has nonetheless had a broad impact. It has been used by 120,000 students in the United States (*www.evidencebasedprograms.org*). The website of Scientific Learning Corporation (*www.scilearn.com*), which markets FFW, calls it a "neuroscience approach to reading intervention" and claims positive results for well over 100 school districts that have implemented FFW. However, an independent review of the technical reports from this corporation found the results to be unconvincing, partly because of the lack of control groups (Wahl, Robinson, & Torgesen, 2003). The total cost of these school-based implementations of FFW is easily in the millions of dollars.

VISUAL TREATMENTS

Visual treatments are used for dyslexia. Like the auditory treatments just discussed, all share the view that remediating a basic sensory deficit will improve a multimodal disorder. What makes this hypothesis implausible is that the phonological and language problems that children with dyslexia have are not restricted to written (or visual) language, but instead are evident in their oral language before the onset of literacy instruction (as reviewed in Chapter 6).

A second theoretical reason to question visual therapies for dyslexia is that the brain, not the eyes, carries out visual information processing. So these theories are fixated on an overly concrete and simplistic answer to a complex problem. Moreover, we currently lack scientific evidence to support the notion that the correction of subtle visual deficits can alter the brain's processing of visual information (AAP, 1998). Cognitive scientists who study the visual system have learned that extraction of relevant information by the brain from visual input is remarkably robust over a wide range of external conditions, including luminance level, degree of contrast, and presence of visual noise. Moreover, skilled readers are remarkably good at letter and word recognition, despite alterations in print or even handwriting. Finally, we also currently lack evidence that dyslexic children differ from nondyslexic children in peripheral vision (AAP, 1998). (Note that by "peripheral vision," I mean those components of the visual system that are outside the brain, not vision in the periphery of the visual field.) For all these reasons, a visual cause or cure for dyslexia is quite implausible theoretically.

The review that follows covers two examples of visual treatments for dyslexia: optometric visual training and tinted lenses. However, the arguments advanced here apply to other visual treatments for dyslexia, such as convergence training, eye patching, and so on.

Optometric Visual Training

As reviewed by Silver (1995), numerous varieties of optometric visual training are offered by optometrists, but all include eye exercises to provide practice in "tracking" (i.e., smooth pursuit and saccadic eye movements) and binocular control of the eyes. Some optometric treatments also include training in visual perception (in which a child has already been engaged every waking hour since birth!) This visual perception training includes form and color discrimination, as well as rapid recognition of tachistoscopically presented images.

Optometric visual training procedures have been repeatedly reviewed by both the AAP (1998; see also Metzger & Werner, 1984) and the American Academy of Ophthalmology (Flax, Solan, & Suchoff, 1983); these reviews concluded that their efficacy has not been established. The best pediatric practices recommended by the AAP (1998) are early detection and treatment of peripheral visual problems in children, such as refractive errors, focusing deficiencies, eye muscle intolerances, and motor fusion deficiencies. Some of these problems require treatment by an ophthalmologist who specializes in the care of children. Once such peripheral visual problems have been detected and treated, there is no further role for vision care and treatment for a child suspected of having a learning disorder such as dyslexia (AAP, 1998).

The AAP (1998) also recommends that pediatricians use validated screening procedures to detect learning disorders in preschool children. For instance, the evidence reviewed in Chapter 6 indicates that measures of letter name and sound knowledge are useful for screening. But screening preschoolers for learning disorders does not appear to be a widespread practice among primary care pediatricians, so training them to use screening procedures for early detection of such disorders could be a very useful change in public policy.

Tinted Lenses

Helen Irlen (1983) proposed a treatment with colored lenses for reading problems caused by what she called "scotopic sensitivity syndrome," which is characterized by (1) photophobia, (2) eye strain, (3) poor visual resolution, (4) a reduced span of focus, (5) impaired depth perception, and (6) poor sustained focus. Notice that the last symptom refers to attention, so this symptom could easily have an alternative explanation. More generally, persons with dyslexia will inevitably find reading to be effortful and may complain that their eyes are tired or that they cannot concentrate, but of course this does not mean that these symptoms *cause* their dyslexia. In Irlen's treatment, a practitioner determines which tint in a lens alleviates a patient's symptoms of scotopic sensitivity, and then has the patient wear the tinted lenses while reading. The claim is that once these scotopic sensitivity symptoms are relieved, the patient's reading will improve.

Irlen (1983) presented her theory at a conference. Before her theory had been tested independently, it quickly became popular (partly because of network TV coverage), and now there are Irlen treatment centers in many American cities. Although Irlen herself was careful to say that her treatment was only relevant for a subset of dyslexic individuals with scotopic sensitivity, in practice Irlen lenses quickly became a widespread treatment for dyslexia.

Nonetheless, the efficacy of this treatment is not supported by independent research (Hoyt, 1990; Solan, 1990) or by the AAP (1998). There is not even a reliable and valid test for scotopic sensitivity (Silver, 1995). If a disorder cannot be reliably diagnosed, then it is impossible to determine whether a treatment alters it.

MOTOR–VESTIBULAR TREATMENTS

Four different treatments are included in this section: SIT, patterning, cerebellar–vestibular treatment, and the Dore program. These various treatments are more theoretically diverse than the auditory or visual treatments, so the criticisms of their theoretical plausibility are treatment-specific. Nonetheless, all four of these treatments share the same general logic outlined earlier: that higher cognitive problems are caused by problems in lower-level skills, and that remediating those skills will remediate the higher-level cognitive problems.

Sensory Integration Therapy

SIT is the therapy developed by Ayres (1979) for sensory integration dysfunction or SMD, which is discussed in Chapter 4 as an unvalidated disorder. Because SIT has been applied to a wide range of disorders, including ASD, developmental coordination disorder (DCD), ID, and other learning disorders, efficacy studies have focused on its application to particular disorders. Although it is not supported as a treatment for these various learning disorders, it could still be efficacious for the symptoms of SMD (i.e., the hypo- and hypersensitivities to sensory stimuli). Unfortunately, its efficacy in that arena has not been tested as much. In what follows, I first describe SIT and then review its efficacy when applied to particular disorders.

SMD is defined by symptoms that are attributed to dysfunction in the vestibular, proprioceptive, and tactile systems. So poor posture and dyspraxia are attributed in sensory integration theory to vestibular dysfunction, even though the standard neurological definition of dyspraxia attributes it to neocortical dysfunction, and even though the vestibular sense is mainly concerned with balance. The proprioceptive system provides sensory inputs from muscles and joints, which are represented cortically in the parietal lobe. Any coordinated movement requires proprioception, because a motor plan to move a body part must take into account its current position in space. In sensory integration theory, proprioceptive dysfunction is hypothesized to underlie motor stereotypics, such as hand flapping or rocking; again, this explanation is neurologically implausible, because the cause of repetitive movements is thought to arise in the executive or motor system. In the theory, problems in the tactile system are thought to underlie hyper- or hyposensitivity to touch. Obviously, other systems must be implicated in nontactile sensory sensitivities.

This brief overview of how sensory integration theory explains the symptoms that SIT treats makes it clear that there is already theoretical implausibility in the explanation of the symptoms. A therapy that is based on an erroneous theory of the symptoms is likely to be ineffective.

SIT is designed to provide a corrective "sensory diet" for these underdeveloped vestibular, proprioceptive, and tactile systems (T. Smith, Mruzek, & Mozingo, 2005). Swinging, rolling, riding on scooter boards, or jumping on a trampoline are treatment activities to provide vestibular stimulation. Proprioceptive stimulation is provided by squeezing a child between pads or pillows, by repeatedly manipulating a joint, or by having the child wear a weighted vest. Tactile stimulation is provided by brushing the child's body or having him or her play with textured toys. The sensory diet for a particular child is adjusted to match that child's particular profile of difficulties.

Like the benefits attributed to some other controversial therapies, the benefits of SIT are claimed to extend to domains of function well beyond those targeted in the treatment. As reviewed by T. Smith et al. (2005), SIT is claimed to improve attention, reading, and language, and to reduce self-injurious behavior.

We now turn to studies of the treatment efficacy of SIT. Chapter 12 has already discussed SIT as an ineffective treatment for DCD. What is important here is that other reviews have found it to be ineffective for the sensory symptoms themselves in such disorders as autism (Dawson & Wathing, 2000) and ID (T. Smith et al., 2005).

Despite this lack of empirical validation, SIT remains very popular among occupational therapists and is widely utilized in both public and private settings in the treatment of children with autism and ID. T. Smith et al. (2005) make recommendations about how other professionals and parents should respond when SIT is prescribed for a child. These recommendations include reviewing the lack of research support for SIT with the professionals prescribing SIT (such as a special education team in a public school), and, if it is still implemented, using objective methods to evaluate the efficacy of SIT in a single-case design (such as an ABAB reversal design).

Patterning

Patterning is an older treatment for children with ID, other learning disorders, and brain injuries, and is reviewed by Silver (1995) and Novella (*www. quackwatch.com/QuackeryRelatedTopics/patterning*). The treatment is based on the old notion that "ontogeny recapitulates phylogeny"—in other words, that the stages of individual human development mirror the stages of evolution, and that developmental problems represent an arrest at an earlier developmental stage. So it is claimed that children with developmental disorders must revisit earlier phylogenetic stages of movement (e.g., crawling) and master them in order to move on in their development. Practicing these earlier forms of movement either actively or passively (if a child cannot perform the movement independently) is thought to impose the proper phylogenetic "pattern" on the brain, allowing development to proceed to the next stage; hence the therapy is called "patterning." This therapy is theoretically implausible, because extensive research on development, learning, and skill acquisition does not support this view of how motor skills develop.

In addition, clinical trials of patterning with children with disabilities have not provided evidence for its efficacy. The AAP (1982) issued a policy statement countering the claims for patterning, and this policy statement has been endorsed by the National Down Syndrome Congress on its website (*www.ndsccenter.org*). Nonetheless, patterning persists.

Cerebellar–Vestibular Treatment

Harold Levinson (1980) holds that vestibular dysfunction causes dyslexia, and that the use of antimotion sickness medication (e.g., Dramamine) is an effective treatment. As noted above in the review of SIT, the functions of the vestibular system do not include higher cognitive functions. Although there is some reputable evidence that the neurobiology of dyslexia includes cerebellar dysfunction (as reviewed in Chapter 6), this is presumably because the cerebellum participates in cognitive processes, such as language, that are causal in the disorder. So the theoretical plausibility of the vestibular treatment theory is extremely weak. Moreover, there is a lack of independent treatment research published in peer-reviewed journals to support this therapy.

Polatajko (1985) did a careful study comparing vestibular function in children with and without learning disabilities and found no differences, as well as no association between levels of vestibular function and academic performance.

Despite these problems, this therapy is still offered at the Levinson Medical Center for Learning Disabilities (*www.dyslexiaonline.com*). In addition, Levinson (1994) criticized mainstream dyslexia research in a book titled *A Scientific Watergate, Dyslexia*.

Dore Treatment

The Dore treatment was developed by a British businessman, Wynford Dore, who wished to help his dyslexic daughter. He was inspired by the just-presented work of Harold Levinson. Like Levinson's treatment, the Dore program targets the cerebellum. The Dore website claims that "the cerebellum is the skill learning centre of the brain," which "works very much like the gearbox within a car. A Ferrari cannot perform to its potential if it has an inadequate gearbox to transfer its potential power into actual performance."

The Dore program is an exercise-based treatment that consists of 10 minutes of doing specified exercises twice a day for several months to a year (*www.dore.co.uk*). A course of treatment is quite expensive, costing up to $4,000 (U.S. currency). The purpose of these exercises is to cure developmental cerebellar delay, which the proponents of this treatment claim is the cause of several of the learning disorders covered in this book, including dyslexia, ADHD, Asperger syndrome, and dyspraxia (i.e., DCD). As discussed earlier, there are good reasons to be skeptical of a treatment that claims to treat multiple disorders. Related Dore treatments are also offered to improve athletic ability.

The theoretical basis of the treatment is that the cerebellum is important not only for motor coordination, but also for higher cognitive functions, such as attention and language skills. Specifically, it is hypothesized to play a crucial role in making both motor and cognitive skills automatic. This is a reasonable premise, since modern neuroimaging studies have found that the cerebellum is activated during cognitive tasks; this research has led cognitive neuroscientists to broaden their conception of cerebellar functions. A careful reader will also recall that structural and functional differences in the cerebellum have been found in neuroimaging studies of the learning disorders that the Dore treatment targets. But the key link in the theoretical rationale for this treatment is the claim that motor exercises will improve *all* cerebellar functions, both motor and cognitive. This is a bold claim, because targeted training of any sort rarely transfers to unrelated skill domains. So, once again, the key question about this treatment is whether there is good empirical evidence that these motor exercises improve skills in the domains of literacy, attention, and social cognition.

The Dore website claims that such empirical evidence exists, citing two papers about one treatment study that were published in the journal *Dyslexia* (Reynolds & Nicolson, 2007; Reynolds, Nicolson, & Hambly, 2003). Because the authors of these two papers are proponents of the Dore treatment, this treatment study is not an independent evaluation. These papers have been extensively criticized by members of the editorial board of *Dyslexia*, six of whom have now resigned in protest over the publication of a treatment study that they considered to be deeply flawed (Bishop, 2007). Although the study was a randomized controlled trial, the control group did not receive any placebo treatment, raising the possibility of placebo effects in the treated group. Moreover, there was only one significant differential pre- versus posttest effect on reading scores, with the treated group demonstrating a greater gain. But, despite randomization, the members of this group had a lower pretest score on this measure, potentially giving them more room to improve. In contrast, on the other reading measures, gains were similar in both groups and thus can be attributed to practice and/or development, not to the treatment. The authors of these two papers found stronger treatment effects on achievement tests administered by the school, but these data were not available for the control group, and so it is impossible to judge whether any gains were due to the treatment specifically.

Therefore, the Dore program is similar to other controversial therapies reviewed here. It claims a scientific basis, but there are questions about its theoretical plausibility; it claims to improve numerous different disorders with the same treatment; and, most importantly, it has not been empirically validated by independent investigators.

OTHER THERAPIES

The therapies reviewed in this section include facilitated communication (FC) and secretin for autism, megavitamins for learning disabilities, and dietary treatments for ADHD.

Facilitated Communication

FC is based on the belief that dyspraxia and other motor impairments prevent people with autism and some other developmental disabilities from communicating, and that all that is needed to reveal their "hidden literacy" is a facilitator who supports their hand or arm while they type on a keyboard.

FC originated in Australia as a treatment for people with CP, who can indeed exhibit a marked discrepancy between their cognitive capacities and their vocal or manual output capacities. Anyone who has witnessed the technology-assisted communication of the famous physicist Stephen Hawking, who has a severe peripheral motor disease (amyotrophic lateral sclerosis or "Lou Gehrig's disease"), can understand the concept of a talented mind locked in an immobile body. So it is certainly true that if a person's communicative impairment is due simply to peripheral incapacity, alternative means of communication will be helpful. One key problem with FC is assuming that the same will be true in such conditions as autism, where the communication impairment is much more fundamental and not just due to peripheral output problems.

Nonetheless, because FC appeared to help people with CP, it was adapted in the early 1990s as a treatment for people with autism by Douglas Biklen, an education professor at Syracuse University. FC then spread rapidly within the autism community in North America and Western Europe, and was soon endorsed by many clinicians working with individuals with autism. Its success was largely based on dramatic videos of sophisticated messages emerging on a keyboard, apparently from the hands of a mute person with autism. It was easy for many to believe that they were watching a treatment miracle, and facilitators themselves sincerely believed that the messages were originating from the disabled person. The success of FC also partly derived from its endorsement by Biklen (1993), an education professor at a prominent university. In 1992, Biklen established the FC Institute at Syracuse University, which is still in operation today.

FC is not theoretically plausible for several reasons. First, as mentioned above, if the communication problem is not just peripheral but instead due to brain dysfunction in social and language networks, then there is unlikely to be a latent communicative potential waiting to be released. Just as some hopeful observers of patients in a persistent vegetative state (e.g., Terri Schiavo) are willing to interpret primitive motor reflexes as intentional or communicative, hopeful parents and clinicians are willing to attribute more communicative intent to children with severe disabilities than the children may actually possess. Indeed, some of the individuals with autism or severe or profound ID who apparently produced sentences or even poetry while receiving FC had never produced anything previously, even with other augmented communication devices. Moreover, these individuals rarely seemed to be even looking at the keyboard while these high-level messages emerged on the computer monitor (Jacobson, Foxx, & Mulick, 2005b). How could someone who had never communicated before and was not looking at the keyboard suddenly produce literate text?

As with any therapy, though, the critical test of FC is empirical. If the facilitated communications were truly generated by a client with disabilities, then similar competence should be evident when a facilitator could not see the keyboard and monitor. Independent studies that manipulated the facilitator's visual access to the keyboard and monitor, or measured facilitator influence in other ways, have consistently shown that the seemingly miraculous messages originate in the *facilitators*, not in the clients with disabilities (Jacobson et al., 2005b). Based on this research, both the AAP (1998) and the American Psychological Association (1994) have concluded that FC lacks efficacy and should be avoided as a treatment for autism.

One may ask why the facilitators believed the messages were coming from the clients with disabilities instead of themselves. This phenomenon of erroneous attribution is similar to what happens with a Ouija board or with automatic writing, and has been thoroughly analyzed by Wegner (2002).

Secretin

Secretin is a peptide hormone that stimulates several organs to release chemicals that aid digestion. Based on the observation that an elevated proportion of children with autism have gastrointestinal symptoms, including inflammation in the gastrointestinal tract, it was hypothesized that there could be deficient levels of secretin in these children. Clinical reports of the usefulness of secretin injections in reducing gastrointestinal symptoms in children with autism appeared, along with claims of improvement in their behavioral symptoms. Like many other therapies considered in this chapter, secretin injections quickly became a widespread treatment, even though reasonable concerns were expressed about possible adverse immune reactions to an injected hormone derived from pigs.

Because of these concerns, and because it is easier to conduct a randomized trial of a medication than a behavioral therapy, a large number of randomized, double-blind, controlled trials of the efficacy of secretin for reducing the symptoms of autism were undertaken (e.g., Coniglio et al., 2001; Dunn-Geier et al., 2000; Unis et al., 2002); these found no measurable effect of secretin. A meta-analysis of these double-blind studies (Esch & Carr, 2004) concluded that the efficacy of secretin as a treatment for the symptoms of autism has not been established empirically.

Megavitamins

As reviewed in Silver (1995), large doses of vitamins were advanced as a treatment for dyslexia and other traditionally defined learning disabilities in 1971. According to Silver (1995), the AAP (1976) concluded that there was no validity to megavitamin treatment for learning disabilities.

Dietary Treatments

The Feingold diet for ADHD was proposed in 1973 by a pediatric allergist, Benjamin Feingold, based on the hypothesis that artificial food additives (including salicylates) caused ADHD. The diet eliminates these additives. Several expert reviews of research on this diet have concluded that its efficacy is unproven (e.g., Wender & Lipton, 1980).

Another dietary treatment for ADHD, widely supported by popular belief, is sugar reduction. Again, this treatment is not empirically supported (Wolraich, Wilson, & White, 1995).

CONCLUSION

I hope that the material in this chapter will help parents and clinicians avoid these controversial therapies for learning disorders and become more skilled at detecting other dubious therapies. Fortunately, research data on therapies are much more accessible today. Appendix B lists useful websites that provide access to research on therapies. Table 15.1 summarizes the controversial therapies reviewed in this chapter.

TABLE 15.1. Summary of Controversial Therapies for Learning Disorders

Autism	Dyslexia	ID	ADHD
Sensory integration therapy (SIT)	SIT	SIT	SIT
Facilitated communication (FC)	Optometric visual training ("eye tracking")	Patterning	Feingold diet
Secretin	Tinted lenses		Sugar-restricted diet
Auditory integration training (AIT)	AIT		
Patterning	Tomatis method		
	Fast ForWord (FFW)		
	Megavitamins		
	Cerebellar–vestibular treatment		

Helpful Resources
for Parents and Teachers

READING DISABILITY/DYSLEXIA

Hall, S. J., & Moats, L. C. (1998). *Straight talk about reading: How parents can make a difference during the early years.* New York: McGraw-Hill.

Shaywitz, S. E. (2003). *Overcoming dyslexia: A new and complete science-based program for reading problems at any level.* New York: Knopf.

ADHD

Barkley, R. A. (2000). *Taking charge of ADHD: The complete, authoritative guide for parents* (rev. ed.). New York: Guilford Press.

Hallowell, E. M., & Ratey, J. J. (1994a). *Driven to distraction: Recognizing and coping with attention deficit disorder from childhood through adulthood.* New York: Pantheon Books.

Hallowell, E. M., & Ratey, J. J. (1994b). *Answers to distraction.* New York: Pantheon Books.

MOOD DISORDERS

Fristad, M. A., & Goldberg Arnold, J. S. (2004). *Raising a moody child: How to cope with depression and bipolar disorder.* New York: Guilford Press.

Papolos, D., & Papolos, J. (2002). *The bipolar child: The definitive and reassuring guide to childhood's most misunderstood disorder* (rev. expanded ed.). New York: Broadway Books.

ANXIETY

Chansky, T. E. (2004). *Freeing your child from anxiety: Powerful, practical solutions to overcome your child's fears, worries, and phobias.* New York: Random House.
Rapee, R. M., Spence, S. H., Cobham, V., & Wignall, A. (2000). *Helping your anxious child: A step-by-step guide for parents.* Oakland, CA: New Harbinger.

MEDICATION

Wilens, T. E. (2009). *Straight talk about psychiatric medications for kids* (rev. ed.). New York: Guilford Press.

BASIC PARENTING

Clark, L., & Robb, J. (2005). *SOS: Help for parents.* Bowling Green, KY: SOS Program & Parents Press.
Forehand, R., & Long, N. (2002). *Parenting the strong-willed child: The clinically proven five-week program for parents of two- to six-year-olds* (rev. and updated ed.). Chicago: Contemporary Books.
Gottman, J. (1997). *Raising an emotionally intelligent child.* New York: Fireside.
Greene, R. W. (1998). *The explosive child: A new approach for understanding and parenting easily frustrated, chronically inflexible children.* New York: HarperCollins.

INTELLECTUAL DISABILITY

Janney, R., & Snell, M. E. (2004). *Modifying schoolwork: Teacher's guide to inclusive practices* (2nd ed.). Baltimore: Brookes.

AUTISM SPECTRUM DISORDER

The Organization for Autism Research has very good downloadable .pdfs (*www.researchautism.org/resources/reading*).

- *A Parent's Guide to Autism Research.* I recommend that parents who are interested in more experimental treatments consult this .pdf to get a good sense of the research and the costs and benefits of newer, more experimental treatments. The world of autism treatment includes some very unusual approaches that have *no* research support and yet are costly and potentially dangerous for children. This guide helps parents to become good consumers.

- *An Educator's Guide to Autism.*
- *An Educator's Guide to Asperger's Syndrome.*
- *A Guide for Transition to Adulthood.*

Children with Autism

Attwood, T. (1998). *Asperger's syndrome: A guide for parents and professionals.* London: Jessica Kingsley.

Baker, B. L., & Brightman, A. (1989). *Steps to independence: A skills training guide for parents and teachers.* Baltimore: Brookes.

Grandin, T., & Barron, S. (2005). *Unwritten rules of social relationships.* Arlington, TX: Future Horizons.

Gutstein, S., & Sheely, R. K. (2002). *Relationship development intervention with young children: Social and emotional development activities for Asperger syndrome, autism, PDD and NLD.* London: Jessica Kingsley.

Hart, C. (1993). *A parent's guide to autism: Answers to the most common questions.* New York: Simon & Schuster.

Hodgdon, L. (1995). *Visual strategies for improving communication.* Troy, MI: Quirk Roberts.

Maurice, C., Green, G., & Luce, C. (1996). *Behavioral intervention for young children with autism.* Austin, TX: PRO-ED.

Mesibov, G., Adams, L., & Klinger, L. (1997). *Autism: Understanding the disorder.* New York: Plenum Press.

National Research Council. (2001). *Educating children with autism.* Washington, DC: National Academy Press.

Siegel, B. (1996). *The world of the autistic child.* New York: Oxford University Press.

Smith, M. J. (2001). *Teaching playskills to children with autistic spectrum disorder.* New York: DRL Books.

Szatmari, P. (2004). *A mind apart.* New York: Guilford Press.

Children and Adolescents with High-Functioning Autism/Asperger Syndrome

A Comprehensive Overview

Klin, A., Volkmar, F. R., & Sparrow, S. S. (2000). *Asperger syndrome.* New York: Guilford Press.

Autobiographical Accounts

Robison, J. E. (2007). *Look me in the eye: My life with Asperger's.* New York: Crown.

Willey, L. H. (1999). *Pretending to be normal: Living with Asperger's syndrome.* London: Jessica Kingsley.

Other Resources

Andron, L. (2001). *Our journey through high functioning autism and Asperger's syndrome.* London: Jessica Kingsley.

Fullerton, A., Stratton, J., Coyne, P., & Gray, C. (1996). *Higher functioning adolescents and young adults with autism: A teacher's guide.* Austin, TX: PRO-ED.

Howlin, P. (1998). *Children with autism and Asperger syndrome: A guide for practitioners and carers.* New York: Wiley.

Ozonoff, S., Dawson, G., & McPartland, J. (2002). *A parent's guide to Asperger syndrome and high-functioning autism.* New York: Guilford Press.

Smith Myles, B., & Adreon, D. (2001). *Asperger syndrome and adolescence: practical solutions for school success.* Shawnee Mission, KS: Autism Asperger.

Smith, Myles, B., & Southwick, J. (2005). *Asperger syndrome and difficult moments* (2nd ed.). Shawnee Mission, KS: Autism Asperger.

Useful Websites

PROFESSIONAL ORGANIZATIONS

American Academy of Child and Adolescent Psychiatry
www.aacap.org
American Academy of Pediatrics
www.aap.org
American Psychological Association
www.apa.org
American Speech–Language–Hearing Association
www.asha.org
Association for Psychological Science
www.psychologicalscience.org
Society for Research in Child Development
www.srcd.org

NONPROFITS FOR SPECIFIC DISORDERS

American Association on Intellectual and Developmental Disabilities
www.aaidd.org
Association for Science in Autism Treatment
www.asatonline.org
Autism Speaks
www.autismspeaks.org
Children and Adults with ADHD
www.chadd.org
International Dyslexia Association
www.interdys.org

EMPIRICAL EVALUATION OF TREATMENTS

The Cochrane Collaboration
  www.cochrane.org
Quackwatch
  www.quackwatch.com
TRIP Database for Evidence Based Medicine
  www.tripdatabase.com

Frequently Used Tests for Learning Disorders

Test/*Composite or subtest*	Abbreviation	Reference	Description	Construct(s) measured
ADHD Rating Scale–IV	—	DuPaul et al. (1998)	Questionnaire measure of DSM-IV symptoms of ADHD	Inattention Hyperactivity–impulsivity
Autism Diagnostic Observation Schedule	ADOS	Lord et al. (1999)	Semistructured play-based interview.	Social and communicative behavior
Beery–Buktenica Test of Visual–Motor Integration	Beery VMI	Beery (1997)	Copying increasingly complex shapes.	Visual–motor integration Visual–spatial skill
Children's Category Test	CCT	Boll (1993)	Nonverbal, multiple-choice problem-solving task administered in sets (with rule changes between sets).	Nonverbal reasoning Problem solving
Clinical Evaluation of Language Fundamentals—Fourth Edition *Core Language*	CELF-4	Semel et al. (2003)	Composite of four oral language subtests. Specific subtests vary by child's age and include such tasks as sentence memory, sentence generation, receptive syntax, and expressive vocabulary.	Syntax Semantics Expressive language Receptive language
Comprehensive Test of Phonological Processing *Elision*	CTOPP	Wagner et al. (1999)	Removing a sound from a word and stating the new word that results.	Phonological awareness
Phoneme Reversal			Reversing phonemes in a sound sequence and stating the word that results.	Phonemic awareness

(continued)

Test/Composite or subtest	Abbreviation	Reference	Description	Construct(s) measured
Comprehensive Test of Phonological Processing (cont.)				
Nonword Repetition			Repeating nonwords	Phonological memory
Rapid Letter Naming			Naming a matrix of letters under time pressure.	Verbal processing speed
Rapid Digit Naming			Naming a matrix of numbers under time pressure.	Verbal processing speed
Delis–Kaplan Executive Function System	D-KEFS	Delis et al. (2001)		
Color–Word Interference			Stroop-like task with word-reading and color-naming baseline conditions. In critical condition, color names are printed in incongruent ink color, and task is to name ink color.	Inhibition
Verbal Fluency (Letter Fluency condition)			Updated version of "FAS" test: Generating as many different words that begin with a particular letter in 60 seconds.	Generating
Trail Making Test			Updated version of Trails A and B with letter-sequencing and number-sequencing baseline conditions. In critical condition, connecting alternating numbers and letters as quickly as possible.	Set shifting Nonverbal processing speed
Goldman–Fristoe Test of Articulation	GFTA	Goldman & Fristoe (1986)	Naming individually presented pictures.	Articulation
Gordon Diagnostic System	Gordon	Gordon (1983)		
Vigilance and distractibility conditions			Watching numbers flashing on a screen, and pushing button only when a particular sequence occurs.	Sustained attention Impulsivity
Gray Oral Reading Test—Fourth Edition	GORT-4	Wiederholt & Bryant (2001)		

Measure	Abbreviation	Citation	Description	Construct
Fluency			Reading paragraphs aloud; scoring includes speed and accuracy.	Reading fluency for connected text
Comprehension			Answering multiple-choice questions about paragraphs.	Reading comprehension
Learning and Behavior Questionnaire *Reading History subscale*	LBQ	Willcutt et al. (in press)	Parent questionnaire measure of early reading history.	Risk for reading problems
Peabody Picture Vocabulary Test, Fourth Edition	PPVT-4	Dunn & Dunn (2007)	Selecting one of four pictures corresponding to a word spoken by the examiner.	Receptive vocabulary
Rey–Osterrieth Complex Figure		Osterrieth (1944); Bernstein & Waber (1996)	Copying a complex geometric figure, then drawing it again from memory.	Visual–spatial skill Organization and planning
Scales of Independent Behavior—Revised	SIB-R	Bruininks et al. (1996)	Questionnaire measure of child's adaptive functioning.	Adaptive functioning
Social Communication Questionnaire	SCQ	Rutter et al. (2003)	Screening tool administered as a parent questionnaire.	Autistic behaviors
Test of Word Reading Efficiency *Sight Word Efficiency*	TOWRE	Torgesen et al. (1999)	Reading as many single words as possible in 45 seconds.	Single-word reading fluency
Phonemic Decoding Efficiency			Reading as many nonwords as possible in 45 seconds.	Phonological coding fluency
Test of Language Development—Primary: Third Edition *Semantics Composite*	TOLD-P:3	Newcomer & Hammill (1997)	Composite of receptive and expressive vocabulary tests.	Semantics
Syntax Composite			Composite of receptive grammar test, expressive morphosyntax test, and sentence repetition test.	Syntax

(continued)

Test/*Composite or subtest*	Abbreviation	Reference	Description	Construct(s) measured
Vineland Adaptive Behavior Scales, Second Edition	Vineland-II	Sparrow et al. (2005)	Semistructured interview with parents about the child's communication, socialization, motor, and daily living skills.	Adaptive functioning
Wechsler Individual Achievement Test	WIAT	Wechsler (1992)		
Written Expression			Writing a short essay in response to standard prompt.	Written composition
Wide Range Assessment of Memory and Learning	WRAML	Sheslow & Adams (1990)		
Sentence Memory			Sentence repetition task.	Verbal short-term memory
Story Memory			Listening to a short story, then retelling it immediately and after a delay.	Verbal memory
Wisconsin Card Sorting Test	WCST	Heaton (1981)	Sorting ambiguous cards according to a changing rule.	Problem solving Inhibition Mental flexibility
Woodcock–Johnson III Tests of Achievement	WJ III	Woodcock et al. (2001)		
Letter Word ID			Reading a list of words.	Single-word reading accuracy
Word Attack			Reading a list of nonwords.	Phonological coding
Spelling			Spelling single words.	Spelling
Math Fluency			Solving simple arithmetic problems under time pressure.	Math fact knowledge Nonverbal processing speed
Calculation			Solving arithmetic and some higher-level math (algebra, calculus) problems.	Mathematical procedures
Applied Problems			Solving math "word problems" read by the examiner.	Mathematical reasoning

References

Abell, F., Krams, M., Ashburner, J., Passingham, R., Friston, K., Frackowiak, R., et al. (1999). The neuroanatomy of autism: A voxel-based whole brain analysis of structural scans. *NeuroReport, 10*(8), 1647–1651.

Achenbach, T. M. (1982). *Developmental psychopathology.* New York: Wiley.

Adams, A.-M., & Gathercole, S. E. (1995). Phonological working memory and speech production in preschool children. *Journal of Speech and Hearing Research, 38*(2), 403.

Alarcon, M., DeFries, J. C., Light, J. G., & Pennington, B. F. (1997). A twin study of mathematics disability. *Journal of Learning Disabilities, 30*(6), 617–623.

Aldridge, M. A., Stone, K. R., Sweeney, M. H., & Bower, T. G. R. (2000). Preverbal children with autism understand the intentions of others. *Developmental Science, 3*(3), 294–301.

Alexander, A. W., & Slinger-Constant, A. M. (2004). Current status of treatments for dyslexia: Critical review. *Journal of Child Neurology, 19*(10), 744–758.

Alexander, D., & Money, J. (1966). Turner's syndrome and Gerstmann's syndrome: Neuropsychologic comparisons. *Neuropsychologia, 4,* 265–273.

Alloway, T. P. (2007). Working memory, reading, and mathematical skills in children with developmental coordination disorder. *Journal of Experimental Child Psychology, 96*(1), 20–36.

Amen, D. G., Paldi, F., & Thisted, R. A. (1993). Brain SPECT imaging. *Journal of the American Academy of Child and Adolescent Psychiatry, 32*(5), 1080–1081.

American Academy of Pediatrics (AAP). (1982). Policy statement: The Doman–Delacto treatment of neurologically handicapped children. *Pediatrics, 70,* 810–812.

American Academy of Pediatrics (AAP). (1998). Policy statement: Auditory integration training and facilitated communication for autism. *Pediatrics, 102*(2), 431–433.

American Psychiatric Association. (1994). *Diagnostic and Statistical Manual of Mental Disorders* (4th ed.). Washington, DC: Author.

293

American Psychiatric Association. (2000). *Diagnostic and statistical manual of mental disorders* (4th ed., text rev.). Washington, DC: Author.

American Psychology Association. (1994). Policy statement: Facilitated communication. Retrieved from *www.apa.org/about/division/cpmscientific.html#5.*

American Psychological Association. (2005). *Policy statement on evidence-based practice in psychology.* Retrieved from *www.apa.org/practice/ebpstatement. pdf.*

American Speech–Language–Hearing Association (ASHA). (2004). *Auditory integration training* [Technical Report]. Retrieved from *www.asha.org/docs/html/ TR2004-00260.*

American Speech–Language–Hearing Association (ASHA). (2005). *(Central) auditory processing disorder* [Technical Report]. Retrieved from *www.asha.org/ docs/html/TR2005-00043.*

Anderson, M. (2001). Annotation: Conceptions of intelligence. *Journal of Child Psychology and Psychiatry, 42*(3), 287–298.

Andrews, W., Liapi, A., Plachez, C., Camurri, L., Zhang, J., Mori, S., et al. (2006). Robo1 regulates the development of major axon tracts and interneuron migration in the forebrain. *Development, 133*(11), 2243–2252.

Aram, D. M., & Nation, J. E. (1980). Preschool language disorders and subsequent language and academic difficulties. *Journal of Communication Disorders, 13*(2), 159–170.

Aron, A. R., & Poldrack, R. A. (2005). The cognitive neuroscience of response inhibition: Relevance for genetic research in attention-deficit/hyperactivity disorder. *Biological Psychiatry, 57*(11), 1285–1292.

Asperger, H. (1991). "Autistic psychopathy" in childhood. (U. Frith, Trans.). In U. Frith (Ed.), *Autism and Asperger syndrome* (pp. 37–92). Cambridge, UK: Cambridge University Press. (Original work published 1944)

Autism and developmental disabilities monitoring network. (2007). Prevalence of autism spectrum disorders. *Centers for Disease Control and Prevention Surveillance Summaries, 56*(SS04), 12–28. Retrieved from *www.cdc.gov/mmwr/ preview/mmwrhtml/SS5601a2.htm.*

Avons, S. E., Wragg, C. A., Cupples, L., & Lovegrove, W. J. (1998). Measures of phonological short-term memory and their relationship to vocabulary development. *Applied Psycholinguistics, 19*(4), 583–601.

Aylward, E. H., Minshew, N. J., Goldstein, G., Honeycutt, N. A., Augustine, A. M., Yates, K. O., et al. (1999). MRI volumes of amygdala and hippocampus in non-mentally retarded autistic adolescents and adults. *Neurology, 53*(9), 2145–2150.

Aylward, E. H., Reiss, A. L., Reader, M. J., Singer, H. S., Brown, J. E., & Denckla, M. B. (1996). Basal ganglia volumes in children with attention-deficit hyperactivity disorder. *Journal of Child Neurology, 11*(2), 112–115.

Aylward, E. H., Richards, T. L., Berninger, V. W., Nagy, W. E., Field, K. M., Grimme, A. C., et al. (2003). Instructional treatment associated with changes in brain activation in children with dyslexia. *Neurology, 61*(2), 212–219.

Ayres, J. (1972). *Sensory integration and learning disorders.* Los Angeles: Western Psychological Services.

Ayres, J. (1979). *Sensory integration and the child.* Los Angeles: Western Psychological Services.

Badcock, D., & Lovegrove, W. (1981). The effects of contrast, stimulus duration, and spatial frequency on visible persistence in normal and specifically disabled readers. *Journal of Experimental Psychology: Human Perception and Performance, 7*(3), 495–505.

Baddeley, A., Gathercole, S., & Papagno, C. (1998). The phonological loop as a language learning device. *Psychological Review, 105*(1), 158–173.

Badian, N. A. (1983). Arithmetic and nonverbal learning. In H. R. Myklebust (Ed.), *Progress in learning disabilities* (Vol. 5, pp. 235–264). New York: Grune & Stratton.

Badian, N. A. (1997). Dyslexia and the double deficit hypothesis. *Annals of Dyslexia, 47,* 69–87.

Bailey, A., Le Couteur, A., Gottesman, I., Bolton, P., Simonoff, E., Yuzda, E., et al. (1995). Autism as a strongly genetic disorder: Evidence from a British twin study. *Psychological Medicine, 25*(1), 63–77.

Bailey, A., Phillips, W., & Rutter, M. (1996). Autism: Towards an integration of clinical, genetic, neuropsychological, and neurobiological perspectives. *Journal of Child Psychology and Psychiatry, 37*(1), 89–126.

Ball, E. W., & Blachman, B. A. (1991). Does phoneme awareness training in kindergarten make a difference in early word recognition and developmental spelling? *Reading Research Quarterly, 26*(1), 49–66.

Barkley, R. A. (1996). Attention-deficit/hyperactivity disorder. In E. J. Mash & R. A. Barkley (Eds.), *Child psychopathology* (pp. 63–112). New York: Guilford Press.

Baron-Cohen, S., Leslie, A. M., & Frith, U. (1985). Does the autistic child have a "theory of mind"? *Cognition, 21*(1), 37–46.

Baron-Cohen, S., Leslie, A. M., & Frith, U. (1986). Mechanical, behavioral and intentional understanding of picture stories in autistic children. *British Journal of Developmental Psychology, 4,* 113–125.

Baron-Cohen, S., Ring, H. A., Bullmore, E. T., Wheelwright, S., Ashwin, C., & Williams, S. C. R. (2000). The amygdala theory of autism. *Neuroscience and Biobehavioral Reviews, 24,* 355–364.

Baron-Cohen, S., Ring, H. A., Wheelwright, S., Bullmore, E. T., Brammer, M. J., Simmons, A., et al. (1999). Social intelligence in the normal and autistic brain: An fMRI study. *European Journal of Neuroscience, 11*(6), 1891–1898.

Baron-Cohen, S., Wheelwright, S., Lawson, J., Griffin, R., Ashwin, C., Billington, J., et al. (2005). Empathizing and systemizing in autism spectrum conditions. In F. R. Volkmar, R. Paul, A. Klin, & D. J. Cohen (Eds.), *Handbook of autism and pervasive developmental disorders* (3rd ed., Vol. 1, pp. 628–639). Hoboken, NJ: Wiley.

Bartlett, C. W., Flax, J. F., Logue, M. W., Vieland, V. J., Bassett, A. S., Tallal, P., et al. (2002). A major susceptibility locus for specific language impairment is located on 13q21. *American Journal of Human Genetics, 71*(1), 45–55.

Bauman, M. L., & Kemper, T. L. (1994). *Neurobiology of autism.* Baltimore: Johns Hopkins University Press.

Baumgardner, T. L., Singer, H. S., Denckla, M. B., Rubin, M. A., Abrams, M. T., Colli, M. J., et al. (1996). Corpus callosum morphology in children with Tourette syndrome and attention deficit hyperactivity disorder. *Neurology, 47*(2), 477–482.

Bayley, N. (2005). *Bayley Scales of Infant and Toddler Development, Third Edition.* San Antonio, TX: Psychological Corporation.

Beery, K. E. (1997). *The Beery–Buktenica Developmental Test of Visual–Motor Integration (VMI).* Cleveland, OH: Modern Curriculum Press.

Beitchman, J. H., Hood, J., & Inglis, A. (1990). Psychiatric risk in children with speech and language disorders. *Journal of Abnormal Child Psychology, 18*(3), 283–296.

Bellini, G., Bravaccio, C., Calamoneri, F., Donatella Cocuzza, M., Fiorillo, P., Gagliano, A., et al. (2005). No evidence for association between dyslexia and DYX1C1 functional variants in a group of children and adolescents from southern Italy. *Journal of Molecular Neuroscience, 27*(3), 311–314.

Bellugi, W., Mills, D., Jernigan, T., Hickok, G., & Galaburda, A. (1999). Linking cognition, brain structure, and brain function in Williams syndrome. In H. Tager-Flusberg (Ed.), *Neurodevelopmental disorders* (pp. 111–136). Cambridge, MA: MIT Press.

Belmont, J. M., & Butterfield, E. C. (1971). Learning strategies as determinants of memory deficiencies. *Cognitive Psychology, 2,* 411–420.

Belmonte, M. K., Allen, G., Beckel-Mitchener, A., Boulanger, L. M., Carper, R. A., & Webb, S. J. (2004). Autism and abnormal development of brain connectivity. *Journal of Neuroscience, 24*(42), 9228–9231.

Bennetto, L., & Pennington, B. F. (1996). The neuropsychology of fragile X syndrome. In R. J. Hagerman & A. Cronister (Eds.), *Fragile X syndrome* (2nd ed., pp. 210–248). Baltimore: Johns Hopkins University Press.

Bennetto, L., & Pennington, B. F. (2002). The neuropsychology of fragile X syndrome. In R. J. Hagerman & A. Cronister (Eds.), *Fragile X syndrome: Diagnosis, treatment, and research* (3rd ed., pp. 210–248). Baltimore: Johns Hopkins University Press.

Bennetto, L., Pennington, B. F., Porter, D., Taylor, A. K., & Hagerman, R. J. (2001). Profile of cognitive functioning in women with the fragile X mutation. *Neuropsychology, 15*(2), 290–299.

Benson, D. F., & Geschwind, N. (1970). Developmental Gerstmann syndrome. *Neurology, 20*(3), 293–298.

Benton, A. L. (1961). The fiction of the "Gerstmann syndrome." Journal of Neurology, Neurosurgery and Psychiatry, 24, 176–181.

Benton, A. L. (1977). Reflections on the Gerstmann syndrome. *Brain and Language, 4,* 45–62.

Benton, A. L. (1992). Gerstmann's syndrome. *Archives of Neurology, 49,* 445–447.

Berch, D. V., & Bender, B. G. (1990). *Sex chromosome abnormalities and human behavior: Psychological studies.* Boulder, CO: Westview Press.

Berger, H. (1926). Ueber Rechenstorungen bei Herderkrankungen des Brosshirns. *Archiv für Psychiatrie and Nervenkrankheiten, 78,* 238–263.

Bernstein, J. H., & Waber, D. P. (1996). *Developmental scoring system for the Rey–Osterrieth Complex Figure.* Odessa, FL: Psychological Assessment Resources.

Bertrand, J., & Mervis, C. B. (1996). Longitudinal analysis of drawings by children with Williams syndrome: Preliminary results. *Visual Arts Research, 22,* 19–34.

Bertrand, J., Mervis, C. B., & Eisenberg, J. D. (1997). Drawing by children with

Williams syndrome: A developmental perspective. *Developmental Neuropsy-chology, 13, 41–67.*

Best, M., & Demb, J. B. (1999). Normal planum temporale asymmetry in dyslexics with a magnocellular pathway deficit. *NeuroReport, 10*(3), 607–612.

Bettelheim, B. (1967). *The empty fortress.* New York: Free Press.

Biederman, J., Faraone, S. V., Keenan, K., Benjamin, J., Krifcher, B., Moore, C., et al. (1992). Further evidence for family-genetic risk factors in attention deficit hyperactivity disorder: Patterns of comorbidity in probands and relatives psychiatrically and pediatrically referred samples. *Archives of General Psychiatry, 49*(9), 728–738.

Biederman, J., Faraone, S. V., Keenan, K., Knee, D., & Tsuang, M. T. (1990). Family-genetic and psychosocial risk factors in DSM-III attention deficit disorder. *Journal of the American Academy of Child and Adolescent Psychiatry, 29*(4), 526–533.

Biklen, D. (1993). *Communication unbound: How facilitated communication is challenging traditional views of autism and ability/disability.* New York: Teachers College Press.

Bird, J., & Bishop, D. V. (1992). Perception and awareness of phonemes in phonologically impaired children. *European Journal of Disorders in Communication, 27*(4), 289–311.

Birren, J. E. (1952). A factorial analysis of the Wechsler Bellevue scale given to an elderly population. *Journal of Consulting Psychology, 16, 399–405.*

Bishop, D. V. (1990). Handedness, clumsiness and developmental language disorders. *Neuropsychologia, 28*(7), 681–690.

Bishop, D. V. (1997). *Uncommon understanding: Development and disorders of language comprehension in children.* Hove, UK: Psychology Press.

Bishop, D. V. (2007). Curing dyslexia and attention-deficit hyperactivity disorder by training motor coordination: Miracle or myth? *Journal of Paediatrics and Child Health, 43, 653–655.*

Bishop, D. V., & Adams, C. (1990). A prospective study of the relationship between specific language impairment, phonological disorders and reading retardation. *Journal of Child Psychology and Psychiatry, 31*(7), 1027–1050.

Bishop, D. V., Adams, C. V., Lehtonen, A., & Rosen, S. (2005). Effectiveness of computerized training of spelling skills in children with language impairments: A comparison of modified and unmodified speech input. *Journal of Research in Reading, 28*(2), 144–157.

Bishop, D. V., Bishop, S. J., Bright, P., James, C., Delaney, T., & Tallal, P. (1999a). Different origin of auditory and phonological processing problems in children with language impairment: Evidence from a twin study. *Journal of Speech, Language and Hearing Research, 42*(1), 155–168.

Bishop, D.V., Carlyon, R. P., Deeks, J. M., & Bishop, S. J. (1999b). Auditory temporal processing impairment: Neither necessary nor sufficient for causing language impairment in children. *Journal of Speech, Language, and Hearing Research, 42*(6), 1295–1310.

Bishop, D. V., & Edmundson, A. (1987). Language-impaired 4-year-olds: Distinguishing transient from persistent impairment. *Journal of Speech and Hearing Disorders, 52*(2), 156–173.

Bishop, D. V., & Snowling, M. J. (2004). Developmental dyslexia and specific language impairment: Same or different? *Psychological Bulletin, 130*(6), 858–886.

Bleuler, E. (1950). *Dementia praecox, or a group within the schizophrenias* (J. Zinkin, Trans.). New York: International Universities Press. (Original work published 1911)

Blondis, T. A. (2004). Neurodevelopmental motor disorders. In D. Dewey & D. E. Tupper (Eds.), *Developmental motor disorders: A neuropsychological perspective* (pp. 113–136). New York: Guilford Press.

Boada, R., & Pennington, B. F. (2006). Deficient implicit phonological representations in children with dyslexia. *Journal of Experimental Child Psychology, 95*(3), 153–193.

Boada, R., Riddle, M., & Pennington, B. F. (2008). Integrating science and practice in education. In C. R. Reynolds & E. Fletcher-Janzen (Eds.), *Neuroscientific and clinical perspectives on the RTI initiative in learning disabilities diagnosis and intervention* (pp. 179–191). Hoboken, NJ: Wiley.

Boets, B., Wouters, J., van Wieringen, A., & Ghesquiere, P. (2006). Auditory temporal information processing in preschool children at family risk for dyslexia: Relations with phonological abilities and developing literacy skills. *Brain and Language, 97*(1), 64–79.

Boetsch, E. A. (1996). *A longitudinal study of the relationship between dyslexia and socioemotional functioning in young children.* Unpublished doctoral dissertation, University of Denver.

Boll, T. (1993). *Children's Category Test.* San Antonio, TX: Psychological Corporation.

Bolton, P., & Griffiths, P. D. (1997). Association of tuberous sclerosis of temporal lobes with autism and atypical autism. *Lancet, 349*(9049), 392–395.

Bolton, P., Macdonald, H., Pickles, A., Rios, P., Goode, S., Crowson, M., et al. (1994). A case–control family history study of autism. *Journal of Child Psychology and Psychiatry, 35*(5), 877–900.

Bookheimer, S. Y. (2000). *fMRI of emotional processing in autism.* Unpublished manuscript, Collaborative Program of Excellence in Autism, Denver, CO.

Borman, G. D., Benson, J., & Overman, T. (2008). *The Scientific Learning Corporation's Fast ForWord computer-based training program in the Baltimore City public schools.* Manuscript submitted for publication.

Bowers, P. G., & Wolf, M. (1993). Theoretical links among naming speed, precise timing mechanisms and orthographic skill in dyslexia. *Reading and Writing: An interdisciplinary Journal, 5*, 69–85.

Bowey, J. A. (2001). Nonword repetition and young children's receptive vocabulary: A longitudinal study. *Applied Psycholinguistics, 22*(3), 441–469.

Bradley, L., & Bryant, P. E. (1983). Categorizing sounds and learning to read: A causal connection. *Nature, 301*(5899), 419–421.

Brainard, S. S., Schreiner, R. A., & Hagerman, R. J. (1991). Cognitive profiles of the carrier fragile X woman. *American Journal of Medical Genetics, 38*(2–3), 505–508.

Brambati, S. M., Termine, C., Ruffino, M., Stella, G., Fazio, F., Cappa, S. F., et al. (2004). Regional reductions of gray matter volume in familial dyslexia. *Neurology, 63*(4), 742–745.

Bronfenbrenner, U., & Ceci, S. J. (1994). Nature–nurture reconceptualized in devel opmental perspective: A bioecological model. *Psychological Review, 101*(4), 568–586.

Brookes, K. J., Mill, J., Guindalini, C., Curran, S., Xu, X., Knight, J., et al. (2006). A common haplotype of the dopamine transporter gene associated with attention-deficit/hyperactivity disorder and interacting with maternal use of alcohol during pregnancy. *Archives of General Psychiatry, 63*(1), 74–81.

Brown, G. T., & Burns, S. A. (2001). The efficacy of neurodevelopmental treatment in pediatrics: A systematic review. *British Journal of Occupational Therapy, 64*, 235–244.

Brown, R., Hobson, R. P., Lee, A., & Stevenson, J. (1997). Are there "autistic-like" features in congenitally blind children? *Journal of Child Psychology and Psychiatry, 38*(6), 693–703.

Brown, W. E., Eliez, S., Memon, V., Rumsey, J. M., White, C. D., & Reiss, A. L. (2001). Preliminary evidence of widespread morphological variations of the brain in dyslexia. *Neurology, 56*(6), 781–783.

Bruininks, R. H. (1978). *Bruininks–Oseretsky test of motor proficiency*. Circle Pines, MN: American Guidance Service.

Bruininks, R. K., Woodcock, R. W., Weatherman, R. F., & Hill, B. K. (1996). *Scales of Independent Behavior—Revised (SIB-R)*. Itasca, IL: Riverside.

Brunswick, N., McCrory, E., Price, C. J., Frith, C. D., & Frith, U. (1999). Explicit and implicit processing of words and pseudowords by adult developmental dyslexics: A search for Wernicke's *Wortschatz? Brain, 122*(Pt. 10), 1901–1917.

Bryden, M. P., & Ley, R. G. (1983). Right-hemisphere involvement in the perception and expression of emotion in normal humans. In K. M. Heilman & P. Satz (Eds.), *The neuropsychology of human emotion* (pp. 6–44). New York: Guilford Press.

Bryson, S. E., & Smith, I. M. (1998). Epidemiology of autism: Prevalence, associated characteristics, and implications for research and service delivery. *Mental Retardation and Developmental Disabilities Research Reviews, 4*, 97–103.

Butterworth, B. (2005). Developmental dyscalculia. In J. I. D. Campbell (Ed.), *Handbook of mathematical cognition* (pp. 455–469). New York: Psychology Press.

Byrne, B., & Fielding-Barnsley, R. (1989). Phonemic awareness and letter knowledge in the child's acquisition of the alphabetic principle. *Journal of Educational Psychology, 81*(3), 313–321.

Byrne, B., Fielding-Barnsley, R., & Ashley, L. (2000). Effects of preschool phoneme identity training after six years: Outcome level distinguished from rate of response. *Journal of Educational Psychology, 92*(4), 659–667.

Byrne, B., & Shea, P. (1979). Semantic and phonetic memory codes in beginning readers. *Memory and Cognition, 7*(5), 333–338.

Cacace, A. T., & McFarland, D. J. (1998). Central auditory processing disorder in school-aged children: A critical review. *Journal of Speech, Language, and Hearing Research, 41*(2), 355–373.

Caltagirone, C., Nocentini, U., & Vicari, S. (1990). Cognitive functions in adult Down's syndrome. *International Journal of Neuroscience, 54*(3–4), 221–230.

Campbell, M. (1988). Fenfluramine treatment of autism. *Journal of Child Psychology and Psychiatry, 29*(1), 1–10.

Cantwell, D. P. (1975). Genetics of hyperactivity. *Journal of Child Psychology and Psychiatry, 16*(3), 261–264.

Carlesimo, G. A., Marotta, L., & Vicari, S. (1997). Long-term memory in mental retardation: Evidence for a specific impairment in subjects with Down's syndrome. *Neuropsychologia, 35*(1), 71–79.

Carpenter, M., Pennington, B. F., & Rogers, S. J. (2001). Understanding of others' intentions in children with autism. *Journal of Autism and Developmental Disorders, 31*(6), 589–599.

Carpenter, P. A., Just, M. A., & Shell, P. (1990). What one intelligence test measures: A theoretical account of the processing in the Raven Progressive Matrices Test. *Psychological Review, 97*(3), 404–431.

Carroll, J. B. (1993). *Human cognitive abilities: A survey of factor analytic studies.* Cambridge, UK: Cambridge University Press.

Casanova, M. F., Araque, J., Giedd, J., & Rumsey, J. M. (2004). Reduced brain size and gyrification in the brains of dyslexic patients. *Journal of Child Neurology, 19*(4), 275–281.

Casey, B. J., Castellanos, F. X., Giedd, J. N., Marsh, W. L., Hamburger, S. D., Schubert, A. B., et al. (1997). Implication of right frontostriatal circuitry in response inhibition and attention-deficit/hyperactivity disorder. *Journal of the American Academy of Child and Adolescent Psychiatry, 36*(3), 374–383.

Caspi, A., McClay, J., Moffitt, T. E., Mill, J., Martin, J., Craig, I. W., et al. (2002). Role of genotype in the cycle of violence in maltreated children. *Science, 297*(5582), 851–854.

Caspi, A., Sugden, K., Moffitt, T. E., Taylor, A., Craig, I. W., Harrington, H., et al. (2003). Influence of life stress on depression: Moderation by a polymorphism in the 5-HTT gene. *Science, 301*(5631), 386–389.

Castellanos, F. X., Giedd, J. N., Marsh, W. L., Hamburger, S. D., Vaituzis, A. C., Dickstein, D. P., et al. (1996). Quantitative brain magnetic resonance imaging in attention-deficit hyperactivity disorder. *Archives of General Psychiatry, 53*(7), 607–616.

Cattell, R. B. (1943). The measurement of adult intelligence. *Psychological Bulletin, 40*, 153–193.

Cattell, R. B. (1963). Theory of fluid and crystallized intelligence: A critical experiment. *Journal of Educational Psychology, 54*, 1–22.

Cattell, R. B., & Horn, J. L. (1978). A check on the theory of fluid and crystallized intelligence with description of new subtest designs. *Journal of Educational Measurement, 15*(3), 139–164.

Centerwall, S. A., & Centerwall, W. R. (1960). A study of children with mongolism reared in the home compared to those reared away from home. *Pediatrics, 25*, 678–685.

Chakrabarti, S., & Fombonne, E. (2001). Pervasive developmental disorders in preschool children. *Journal of the American Medical Association, 285*(24), 3093–3099.

Chambless, D. L., Baker, M. J., Baucom, D. H., Beutler, L. E., Calhoun, K. S., Crits-Christoph, P., et al. (1998). Update on empirically validated treatments, II. *The Clinical Psychologist, 51*(1), 3–16.

Chapman, R. S. (1999). Language and cognitive development in children and adolescents with Down syndrome. In J. F. Miller, L. A. Leavitt, & M. Leddy (Eds.), *Improving the communication of people with Down syndrome* (pp. 41–60). Baltimore: Brookes.

Chess, S. (1977). Follow-up report on autism in congenital rubella. *Journal of Autism and Childhood Schizophrenia, 7,* 69–81.

Chhabildas, N., Pennington, B. F., & Willcutt, E. G. (2001). A comparison of the neuropsychological profiles of the DSM-IV subtypes of ADHD. *Journal of Abnormal Child Psychology, 29*(6), 529–540.

Christensen, L. L., & Nielsen, J. (1981). A neuropsychological investigation of 17 women with Turner's syndrome. In W. Schmid & J. Nielsen (Eds.), *Human behavior and genetics* (pp. 151–166). Amsterdam: Elsevier/North-Holland.

Clark, C., Klonoff, H., & Hadyen, M. (1990). Regional cerebral glucose metabolism in Turner syndrome. *Canadian Journal of Neurological Science, 17,* 140–144.

Cohen, H. (1966). Psychological test findings in adolescents having ovarian dysgenesis. *Psychological Medicine, 24,* 249–256.

Cohen, I. L., Vietze, P. M., Sudhalter, V., Jenkins, E. C., & Brown, W. T. (1989). Parent–child dyadic gaze patterns in fragile X males and in non-fragile X males with autistic disorder. *Journal of Child Psychology and Psychiatry, 30*(6), 845–856.

Cohen, J. D. (2003). *Organization and function of the prefrontal cortex: Neuroimaging and computational modeling.* Paper presented at the John Merck Fund Summer Institute on the Biology of Developmental Disabilities, Princeton University.

Cohen, J. D., & Servan-Schreiber, D. (1992). Context, cortex, and dopamine: A connectionist approach to behavior and biology in schizophrenia. *Psychological Review, 99,* 45–77.

Cohen, W., Hodson, A., O'Hare, A., Boyle, J., Durrani, T., McCartney, E., et al. (2005). Effects of computer-based intervention through acoustically modified speech (Fast ForWord) in severe mixed receptive–expressive language impairment: Outcomes from a randomized controlled trial. *Journal of Speech, Language, and Hearing Research, 48*(3), 715–729.

Coniglio, S. J., Lewis, J. D., Lang, C., Burns, T. G., Subhani-Siddique, R., Weintraub, A., et al. (2001). A randomized, double-blind, placebo-controlled trial of single-dose intravenous secretin as treatment for children with autism. *Journal of Pediatrics, 138*(5), 649–655.

Constantino, J. N., & Todd, R. D. (2003). Autistic traits in the general population: A twin study. *Archives of General Psychiatry, 60*(5), 524–530.

Coonrod, E. E., & Stone, W. L. (2005). Screening for autism in young children. In F. R. Volkmar, R. Paul, A. Klin, & D. J. Cohen (Eds.), *Handbook of autism and pervasive developmental disorders* (3rd ed., Vol. 2, pp. 707–729). Hoboken, NJ: Wiley.

Cope, N. A., Harold, D., Hill, G., Moskvina, V., Stevenson, J., Holmans, P., et al. (2005a). Strong evidence that KIAA0319 on chromosome 6p is a susceptibility gene for developmental dyslexia. *American Journal of Human Genetics, 76*(4), 581–591.

Cope, N. A., Hill, G., van den Bree, M., Harold, D., Moskvina, V., Green, E. K., et al. (2005b). No support for association between dyslexia susceptibility 1 candidate 1 and developmental dyslexia. *Molecular Psychiatry, 10*(3), 237–238.

Corina, D. P., Richards, T. L., Serafini, S., Richards, A. L., Steury, K., Abbott, R. D., et al. (2001). fMRI auditory language differences between dyslexic and able reading children. *NeuroReport, 12*(6), 1195–1201.

Courchesne, E. (2004). Brain development in autism: Early overgrowth followed by premature arrest of growth. *Mental Retardation and Developmental Disabilities Research Review, 10*(2), 106–111.

Courchesne, E., Carper, R., & Akshoomoff, N. (2003). Evidence of brain overgrowth in the first year of life in autism. *Journal of the American Medical Association, 290*(3), 337–344.

Courchesne, E., & Pierce, K. (2005). Why the frontal cortex in autism might be talking only to itself: Local over-connectivity but long-distance disconnection. *Current Opinion in Neurobiology, 15*(2), 225–230.

Courchesne, E., Yeung-Courchesne, R., Press, G. A., Hesselink, J. R., & Jernigan, T. L. (1988). Hypoplasia of cerebellar vermal lobules VI and VII in autism. *New England Journal of Medicine, 318*(21), 1349–1354.

Cox, A., Klein, K., Charman, T., Baird, G., Baron-Cohen, S., Swettenham, J., et al. (1999). Autism spectrum disorders at 20 and 42 months of age: Stability of clinical and ADI-R diagnosis. *Journal of Child Psychology and Psychiatry, 40*(5), 719–732.

Critchley, H. D., Daly, E. M., Bullmore, E. T., Williams, S. C., Van Amelsvoort, T., Robertson, D. M., et al. (2000). The functional neuroanatomy of social behaviour: Changes in cerebral blood flow when people with autistic disorder process facial expressions. *Brain, 123*(Pt. 11), 2203–2212.

Crnic, L. S., & Pennington, B. (2000). Down syndrome: Neuropsychology and animal models. In C. Rovee-Collier, L. P. Lipsitt, & H. Hayne (Eds.), *Progress in infancy research* (Vol. 1, pp. 69–111). Mahwah, NJ: Erlbaum.

Croen, L. A., Grether, J. K., Hoogstrate, J., & Selvin, S. (2002). The changing prevalence of autism in California. *Journal of Autism and Developmental Disorders, 32*(3), 207–215.

Cronbach, L. J., & Meehl, P. E. (1955). Construct validity in psychological tests. *Psychological Bulletin, 52*(4), 281–302.

Csibra, G., Gergely, G., Biro, S., Koos, O., & Brockbank, M. (1999). Goal attribution without agency cues: The perception of 'pure reason' in infancy. *Cognition, 72*(3), 237–267.

Cunningham, A. E. (1990). Explicit versus implicit instruction in phonemic awareness. *Journal of Experimental Child Psychology, 50*(3), 429–444.

Cunningham, A. E., & Stanovich, K. E. (1998). The impact of print exposure on word recognition. In J. L. Metsala & L. C. Ehri (Eds.), *Word recognition in beginning literacy* (pp. 235–262). Mahwah, NJ: Erlbaum.

Curtis, M. E. (1980). Development of components of reading skill. *Journal of Educational Psychology, 72*, 656–669.

D'Angiulli, A., & Siegel, L. S. (2003). Cognitive functioning as measured by the WISC-R: Do children with learning disabilities have distinctive patterns of performance? *Journal of Learning Disabilities, 36*(1), 48–58.

Daneman, M., & Case, R. (1981). Syntactic form, semantic complexity, and short-term memory: Influences on children's acquisition of new linguistic structures. *Developmental Psychology, 17*(4), 367–378.

Dawes, R. M. (1994). *House of cards: Psychology and psychotherapy built on myth.* New York: Free Press.

Dawson, G., Carver, L., Meltzoff, A. N., Panagiotides, H., McPartland, J., & Webb, S. J. (2002a). Neural correlates of face and object recognition in young children with autism spectrum disorder, developmental delay, and typical development. *Child Development, 73*(3), 700–717.

Dawson, G., Munson, J., Estes, A., Osterling, J., McPartland, J., Toth, K., et al. (2002b). Neurocognitive function and joint attention ability in young children with autism spectrum disorder versus developmental delay. *Child Development, 73*(2), 345–358.

Dawson, G., & Osterling, J. (1997). Early intervention in autism: Effectiveness and common elements of current approaches. In M. J. Guralnick (Ed.), *The effectiveness of early intervention* (pp. 307–325). Baltimore: Brookes.

Dawson, G., & Wathing, R. (2000). Interventions to facilitate auditory, visual, and motor integration in autism: A review of the evidence. *Journal of Developmental Disabilities, 30*, 415–421.

De Fosse, L., Hodge, S. M., Makris, N., Kennedy, D. N., Caviness, V. S., Jr., McGrath, L., et al. (2004). Language–association cortex asymmetry in autism and specific language impairment. *Annals of Neurology, 56*(6), 757–766.

DeFries, J. C., & Gillis, J. J. (1993). Genetics of reading disability. In R. Plomin & G. E. McClearn (Eds.), *Nature, nurture, and psychology* (pp. 121–145). Washington DC: American Psychological Association.

Dehaene, S. (2003). Acalculia and number processing disorders. In T. E. Feinberg & M. J. Farah (Eds.), *Behavioral neurology and neuropsychology* (2nd ed., pp. 207–215). New York: McGraw-Hill.

Delis, D. C., Kaplan, E., & Kramer, J. H. (2001). *Delis–Kaplan Executive Function System.* San Antonio, TX: Psychological Corporation.

Denckla, M. B. (1979). Childhood disabilities. In K. M. Heilman & E. Valenstein (Eds.), *Clinical neuropsychology* (pp. 535–573). New York: Oxford University Press.

Denckla, M. B. (1983). The neuropsychology of social-emotional learning disabilities. *Archives of Neurology, 40*(8), 461–462.

Denckla, M. B., & Rudel, R. G. (1976). Rapid 'automatized' naming (R.A.N.): Dyslexia differentiated from other learning disabilities. *Neuropsychologia, 14*(4), 471–479.

Detterman, D. K., & Daniel, M. H. (1989). Correlations of mental tests with each other and with cognitive variables are highest for low IQ groups. *Intelligence, 13*, 349–359.

Deutsch, G. K., Dougherty, R. F., Bammer, R., Siok, W. T., Gabrieli, J. D., & Wandell, B. (2005). Children's reading performance is correlated with white matter structure measured by diffusion tensor imaging. *Cortex, 41*(3), 354–363.

Devenny, D. A., Hill, A. L., Patxot, O., Silverman, W. P., & Wisniewski, K. E. (1992). Aging in higher functioning adults with Down's syndrome: An interim report in a longitudinal study. *Journal of Intellectual Disability Research, 36*(3), 241–250.

Dewey, D., & Bottos, S. (2004). Neuroimaging of developmental motor disorders. In D. Dewey & D. E. Tupper (Eds.), *Developmental motor disorders: A neuropsychological perspective* (pp. 26–43). New York: Guilford Press.

Dewey, D., Cantell, M., & Crawford, S. G. (2007). Motor and gestural performance in children with autism spectrum disorders, developmental coordination disorder, and/or attention deficit hyperactivity disorder. *Journal of the International Neuropsychological Society, 13*(2), 246–256.

Dingman, H. F., & Tarjan, G. (1960). Mental retardation and the normal distribution curve. *American Journal of Mental Deficiency, 64,* 991–994.

Down, J. L. N. (1866). Observations on ethnic classification of idiots. *Mental Science, 13,* 121–128.

Dugdale, R. L. (1877). *The Jukes.* New York: Putnam.

Dunn-Geier, J., Ho, H. H., Auersperg, E., Doyle, D., Eaves, L., Matsuba, C., et al. (2000). Effect of secretin on children with autism: A randomized controlled trial. *Developmental Medicine and Child Neurology, 42*(12), 796–802.

Dunn, L. M., & Dunn, D. M. (2007). *Peabody Picture Vocabulary Test, Fourth Edition (PPVT-4).* Bloomington, MN: Pearson Assessments.

Dunst, C. J. (1990). Sensorimotor development of infants with Down syndrome. In D. Cicchetti & M. Beeghly (Eds.), *Children with Down syndrome* (pp. 180–230). New York: Cambridge University Press.

DuPaul, G. J., Power, T. J., Anastopoulos, A. D., & Reid, R. (1998). *ADHD Rating Scale–IV: Checklists, norms, and clinical interpretation.* New York: Guilford Press.

Dupont, A., Vaeth, M., & Videbech, P. (1986). Mortality and life expectancy of Down's syndrome in Denmark. *Journal of Mental Deficiency Research, 30*(2), 111–120.

Durston, S., & Konrad, K. (2007). Integrating genetic, psychopharmacological and neuroimaging studies: A converging methods approach to understanding the neurobiology of ADHD. *Developmental Review, 27*(3), 374–395.

Dykens, E. M., Hodapp, R. M., & Leckman, J. F. (1987). Strengths and weaknesses in the intellectual functioning of males with fragile X syndrome. *American Journal of Mental Deficiency, 92*(2), 234–236.

Eckert, M. A., Leonard, C. M., Richards, T. L., Aylward, E. H., Thomson, J., & Berninger, V. W. (2003). Anatomical correlates of dyslexia: Frontal and cerebellar findings. *Brain, 126*(Pt. 2), 482–494.

Eckert, M. A., Leonard, C. M., Wilke, M., Eckert, M., Richards, T., & Richards, A. (2005). Anatomical signatures of dyslexia in children: Unique information from manual and voxel based morphometry brain measures. *Cortex, 41*(3), 304–315.

Eden, G. F., VanMeter, J. W., Rumsey, J. M., Maisog, J. M., Woods, R. P., & Zeffiro, T. A. (1996). Abnormal processing of visual motion in dyslexia revealed by functional brain imaging. *Nature, 382*(6586), 66–69.

Einfeld, S., Maloney, H., & Hall, W. (1989). Autism is not associated with the fragile X syndrome. *American Journal of Medical Genetics, 34*(2), 187–193.

Eley, T. C., Bishop, D. V., Dale, P. S., Oliver, B., Petrill, S. A., Price, T. S., et al. (1999). Genetic and environmental origins of verbal and performance components of cognitive delay in 2-year-olds. *Developmental Psychology, 35*(4), 1122–1131.

Eliez, S., Rumsey, J. M., Giedd, J. N., Schmitt, J. E., Patwardhan, A. J., & Reiss, A. L. (2000). Morphological alteration of temporal lobe gray matter in dyslexia: An MRI study. *Journal of Child Psychology and Psychiatry, 41*(5), 637–644.

Ellis, N. R. (1963). The stimulus trace and behavioral inadequacy. In N. R. Ellis (Ed.), *Handbook of mental deficiency: Psychological theory and research* (pp. 134–158). New York: McGraw-Hill.

Ellis, N. R., Woodley-Zanthos, P., & Dulaney, C. L. (1989). Memory for spatial location in children, adults, and mentally retarded persons. *American Journal of Mental Retardation, 93*(5), 521–526.

Elman, J. L., Bates, E. A., Johnson, M. C., Karmiloff-Smith, A., Parisi, D., & Plunkett, K. (1996). *Rethinking innateness.* Cambridge, MA: MIT Press.

Epstein, C. J. (1989). Down syndrome. In C. R. Scriver, A. L. Beaudet, W. S. Sly, & P. Valle (Eds.), *The metabolic basis of inherited disease* (pp. 291–396). New York: McGraw-Hill.

Esch, B. E., & Carr, J. E. (2004). Secretin as a treatment for autism: A review of the evidence. *Journal of Autism and Developmental Disorders, 34*(5), 543–556.

Etcoff, N. L. (1984). Selective attention to facial identity and facial emotion. *Neuropsychologia, 22*(3), 281–295.

Evidence-Based Medicine Working Group. (1992). Evidence-based medicine: A new approach to teaching the practice of medicine. *Journal of the American Medical Association, 268,* 2420–2425.

Ewart, A. K., Jin, W., Atkinson, D., Morris, C. A., & Keating, M. T. (1994). Supravalvular aortic stenosis associated with a deletion disrupting the elastin gene. *Journal of Clinical Investigation, 93*(3), 1071–1077.

Ewart, A. K., Morris, C. A., Atkinson, D., Jin, W., Sternes, K., Spallone, P., et al. (1993a). Hemizygosity at the elastin locus in a developmental disorder, Williams syndrome. *Nature Genetics, 5*(1), 11–16.

Ewart, A. K., Morris, C. A., Ensing, G. J., Loker, J., Moore, C., Leppert, M., et al. (1993b). A human vascular disorder, supravalvular aortic stenosis, maps to chromosome 7. *Proceedings of the National Academy of Sciences USA, 90*(8), 3226–3230.

Fagerheim, T., Raeymaekers, P., Tonnessen, F. E., Pedersen, M., Tranebjaerg, L., & Lubs, H. A. (1999). A new gene (DYX3) for dyslexia is located on chromosome 2. *Journal of Medical Genetics, 36*(9), 664–669.

Farah, M. J. (2003). Computational modeling in behavioral neurology and neuropsychology. In T. E. Feinberg & J. J. Farah (Eds.), *Behavioral neurology and neuropsychology* (pp. 135–143). New York: McGraw-Hill.

Faraone, S. V., Biederman, J., Chen, W. J., Kricher, B., Moore, C., Sprich, S., et al. (1992). Segregation analysis of attention deficit hyperactivity disorder: Evidence for single major gene transmission. *Psychiatric Genetics, 2,* 257–275.

Faraone, S. V., Biederman, J., Keenan, K., & Tsuang, M. T. (1991). A family-genetic study of girls with DSM-III attention deficit disorder. *American Journal of Psychiatry, 148*(1), 112–117.

Faraone, S. V., Perlis, R. H., Doyle, A. E., Smoller, J. W., Goralnick, J. J., Holmgren, M. A., et al. (2005). Molecular genetics of attention-deficit/hyperactivity disorder. *Biological Psychiatry, 57*(11), 1313–1323.

Faraone, S. V., Spencer, T., Aleardi, M., Pagano, C., & Biederman, J. (2004). Meta-analysis of the efficacy of methylphenidate for treating adult attention-deficit/hyperactivity disorder. *Journal of Clinical Psychopharmacology, 24*(1), 24–29.

Farmer, M. E., & Klein, R. M. (1995). The evidence for a temporal processing deficit linked to dyslexia: A review. *Psychonomic Bulletin and Review, 2*(4), 460–493.

Fawcett, A. J., Nicolson, R. I., & Dean, P. (1996). Impaired performance of children with dyslexia on a range of cerebellar tasks. *Annals of Dyslexia, 46,* 259–283.

Fein, D., Pennington, B., Markowitz, P., Braverman, M., & Waterhouse, L. (1986). Toward a neuropsychological model of infantile autism: Are the social deficits primary? *Journal of the American Academy of Child Psychiatry, 25*(2), 198–212.

Ferguson, H. B., & Rappaport, J. L. (1983). Nosological issues and biological validation. In M. Rutter (Ed.), *Developmental neuropsychiatry* (pp. 369–384). New York: Guilford Press.

Filipek, P. A., Kennedy, D. N., & Caviness, V. S. (1992). Neuroimaging in child neuropsychology. In I. Rapin & S. Segalowitz (Eds.), *Handbook of neuropsychology* (Vol. 6, pp. 301–328). Amsterdam: Elsevier Science.

Filipek, P. A., Semrud-Clikeman, M., Steingard, R. J., Renshaw, P. F., Kennedy, D. N., & Biederman, J. (1997). Volumetric MRI analysis comparing subjects having attention-deficit hyperactivity disorder with normal controls. *Neurology, 48*(3), 589–601.

Fisher, S. E., & DeFries, J. C. (2002). Developmental dyslexia: Genetic dissection of a complex cognitive trait. *Nature Reviews Neuroscience, 3*(10), 767–780.

Fisher, S. E., & Francks, C. (2006). Genes, cognition and dyslexia: Learning to read the genome. *Trends in Cognitive Sciences, 10*(6), 250–257.

Fitzhugh, K., Fitzhugh, L., & Reitan, R. (1967). Influence of age on measures of problem solving and experimental background in subjects with long-standing cerebral dysfunction. *Journal of Gerontology, 19,* 132–134.

Flannery, K. A., Liederman, J., Daly, L., & Schultz, J. (2000). Male prevalence for reading disability is found in a large sample of black and white children free from ascertainment bias. *Journal of the International Neuropsychological Society, 6*(4), 433–442.

Flax, N., Solan, H. A., & Suchoff, I. B. (1983). Optometry and dyslexia. *Journal of the American Optometry Association, 27,* 593–594.

Fletcher, J. M. (1985). External validation of learning disability typologies. In B. P. Rourke (Ed.), *Neuropsychology of learning disabilities* (pp. 187–211). New York: Guilford Press.

Fletcher, J. M., Foorman, B. R., Shaywitz, S. E., & Shaywitz, B. A. (1999). Conceptual and methodological issues in dyslexia research: A lesson for developmental disorders. In H. Tager-Flusberg (Ed.), *Neurodevelopmental disorders* (pp. 271–305). Cambridge, MA: MIT Press.

Folstein, S., & Rutter, M. (1977). Genetic influences and infantile autism. *Nature, 265*(5596), 726–728.

Folstein, S. E., & Rutter, M. L. (1988). Autism: Familial aggregation and genetic implications. *Journal of Autism and Developmental Disorders, 18*(1), 3–30.

Fortna, A., Kim, Y., MacLaren, E., Marshall, K., Hahn, G., Meltesen, L., et al. (2004). Lineage-specific gene duplication and loss in human and great ape evolution. *PLoS Biology, 2*(7), 937–954.

Foster, J. C., & Taylor, C. A. (1920). The applicability of mental tests to persons over 50. *Journal of Applied Psychology, 4*, 39–58.

Fowler, A. E. (1991). How early phonological development might set the stage for phoneme awareness. In S. A. Brady & D. P. Shankweiler (Eds.), *Phonological processes in literacy: A tribute to Isabelle Y. Liberman* (pp. 97–118). Hillsdale, NJ: Erlbaum.

Fowler, A. E. (1998). Language in mental retardation: Associations with and dissociations from general cognition. In J. A. Burack, R. M. Hodapp, & E. Zigler (Eds.), *Handbook of mental retardation and development* (pp. 290–333). Cambridge, UK: Cambridge University Press.

Fowler, A. E., Gelman, R., & Gleitman, L. R. (1994). The course of language learning in children with Down syndrome: Longitudinal and language level comparisons with young normally developing children. In H. Tager-Flusberg (Ed.), *Constraints on language acquisition* (pp. 91–140). Hillsdale, NJ: Erlbaum.

Fowler, A. E., & Swainson, B. (2004). Relationships of naming skills to reading, memory, and receptive vocabulary: Evidence for imprecise phonological representations of words by poor readers. *Annals of Dyslexia, 54*(2), 247–280.

Francks, C., Paracchini, S., Smith, S. D., Richardson, A. J., Scerri, T. S., Cardon, L. R., et al. (2004). A 77-kilobase region of chromosome 6p22.2 is associated with dyslexia in families from the United Kingdom and from the United States. *American Journal of Human Genetics, 75*(6), 1046–1058.

Frangiskakis, J. M., Ewart, A. K., Morris, C. A., Mervis, C. B., Bertrand, J., Robinson, B. F., et al. (1996). LIM-kinase1 hemizygosity implicated in impaired visuospatial constructive cognition. *Cell, 86*(1), 59–69.

Frank, M. J. (2005). Dynamic dopamine modulation in the basal ganglia: A neurocomputational account of cognitive deficits in medicated and non-medicated parkinsonism. *Journal of Cognitive Neuroscience, 17*, 51–72.

Freund, L. S., & Reiss, A. L. (1991). Cognitive profiles associated with the fra(X) syndrome in males and females. *American Journal of Medical Genetics, 38*(4), 542–547.

Friedman, N. P., Miyake, A., Corley, R. P., Young, S. E., DeFries, J. C., & Hewitt, J. K. (2006). Not all executive functions are related to intelligence. *Psychological Science, 17*(2), 172–179.

Frith, U., & Happé, F. (1994). Autism: Beyond "theory of mind." *Cognition, 50*, 115–132.

Fry, A. F., & Hale, S. (1996). Processing speed, working memory, and fluid intelligence. *Psychological Science, 7*(4), 237–241.

Fuster, J. M. (1989). *The prefrontal cortex: Anatomy, physiology and neuropsychology of the frontal lobe* (2nd ed.). New York: Raven Press.

Galaburda, A. M., Menard, M. T., & Rosen, G. D. (1994). Evidence for aberrant auditory anatomy in developmental dyslexia. *Proceedings of the National Academy of Sciences USA, 91*(17), 8010–8013.

Galaburda, A. M., Sherman, G. F., Rosen, G. D., Aboitiz, F., & Geschwind, N. (1985). Developmental dyslexia: Four consecutive patients with cortical anomalies. *Annals of Neurology, 18*(2), 222–233.

Galvez, R., Smith, R. L., & Greenough, W. T. (2005). Olfactory bulb mitral cell dendritic pruning abnormalities in a mouse model of the fragile-X mental retardation syndrome: Further support for FMRP's involvement in dendritic development. *Brain Research: Developmental Brain Research, 157*(2), 214–216.

Garber, K., Smith, K. T., Reines, D., & Warren, S. T. (2006). Transcription, translation and fragile X syndrome. *Current Opinion in Genetics and Development, 16*(3), 270–275.

Garron, D. (1977). Intelligence among persons with Turner's syndrome. *Behavior Genetics, 7*, 105–127.

Gathercole, S. E., & Baddeley, A. D. (1989). Evaluation of the role of phonological STM in the development of vocabulary in children: A longitudinal study. *Journal of Memory and Language, 28*(2), 200–213.

Gathercole, S. E., & Baddeley, A. D. (1990a). Phonological memory deficits in language disordered children: Is there a causal connection? Journal of Memory and Language, 29(3), 336–360.

Gathercole, S. E., & Baddeley, A. D. (1990b). The role of phonological memory in vocabulary acquisition: A study of young children learning new names. *British Journal of Developmental Psychology, 81*, 439–454.

Gathercole, S. E., Willis, C. S., Emslie, H., & Baddeley, A. D. (1992). Phonological memory and vocabulary development during the early school years: A longitudinal study. *Developmental Psychology, 28*(5), 887–898.

Gauger, L. M., Lombardino, L. J., & Leonard, C. M. (1997). Brain morphology in children with specific language impairment. *Journal of Speech, Language, and Hearing Research, 40*(6), 1272–1284.

Gayan, J., & Olson, R. K. (2001). Genetic and environmental influences on orthographic and phonological skills in children with reading disabilities. *Developmental Neuropsychology, 20*(2), 483–507.

Gazzaniga, M. S., Ivry, R. B., & Magnun, G. R. (2002). *Cognitive neuroscience: The biology of the mind* (2nd ed.). New York: Norton.

Geary, D. C. (1994). *Children's mathematical development: Research and practical applications*. Washington, DC: American Psychological Association.

Geary, D. C., Hamson, C. O., & Hoard, M. K. (2000). Numerical and arithmetical cognition: A longitudinal study of process and concept deficits in children with learning disability. *Journal of Experimental Child Psychology, 77*, 236–263.

Geary, D. C., Hoard, M. K., Byrd-Craven, J., & DeSoto, M. C. (2004). Strategy choices in simple and complex addition: Contributions of working memory and counting knowledge for children with mathematical disability. *Journal of Experimental Child Psychology, 88*(2), 121–151.

Gelman, R., & Gallistel, C. R. (1986). *The child's understanding of number* (2nd.). Cambridge, MA: Harvard University Press.

Georgiewa, P., Rzanny, R., Hopf, J. M., Knab, R., Glauche, V., Kaiser, W. A., et al. (1999). fMRI during word processing in dyslexic and normal reading children. *NeuroReport, 10*(16), 3459–3465.

Gernsbacher, M. A., Sauer, E. A., Geye, H. M., Schweigert, E. K., & Goldsmith, H. (2008). Infant and toddler oral- and manual-motor skills predict later speech fluency in autism. *Journal of Child Psychology and Psychiatry, 49*(1), 43–50.

Gibson, D. (1978). *Down syndrome: The psychology of mongolism.* Cambridge, UK: Cambridge University Press.

Giedd, J. N., Castellanos, F. X., Casey, B. J., Kozuch, P., King, A. C., Hamburger, S. D., et al. (1994). Quantitative morphology of the corpus callosum in attention deficit hyperactivity disorder. *American Journal of Psychiatry, 151*(5), 665–669.

Gilger, J., Pennington, B., & DeFries, J. (1991). Risk for reading disability as a function of parental history in three family studies. *Reading and Writing: An Interdisciplinary Journal, 3*, 205–217.

Gillam, R. B., Loeb, D. F., Hoffman, L. M., Bohman, T., Champlin, C. A., Thibodeau, L., et al. (2008). The efficacy of Fast ForWord Language intervention in school-age children with language impairment: A randomized controlled trial. *Journal of Speech, Language, and Hearing Research, 51*(1), 97–119.

Gittelman, R., Mannuzza, S., Shenker, R., & Gonagura, N. (1985). Hyperactive boys almost grown up. *Archives of General Psychiatry, 42*, 937–947.

Goddard, H. H. (1912). *The Kallikak family: A study in the heredity of feeble-mindedness.* New York: Macmillan.

Goldman, R., & Fristoe, M. (1986). *The Goldman–Fristoe Test of Articulation.* Circle Pines, MN: American Guidance Service.

Gordon, M. (1983). *Gordon Diagnostic System.* DeWitt, NY: Gordon Systems.

Grandin, T. (1995). *Thinking in pictures.* New York: Doubleday.

Gravel, J. S. (1994). Auditory integrative training: Placing the burden of proof. *American Journal of Speech and Language Pathology, 3*, 25–29.

Greer, N., Mosser, G., Logan, G., & Halaas, G. W. (2000). A practical approach to evidence grading. *Joint Commission Journal on Quality Improvement, 26*, 700–712.

Griffith, E. M., Pennington, B. F., Wehner, E. A., & Rogers, S. J. (1999). Executive functions in young children with autism. *Child Development, 70*(4), 817–832.

Griffiths, R. (1967). *The abilities of babies.* London: London University Press.

Groopman, J. (2007, January 29). What's the trouble? *The New Yorker,* pp. 36–41.

Gross-Tsur, V., Manor, O., & Shalev, R. S. (1996). Developmental dyscalculia: Prevalence and demographic features. *Developmental Medicine and Child Neurology, 38*(1), 25–33.

Gualtieri, C. T., & Hicks, R. E. (1985). Neuropharmacology of methylphenidate and a neural substrate for childhood hyperactivity. *Psychiatric Clinics of North America, 8*(4), 875–892.

Haaga, D. A., Dyck, M. J., & Ernst, D. (1991). Empirical status of cognitive theory of depression. *Psychological Bulletin, 110*(2), 215–236.

Habib, M., Rey, V., Daffaure, V., Camps, R., Espesser, R., & Demonet, J. F. (2002). Phonological training in dyslexics using temporally modified speech: A three-step pilot investigation. *International Journal of Language and Communication Disorders, 37*, 289–308.

Hadjikhani, N., Joseph, R. M., Snyder, J., Chabris, C. F., Clark, J., Steele, S., et al. (2004). Activation of the fusiform gyrus when individuals with autism spectrum disorder view faces. *NeuroImage, 22*(3), 1141–1150.

Hagerman, R. J. (1987). Fragile X syndrome. *Current Problems in Pediatrics, 17*(11), 621–674.

Hagerman, R. J. (1996). Physical and behavioral phenotype. In R. J. Hagerman & A. Cronister (Eds.), *Fragile X syndrome: Diagnosis, treatment, and research* (2nd ed., pp. 3–87). Baltimore: Johns Hopkins University Press.

Hagerman, R. J. (1999). Clinical and molecular aspects of fragile X syndrome. In R. H. Tager-Flusberg (Ed.), *Neurodevelopmental disorders* (pp. 27–42). Cambridge, MA: MIT Press.

Hagerman, R. J., Jackson, C., Amiri, K., Silverman, A. C., O'Connor, R., & Sobesky, W. (1992). Girls with fragile X syndrome: Physical and neurocognitive status and outcome. *Pediatrics, 89*(3), 395–400.

Hagerman, R. J., Kemper, M., & Hudson, M. (1985). Learning disabilities and attentional problems in boys with the fragile X syndrome. *American Journal of Diseases of Children, 139*(7), 674–678.

Hallenbeck, B. A., & Kauffman, J. M. (1994). United States. In K. Mazurek & M. A. Winzer (Eds.), *Comparative studies in special education* (pp. 403–419). Washington, DC: Gallaudet University Press.

Hallgren, B. (1950). Specific dyslexia: A clinical and genetic study. *Acta Psychiatrica et Neurologica Scandinavica, 65*(Suppl. 1), 1–287.

Hannula-Jouppi, K., Kaminen-Ahola, N., Taipale, M., Eklund, R., Nopola-Hemmi, J., Kaariainen, H., et al. (2005). The axon guidance receptor gene ROBO1 is a candidate gene for developmental dyslexia. *PLoS Genetics, 1*(4), e50.

Hanson, D. M., Jackson, A. W., III, & Hagerman, R. J. (1986). Speech disturbances (cluttering) in mildly impaired males with the Martin–Bell/fragile X syndrome. *American Journal of Medical Genetics, 23*(1–2), 195–206.

Happé, F. (1997). Central coherence and theory of mind in autism: Reading homographs in context. *British Journal of Developmental Psychology, 15*(1), 1–12.

Happé, F. (2005). The weak central coherence account of autism. In F. R. Volkmar, R. Paul, A. Klin, & D. J. Cohen (Eds.), *Handbook of autism and pervasive developmental disorders* (3rd ed., Vol. 1, pp. 640–649). Hoboken, NJ: Wiley.

Harm, M. W., & Seidenberg, M. S. (1999). Phonology, reading acquisition, and dyslexia: Insights from connectionist models. *Psychological Review, 106*(3), 491–528.

Harm, M. W., & Seidenberg, M. S. (2004). Computing the meanings of words in reading: Cooperative division of labor between visual and phonological processes. *Psychological Review, 111*(3), 662–720.

Harold, D., Paracchini, S., Scerri, T., Dennis, M., Cope, N., Hill, G., et al. (2006). Further evidence that the KIAA0319 gene confers susceptibility to developmental dyslexia. *Molecular Psychiatry, 11*(12), 1085–1091.

Hartley, S. L., Horrell, S. V., & Maclean, W. E., Jr. (2007). Science to practice in intellectual disability: The role of empirically supported treatments. In J. W. Jacobson, J. A. Mulick, & J. Rojahn (Eds.), *Handbook of intellectual and developmental disabilities* (pp. 425–443). New York: Springer.

Hartung, C. M., Freidman Crawford, M., Willcutt, E. G., & Pennington, B. F. (2008). *Gender differences in DSM-IV ADHD*. Manuscript submitted for publication.

Hartung, C. M., Willcutt, E. G., Lahey, B. B., Pelham, W. E., Loney, J., Stein, M. A., et al. (2002). Sex differences in young children who meet criteria for attention deficit hyperactivity disorder. *Journal of Clinical Child and Adolescent Psychology, 31*(4), 453–464.

Hatcher, P. J., Hulme, C., & Ellis, A. W. (1994). Ameliorating early reading failure by integrating the teaching of reading and phonological skills: The phonological linkage hypothesis. *Child Development, 65*(1), 41–57.

Hatcher, P. J., Hulme, C., & Snowling, M. J. (2004). Explicit phoneme training combined with phonic reading instruction helps young children at risk of reading failure. *Journal of Child Psychology and Psychiatry, 45*(2), 338–358.

Hattori, M., Fujiyama, A., Taylor, T. D., Watanabe, H., Yada, T., Park, H. S., et al. (2000). The DNA sequence of human chromosome 21. *Nature, 405*(6784), 311–319.

Haworth, C. M., Kovas, Y., Petrill, S. A., & Plomin, R. (2007). Developmental origins of low mathematics performance and normal variation in twins from 7 to 9 years. *Twin Research and Human Genetics, 10*(1), 106–117.

Heath, S. M., & Hogben, J. H. (2004). Cost-effective prediction of reading difficulties. *Journal of Speech, Language, and Hearing Research, 47*(4), 751–765.

Heaton, R. K. (1981). *Wisconsin Card Sorting Test manual*. Odessa, FL: Psychological Assessment Resources.

Hebb, D. O. (1942). The effect of early and late brain injury upon test scores, and the nature of normal adult intelligence. *Proceedings of the American Philosophical Society, 85*, 275–292.

Hebb, D. O. (1949). *The organization of behavior*. New York: Wiley.

Hecaen, H., & Albert, M. L. (1978). *Human neuropsychology*. New York: Wiley-Interscience.

Hecaen, H., Angelergues, R., & Houillier, S. (1961). Les variétés cliniques des acalculies au cours des lésions retro-rolandiques: Approache statistique du problème. *Revue Neurologique, 105*, 85–103.

Heiervang, E., Hugdahl, K., Steinmetz, H., Inge Smievoll, A., Stevenson, J., Lund, A., et al. (2000). Planum temporale, planum parietale and dichotic listening in dyslexia. *Neuropsychologia, 38*(13), 1704–1713.

Henderson, S. E., & Hall, D. (1982). Concomitants of clumsiness in young school-children. *Developmental Medicine and Child Neurology, 24*(4), 448–460.

Henderson, S. E., & Sugden, D. A. (1992). *Movement assessment battery for children*. London: The Psychological Corporation.

Henschen, S. E. (1925 [originally published in 1919]). Clinical and anatomical contributions on brain pathology. *Archives of Neurology and Psychiatry, 13*, 226–249.

Herman, A. E., Galaburda, A. M., Fitch, R. H., Carter, A. R., & Rosen, G. D. (1997). Cerebral microgyria, thalamic cell size and auditory temporal processing in male and female rats. *Cerebral Cortex, 7*(5), 453–464.

Hill, E. L., & Frith, U. (2003). *Understanding autism: Insights from mind and brain.* New York: Oxford University Press.

Hines, S., & Bennett, F. (1996). Effectiveness of early intervention for children with Down syndrome. *Mental Retardation and Developmental Disabilities Research Reviews, 2*(2), 96–101.

Hinshelwood, J. (1907). Four cases of congenital word-blindness occurring in the same family. *British Medical Journal, 21,* 1229–1232.

Hoare, D., & Larkin, D. (1991). Kinaesthetic abilities of clumsy children. *Developmental Medicine and Child Neurology, 33*(8), 671–678.

Hobson, R. P. (1989). Beyond cognition: A theory of autism. In G. Dawson (Ed.), *Autism: Nature, diagnosis, and treatment* (pp. 22–48). New York: Guilford Press.

Hobson, R. P. (1993). Understanding persons: The role of affect. In S. Baron-Cohen, H. Tager-Flusberg, & D. J. Cohen (Eds.), *Understanding other minds* (pp. 204–227). Oxford: Oxford University Press.

Hodapp, R. M., Burack, J. A., & Zigler, E. (1998). Developmental approaches to mental retardation: A short introduction. In J. A. Burack, R. M. Hodapp, & E. Zigler (Eds.), *Handbook of mental retardation and development* (pp. 3–19). Cambridge, UK: Cambridge University Press.

Hodapp, R. M., & Dykens, E. M. (1996). Mental retardation. In R. J. Mash & R. A. Barkley (Eds.), *Child psychopathology* (pp. 362–389). New York: Guilford Press.

Hodapp, R. M., Leckman, J. F., Dykens, E. M., Sparrow, S. S., Zelinsky, D. G., & Ort, S. I. (1992). K-ABC profiles in children with fragile X syndrome, Down syndrome, and nonspecific mental retardation. *American Journal of Mental Retardation, 97*(1), 39–46.

Hodapp, R. M., & Zigler, E. (1990). Applying the developmental perspective to individuals with Down syndrome. In D. Cicchetti & M. Beeghly (Eds.), *Children with Down syndrome* (pp. 1–28). New York: Cambridge University Press.

Hoffmann, H. (1845). *Der Struwwelpeler: Oder lustige Geschichlen unddrollige Bilder.* Leipzig: Insel-Verdag.

Hook, P. E., Macaruso, P., & Jones, S. (2001). Efficacy of Fast ForWord training on facilitating acquisition of reading skills by children with reading difficulties: A longitudinal study. *Annals of Dyslexia, 51,* 75–96.

Hoover, W. A., & Gough, P. B. (1990). The simple view of reading. *Reading and Writing: An interdisciplinary Journal, 2,* 127–160.

Horn, J. L., & Noll, J. (1997). Human cognitive capabilities: Gf-Gc theory. In D. P. Flanagan, J. L. Genshaft, & P. L. Harrison (Eds.), *Contemporary intellectual assessment: Theories, tests, and issues* (pp. 53–91). New York: Guilford Press.

Howard, W. L., & Silvestri, S. M. (2005). The neutralization of special education. In J. W. Jacobson, R. M. Foxx & J. A. Mulick (Eds.), *Controversial therapies for developmental disorders* (pp. 193–214). Mahwah, NJ: Erlbaum.

Hoyt, C. C. (1990). Irlen lenses and reading difficulties. *Journal of Learning Disabilities, 23,* 624–626.

Hsiung, G. Y., Kaplan, B. J., Petryshen, T. L., Lu, S., & Field, L. L. (2004). A dyslexia susceptibility locus (DYX7) linked to dopamine D4 receptor (DRD4) region on chromosome 11p15.5. *American Journal of Medical Genetics: B. Neuropsychiatric Genetics, 125*(1), 112–119.

Hugdahl, K., Gundersen, H., Brekke, C., Thomsen, T., Rimol, L. M., Ersland, L., et al. (2004). fMRI brain activation in a finnish family with specific language impairment compared with a normal control group. *Journal of Speech, Language, and Hearing Research, 47*(1), 162–172.

Hugdahl, K., Heiervang, E., Ersland, L., Lundervold, A., Steinmetz, H., & Smievoll, A. I. (2003). Significant relation between MR measures of planum temporale area and dichotic processing of syllables in dyslexic children. *Neuropsychologia, 41*(6), 666–675.

Hulme, C. (1988). The implausibility of low-level visual deficits as a cause of children's reading difficulties. *Cognitive Neuropsychology, 5*(3), 369–374.

Hulme, C., & Mackenzie, S. (1992). *Working memory and severe learning difficulties.* Hove, UK: Erlbaum.

Hulslander, J., Talcott, J., Witton, C., DeFries, J., Pennington, B., Wadsworth, S., et al. (2004). Sensory processing, reading, IQ, and attention. *Journal of Experimental Child Psychology, 88*(3), 274–295.

Humphreys, P., Kaufmann, W. E., & Galaburda, A. M. (1990). Developmental dyslexia in women: Neuropathological findings in three patients. *Annals of Neurology, 28*(6), 727–738.

Hynd, G. W., Hern, K. L., Novey, E. S., Eliopulos, D., Marshall, R., Gonzalez, J. J., et al. (1993). Attention deficit-hyperactivity disorder and asymmetry of the caudate nucleus. *Journal of Child Neurology, 8*(4), 339–347.

Hynd, G. W., Semrud-Clikeman, M., Lorys, A. R., Novey, E. S., & Eliopulos, D. (1990). Brain morphology in developmental dyslexia and attention deficit disorder/hyperactivity. *Archives of Neurology, 47*(8), 919–926.

Hynd, G. W., Semrud-Clikeman, M., Lorys, A. R., Novey, E. S., Eliopulos, D., & Lyytinen, H. (1991). Corpus callosum morphology in attention deficit-hyperactivity disorder: Morphometric analysis of MRI. *Journal of Learning Disabilities, 24*(3), 141–146.

International Molecular Genetic Study of Autism Consortium. (1998). A full genome screen for autism with evidence for linkage to a region on chromosome 7q. *Human Molecular Genetics, 7*, 571–578.

Irlen, H. (1983). *Successful treatment of learning disabilities.* Paper presented at the 91st Annual Convention of the American Psychological Association, Anaheim, CA.

Jacobson, J. W., Foxx, R. M., & Mulick, J. A. (Eds.). (2005a). *Controversial therapies for developmental disabilities.* Mahwah, NJ: Erlbaum.

Jacobson, J. W., Foxx, R. M., & Mulick, J. A. (2005b). Facilitated communication: The ultimate fad treatment. In J. W. Jacobson, R. M. Foxx, & J. A. Mulick (Eds.), *Controversial therapies for developmental disabilities: Fad, fashion, and science in professional practice* (pp. 363–383). Mahwah, NJ: Erlbaum.

Jacquemont, S., Hagerman, R. J., Hagerman, P. J., & Leehey, M. A. (2007). Fragile-X syndrome and fragile X-associated tremor/ataxia syndrome: Two faces of FMR1. *The Lancet Neurology, 6*(1), 45–55.

Jernigan, T. L., Bellugi, U., Sowell, E., Doherty, S., & Hesselink, J. R. (1993).

Cerebral morphologic distinctions between Williams and Down syndromes. *Archives of Neurology, 50*(2), 186–191.

Joanisse, M. F., & Seidenberg, M. S. (2003). Phonology and syntax in specific language impairment: Evidence from a connectionist model. *Brain and Language, 86*(1), 40–56.

Johnson, M. H. (2005). *Developmental cognitive neuroscience* (2nd ed.). Oxford: Blackwell.

Jones, H. E. (1959). Intelligence and problem solving. In J. E. Birren (Ed.), *Handbook of aging and the individual* (pp. 700–738). Chicago: University of Chicago Press.

Jucaite, A., Fernell, E., Forssberg, H., & Hadders-Algra, M. (2003). Deficient coordination of associated postural adjustments during a lifting task in children with neurodevelopmental disorders. *Developmental Medicine and Child Neurology, 45*(11), 731–742.

Kadesjo, B., & Gillberg, C. (1998). Attention deficits and clumsiness in Swedish 7-year-old children. *Developmental Medicine and Child Neurology, 40*(12), 796–804.

Kahn, R. S., Khoury, J., Nichols, W. C., & Lanphear, B. P. (2003). Role of dopamine transporter genotype and maternal prenatal smoking in childhood hyperactive–impulsive, inattentive, and oppositional behaviors. *Journal of Pediatrics, 143*(1), 104–110.

Kail, R. (1991). Development of processing speed in childhood and adolescence. *Advances in Child Development and Behavior, 23*, 151–185.

Kamhi, A. G., & Beasley, D. A. (1985). Central auditory processing disorder: Is it a meaningful construct or a twentieth century unicorn? *Journal of Communication Disorders, 9*, 5–13.

Kanner, L. (1943). Autistic disturbances of affective contact. *Nervous Child, 2*, 217–250.

Kaplan, B. J., Dewey, D., Crawford, S. G., & Fisher, G. C. (1998). Deficits in long-term memory are not characteristic of attention deficit hyperactivity disorder. *Journal of Clinical and Experimental Neuropsychology, 20*(4), 518–528.

Kasari, C., Sigman, M., Mundy, P., & Yirmiya, N. (1990). Affective sharing in the context of joint attention interactions of normal, autistic, and mentally retarded children. *Journal of Autism and Developmental Disorders, 20*(1), 87–100.

Katschmarsky, S., Cairney, S., Maruff, P., Wilson, P. H., & Currie, J. (2001). The ability to execute saccades on the basis of efference copy: Impairments in double-step saccade performance in children with developmental co-ordination disorder. *Experimental Brain Research, 136*(1), 73–78.

Kaufmann, L., Handl, P., & Thony, B. (2003). Evaluation of a numeracy intervention program focusing on basic numerical knowledge and conceptual knowledge: A pilot study. *Journal of Learning Disabilities, 36*(6), 564–573.

Keenan, J. M., Betjemann, R. S., Wadsworth, S. J., DeFries, J. C., & Olson, R. K. (2006). Genetic and environmental influences on reading and listening comprehension. *Journal of Research in Reading, 29*, 79–91.

Kemper, M. B., Hagerman, R. J., Ahmad, R. S., & Mariner, R. (1986). Cognitive profiles and the spectrum of clinical manifestations in heterozygous fra (X) females. *American Journal of Medical Genetics, 23*(1–2), 139–156.

Kemper, M. B., Hagerman, R. J., & Altshul-Stark, D. (1988). Cognitive profiles of boys with the fragile X syndrome. *American Journal of Medical Genetics, 30*(1–2), 191–200.

Kenney, M. K., Barac-Cikoja, D., Finnegan, K., Jeffries, N., & Ludlow, C. L. (2006). Speech perception and short-term memory deficits in persistent developmental speech disorder. *Brain and Language, 96*(2), 178–190.

Kerr, J. (1897). School hygiene, in its mental, moral, and physical aspects: Howard Medical Prize Essay. *Journal of the Royal Statistical Society, 60,* 613–680.

Kesslak, J. P., Nagata, S. F., Lott, I., & Nalcioglu, O. (1994). Magnetic resonance imaging analysis of age-related changes in the brains of individuals with Down's syndrome. *Neurology, 44*(6), 1039–1045.

Kinsbourne, M., & Warrington, E. K. (1963). The developmental Gerstmann syndrome. *Archives of Neurology, 8,* 490–501.

Klein, B. P., & Mervis, C. B. (1999). Contrasting patterns of cognitive abilities of 9- and 10-year-olds with Williams syndrome or Down syndrome. *Developmental Neuropsychology, 16*(2), 177–196.

Klin, A., Jones, W., Schultz, R. T., & Volkmar, F. R. (2005). The enactive mind—from actions to cognition: Lessons from autism. In F. R. Volkmar, R. Paul, A. Klin, & D. J. Cohen (Eds.), *Handbook of autism and pervasive developmental disorders* (3rd ed., Vol. 1, pp. 345–360). Hoboken, NJ: Wiley.

Klin, A., Volkmar, F. R., Sparrow, S. S., Cicchetti, D. V., & Rourke, B. P. (1995). Validity and neuropsychological characterization of Asperger syndrome: Convergence with nonverbal learning disabilities syndrome. *Journal of Child Psychology and Psychiatry, 36*(7), 1127–1140.

Klingberg, T., Fernell, E., Olesen, P. J., Johnson, M., Gustafsson, P., Dahlstrom, K., et al. (2005). Computerized training of working memory in children with ADHD: A randomized, controlled trial. *Journal of the American Academy of Child and Adolescent Psychiatry, 44*(2), 177–186.

Klingberg, T., Hedehus, M., Temple, E., Salz, T., Gabrieli, J. D., Moseley, M. E., et al. (2000). Microstructure of temporo-parietal white matter as a basis for reading ability: Evidence from diffusion tensor magnetic resonance imaging. *Neuron, 25*(2), 493–500.

Klinger, L. G., & Dawson, G. (1996). Autistic disorder. In E. J. Mash & R. A. Barkley (Eds.), *Child psychopathology* (pp. 311–339). New York: Guilford Press.

Knopik, V. S., & DeFries, J. C. (1999). Etiology of covariation between reading and mathematics performance: A twin study. *Twin Research and Human Genetics, 2*(3), 226–234.

Kobayashi, R., Murata, T., & Yoshinaga, K. (1992). A follow-up study of 201 children with autism in Kyushu and Yamaguchi areas, Japan. *Journal of Autism and Developmental Disorders, 22*(3), 395–411.

Koenig, M., & Gunter, C. (2005). Fads in speech–language pathology. In J. W. Jacobson, R. M. Foxx, & J. A. Mulick (Eds.), *Controversial therapies for developmental disorders* (pp. 215–234). Mahwah, NJ: Erlbaum.

Kolb, B., & Whishaw, I. Q. (1990). *Fundamentals of human neuropsychology* (3rd ed.). New York: Freeman.

Koontz, K. L., & Berch, D. B. (1996). Identifying simple numerical stimuli: Processing inefficiencies exhibited by arithmetic learning disabled children. *Mathematical Cognition, 2*(1), 1–23.

Kosc, L. (1974). Developmental dyscalculia. *Journal of Learning Disabilities, 7*, 159–162.

Koyama, T., Tachimori, H., Osada, H., Takeda, T., & Kurita, H. (2007). Cognitive and symptom profiles in Asperger's syndrome and high-functioning autism. *Psychiatry and Clinical Neuroscience, 61*(1), 99–104.

Laasonen, M., Service, E., & Virsu, V. (2001). Temporal order and processing acuity of visual, auditory, and tactile perception in developmentally dyslexic young adults. *Cognitive, Affective, and Behavioral Neuroscience, 1*(4), 394–410.

Lachiewicz, A. M., Spiridigliozzi, G. A., Gullion, C. M., Ransford, S. N., & Rao, K. (1994). Aberrant behaviors of young boys with fragile X syndrome. *American Journal of Mental Retardation, 98*(5), 567–579.

Lai, C. S., Fisher, S. E., Hurst, J. A., Vargha-Khadem, F., & Monaco, A. P. (2001). A forkhead-domain gene is mutated in a severe speech and language disorder. *Nature, 413*(6855), 519–523.

Lainhart, J. E., Piven, J., Wzorek, M., Landa, R., Santangelo, S. L., Coon, H., et al. (1997). Macrocephaly in children and adults with autism. *Journal of the American Academy of Child and Adolescent Psychiatry, 36*(2), 282–290.

Lamb, J. A., Moore, J., Bailey, A., & Monaco, A. P. (2000). Autism: Recent molecular genetic advances. *Human Molecular Genetics, 9*(6), 861–868.

Landerl, K., Bevan, A., & Butterworth, B. (2004). Developmental dyscalculia and basic numerical capacities: A study of 8–9-year-old students. *Cognition, 93*(2), 99–125.

Law, J., Garrett, Z., & Nye, C. (2003). Speech and language therapy interventions for children with primary speech and language delay or disorder. *Cochrane Database Systems Review, 3*, CD004110.

Laws, G., & Gunn, D. (2004). Phonological memory as a predictor of language comprehension in Down syndrome: A five-year follow-up study. *Journal of Child Psychology and Psychiatry, 45*(2), 326–337.

Leitao, S., Hogben, J., & Fletcher, J. (1997). Phonological processing skills in speech and language impaired children. *European Journal of Disorders of Communication, 32*(2), 91–111.

Lejeune, J., Gauthier, M., & Turpin, R. (1959). [Human chromosomes in tissue cultures.]. *Comptes Rendus Hebdomadaires des Seances de l'Academie des Sciences, 248*(4), 602–603.

Leonard, C. M., Eckert, M. A., Lombardino, L. J., Oakland, T., Kranzler, J., Mohr, C. M., et al. (2001). Anatomical risk factors for phonological dyslexia. *Cerebral Cortex, 11*(2), 148–157.

Leonard, C. M., Lombardino, L. J., Walsh, K., Eckert, M. A., Mockler, J. L., Rowe, L. A., et al. (2002). Anatomical risk factors that distinguish dyslexia from SLI predict reading skill in normal children. *Journal of Communication Disorders, 35*(6), 501–531.

Leonard, L. B. (1995). Phonological impairment. In P. Fletcher & B. MacWhinney (Eds.), *The handbook of child language* (pp. 573–602). Oxford: Blackwell.

Leonard, L. B. (2000). *Children with specific language impairment.* Cambridge, MA: MIT Press.

Levin, H. S., Eisenberg, H. M., & Benton, A. L. (1991). *Frontal lobe function and dysfunction.* New York: Oxford University Press.

Levinson, H. N. (1980). *A solution to the riddle of dyslexia.* New York: Springer-Verlag.

Levinson, H. N. (1994). *A scientific Watergate, dyslexia.* Lake Success, NY: Stonebridge.

Levy, L. M., Levy, R. I., & Grafman, J. (1999). Metabolic abnormalities detected by 1H-MRS in dyscalculia and dysgraphia. *Neurology, 53,* 639–641.

Lewis, B. A., Cox, N. J., & Byard, P. J. (1993). Segregation analysis of speech and language disorders. *Behavior Genetics, 23*(3), 291–297.

Lewis, B. A., & Freebairn, L. (1992). Residual effects of preschool phonology disorders in grade school, adolescence, and adulthood. *Journal of Speech and Hearing Research, 35*(4), 819–831.

Lewis, C., Hitch, G. J., & Walker, P. (1994). The prevalence of specific arithmetic difficulties and specific reading difficulties in 9- to 10-year-old boys and girls. *Journal of Child Psychology and Psychiatry, 35*(2), 283–292.

Liberman, I. Y., Shankweiler, D., Orlando, C., Harris, K. S., & Berti, F. B. (1971). Letter confusions and reversals of sequence in the beginning reader: Implications for Orton's theory of developmental dyslexia. *Cortex, 7*(2), 127–142.

Light, J. G., & DeFries, J. C. (1995). Comorbidity of reading and mathematics disabilities: Genetic and environmental etiologies. *Journal of Learning Disabilities, 28*(2), 96–106.

Light, J. G., Defries, J. C., & Olson, R. K. (1998). Multivariate behavioral genetic analysis of achievement and cognitive measures in reading-disabled and control twin pairs. *Human Biology, 70*(2), 215–237.

Lindamood, C. H., & Lindamood, P. C. (1998). *Lindamood Phoneme Sequencing Program (LiPS).* Austin, TX: PRO-ED.

Livingstone, M. S., Rosen, G. D., Drislane, F. W., & Galaburda, A. M. (1991). Physiological and anatomical evidence for a magnocellular defect in developmental dyslexia. *Proceedings of the National Academy of Sciences USA, 88*(18), 7943–7947.

Logdberg, B., & Brun, A. (1993). Prefrontal neocortical disturbances in mental retardation. *Journal of Intellectual Disability Research, 37*(Pt. 5), 459–468.

Lord, C., Rutter, M., DiLavore, P. C., & Risi, S. (1999). *Autism Diagnostic Observation Schedule (ADOS).* Los Angeles: Western Psychological Services.

Lord, C., Rutter, M., & Le Couteur, A. (1994). Autism Diagnostic Interview— Revised: A revised version of a diagnostic interview for caregivers of individuals with possible pervasive developmental disorders. *Journal of Autism and Developmental Disorders, 24*(5), 659–685.

Lou, H. C., Henriksen, L., & Bruhn, P. (1984). Focal cerebral hypoperfusion in children with dysphasia and/or attention deficit disorder. *Archives of Neurology, 41*(8), 825–829.

Lou, H. C., Henriksen, L., Bruhn, P., Borner, H., & Nielsen, J. B. (1989). Striatal dysfunction in attention deficit and hyperkinetic disorder. *Archives of Neurology, 46*(1), 48–52.

Lovaas, O. I. (1987). Behavioral treatment and normal educational and intellectual functioning in young autistic children. *Journal of Consulting and Clinical Psychology, 55*(1), 3–9.

Lundberg, I., Frost, J., & Petersen, O. P. (1988). Effects of an extensive program for stimulating phonological awareness in preschool children. *Reading Research Quarterly, 23*(3), 263–284.

Luria, A. (1961). *The role of speech in the regulation of normal and abnormal behavior.* New York: Pergamon Press.

Luria, A. (1966). *Higher cortical functions in man.* New York: Basic Books.

MacDermot, K. D., Bonora, E., Sykes, N., Coupe, A. M., Lai, C. S., Vernes, S. C., et al. (2005). Identification of FOXP2 truncation as a novel cause of developmental speech and language deficits. *American Journal of Human Genetics, 76*(6), 1074–1080.

Madsen, K. M., Hviid, A., Vestergaard, M., Schendel, D., Wohlfahrt, J., Thorsen, P., et al. (2002). [MMR vaccination and autism—a population-based follow-up study]. *New England Journal of Medicine, 347*, 1477–1482.

Maes, B., Fryns, J. P., Van Walleghem, M., & Van den Berghe, H. (1993). Fragile-X syndrome and autism: A prevalent association or a misinterpreted connection? *Genetic Counseling, 4*(4), 245–263.

Mahler, M. (1952). On child psychosis and schizophrenia: Autistic and symbiotic infantile psychosis. *Psychoanalytic Study of the Child, 7*, 286–305.

Mandich, A., Buckolz, E., & Polatajko, H. (2002). On the ability of children with developmental coordination disorder (DCD) to inhibit response initiation: The Simon effect. *Brain and Cognition, 50*(1), 150–162.

Mangan, P. A. (1992). *Spatial memory abilities and abnormal development of the hippocampus formation in Down syndrome.* Unpublished manuscript, University of Arizona.

Mangeot, S. D., Miller, L. J., McIntosh, D. N., McGrath-Clarke, J., Simon, J., Hagerman, R. J., et al. (2001). Sensory modulation dysfunction in children with attention-deficit-hyperactivity disorder. *Developmental Medicine and Child Neurology, 43*(6), 399–406.

Manor, O., Shalev, R. S., Joseph, A., & Gross-Tsur, V. (2001). Arithmetic skills in kindergarten children with developmental language disorders. *European Journal of Pediatric Neurology, 5*(2), 71–77.

Marcell, M. M., & Weeks, S. L. (1988). Short-term memory difficulties and Down's syndrome. *Journal of Mental Deficiency Research, 32*(Pt. 2), 153–162.

Marino, C., Giorda, R., Luisa Lorusso, M., Vanzin, L., Salandi, N., Nobile, M., et al. (2005). A family-based association study does not support DYX1C1 on 15q21.3 as a candidate gene in developmental dyslexia. *European Journal of Human Genetics, 13*(4), 491–499.

Marshall, C. M., Snowling, M. J., & Bailey, P. J. (2001). Rapid auditory processing and phonological ability in normal readers and readers with dyslexia. *Journal of Speech, Language, and Hearing Research, 44*(4), 925–940.

Martin, F., & Lovegrove, W. (1984). The effects of field size and luminance on contrast sensitivity differences between specifically reading disabled and normal children. *Neuropsychologia, 22*(1), 73–77.

Martin, N. C., Piek, J. P., & Hay, D. (2006). DCD and ADHD: A genetic study of their shared etiology. *Human Movement Science, 25*(1), 110–124.

Maruff, P., Purcell, R., Tyler, P., Pantelis, C., & Currie, J. (1999). Abnormalities of internally generated saccades in obsessive–compulsive disorder. *Psychological Medicine, 29*(6), 1377–1385.

Mataro, M., Garcia-Sanchez, C., Junque, C., Estevez-Gonzalez, A., & Pujol, J. (1997). Magnetic resonance imaging measurement of the caudate nucleus in adolescents with attention-deficit hyperactivity disorder and its relationship with neuropsychological and behavioral measures. *Archives of Neurology, 54*(8), 963–968.

Matson, J. L., & Laud, R. B. (2007). Assessment and treatment psychopathology among people with developmental delays. In J. W. Jacobson, J. A. Mulick, & J. Rojahn (Eds.), *Handbook of intellectual and developmental disabilities* (pp. 507–539). New York: Springer.

Mattes, J. A. (1989). The role of frontal lobe dysfunction in childhood hyperkinesis. *Comprehensive Psychiatry, 21*, 358–369.

Mazurek, K., & Winzer, M. R. (1994). *Comparative studies in special education.* Washington, DC: Gallaudet University Press.

Mazzocco, M. M., Hagerman, R. J., Cronister-Silverman, A., & Pennington, B. F. (1992). Specific frontal lobe deficits among women with the fragile X gene. *Journal of the American Academy of Child and Adolescent Psychiatry, 31*(6), 1141–1148.

Mazzocco, M. M., Pennington, B. F., & Hagerman, R. J. (1993). The neurocognitive phenotype of female carriers of fragile X: Additional evidence for specificity. *Journal of Developmental and Behavioral Pediatrics, 14*(5), 328–335.

McCandliss, B. D., Cohen, L., & Dehaene, S. (2003). The visual word form area: Expertise for reading in the fusiform gyrus. *Trends in Cognitive Sciences, 7*(7), 293–299.

McCauley, E., Kay, T., Ito, J., & Treder, R. (1987). The Turner syndrome: Cognitive deficits, affective discrimination, and behavior problems. *Child Development, 58*(2), 464–473.

McCrory, E., Frith, U., Brunswick, N., & Price, C. (2000). Abnormal functional activation during a simple word repetition task: A PET study of adult dyslexics. *Journal of Cognitive Neuroscience, 12*(5), 753–762.

McCrory, E. J., Mechelli, A., Frith, U., & Price, C. J. (2005). More than words: A common neural basis for reading and naming deficits in developmental dyslexia? *Brain, 128*(Pt. 2), 261–267.

McEachin, J. J., Smith, T., & Lovaas, O. I. (1993). Long-term outcome for children with autism who received early intensive behavioral treatment. *American Journal of Mental Retardation, 97*(4), 359–372. (Discussion, 373–391.)

McGlone, J. (1985). Can spatial deficits in Turner's syndrome be explained by focal CNS dysfunction or atypical speech lateralization? *Journal of Clinical and Experimental Neuropsychology, 7*(4), 375–394.

McGrath, L. M., Pennington, B. F., Willcutt, E. G., Boada, R., Shriberg, L. D., & Smith, S. D. (2007). Gene × environment interactions in speech sound disorder predict language and preliteracy outcomes. *Development and Psychopathology, 19*(4), 1047–1072.

McGrath, L. M., Smith, S. D., & Pennington, B. F. (2006). Breakthroughs in the search for dyslexia candidate genes. *Trends in Molecular Medicine, 12*(7), 333–341.

McIntosh, D. N., Miller, L. J., Shyu, V., & Hagerman, R. J. (1999). Sensory-modulation disruption, electrodermal responses, and functional behaviors. *Developmental Medicine and Child Neurology, 41*(9), 608–615.

McIntosh, D. N., Reichmann-Decker, A., Winkielman, P., & Wilbarger, J. L. (2006). When the social mirror breaks: Deficits in automatic, but not voluntary mimicry of emotional facial expressions in autism. *Developmental Science, 9*(3), 295–302.

Meehl, P. E. (1973). Some methodological reflections on the difficulties of psychoanalytic research. *Psychological Issues, 8*(2), 104–117.

Meltzoff, A. (1995). Understanding the intentions of others: Re-enactment of intended acts by 18-month-old children. *Developmental Psychology, 31*, 1–16.

Meltzoff, A., & Gopnik, A. (1993). The role of imitation in understanding persons and developing a theory of mind. In S. Baron-Cohen (Ed.), *Understanding other minds* (pp. 335–366). Oxford: Oxford University Press.

Meng, H., Hager, K., Held, M., Page, G. P., Olson, R. K., Pennington, B. F., et al. (2005a). TDT-association analysis of EKN1 and dyslexia in a Colorado twin cohort. *Human Genetics, 118*(1), 87–90.

Meng, H., Smith, S. D., Hager, K., Held, M., Liu, J., Olson, R. K., et al. (2005b). DCDC2 is associated with reading disability and modulates neuronal development in the brain. *Proceedings of the National Academy of Sciences USA, 102*(47), 17053–17058.

Mervis, C. B. (1999). The Williams syndrome cognitive profile: Strengths, weaknesses, and interrelations among auditory short term memory, language, and visuospatial constructive cognition. In R. Fivush, W. Hirst, & E. Winograd (Eds.), *Essays in honor of Ulric Neisser* (pp. 193–227). Mahwah, NJ: Erlbaum.

Mervis, C. B., & Bertrand, J. (1997). Developmental relations between cognition and language: Evidence from Williams syndrome. In L. B. Adamson & M. A. Romski (Eds.), *Communication and language acquisition: Discoveries from atypical development* (pp. 148–158). Baltimore: Brookes.

Mervis, C. B., & Klein-Tasman, B. P. (2000). Williams syndrome: Cognition, personality, and adaptive behavior. *Mental Retardation and Developmental Disabilities Research Review, 6*(2), 148–158.

Mervis, C. B., Robinson, B. F., Bertrand, J., Morris, C. A., Klein-Tasman, B. P., & Armstrong, S. C. (2000). The Williams syndrome cognitive profile. *Brain and Cognition, 44*(3), 604–628.

Merzenich, M. M., Jenkins, W. M., Johnston, P., Schreiner, C., Miller, S. L., & Tallal, P. (1996). Temporal processing deficits of language-learning impaired children ameliorated by training. *Science, 271*(5245), 77–81.

Metsala, J. L. (1997a). An examination of word frequency and neighborhood density in the development of spoken-word recognition. *Memory and Cognition, 25*(1), 47–56.

Metsala, J. L. (1997b). Spoken word recognition in reading disabled children. *Journal of Educational Psychology, 89*(1), 159–169.

Metsala, J. L., & Walley, A. C. (1998). Spoken vocabulary growth and the segmental restructuring of lexical representations: Precursors to phonemic awareness and early reading ability. In J. L. Metsala & L. C. Ehri (Eds.), *Word recognition in beginning literacy* (pp. 89–120). Mahwah, NJ: Erlbaum.

Metzger, R. I., & Werner, D. B. (1984). Use of visual training for reading disabilities. *Pediatrics, 73*, 824–829.

Michaud, L. J. (2004). Prescribing therapy services for children with motor disabilities. *Pediatrics, 113*(6), 1836–1838.

Miyake, A., Friedman, N. P., Emerson, M. J., Witzki, A. H., Howerter, A., & Wager, T. D. (2000). The unity and diversity of executive functions and their contributions to complex "frontal lobe" tasks: A latent variable analysis. *Cognitive Psychology, 41*(1), 49–100.

Mock, D. R., & Kauffman, J. M. (2005). The delusion of full inclusion. In J. W. Jacobson, R. M. Foxx, & J. A. Mulick (Eds.), *Controversial therapies for developmental disabilities* (pp. 113–128). Mahwah, NJ: Erlbaum.

Mody, M., Studdert-Kennedy, M., & Brady, S. (1997). Speech perception deficits in poor readers: Auditory processing or phonological coding? *Journal of Experimental Child Psychology, 64*(2), 199–231.

Money, J. (1973). Turner's syndrome and parietal lobe functions. *Cortex, 9*, 387–393.

Moody, E. J., & McIntosh, D. N. (2006). Mimicry and autism: Bases and consequences of rapid, automatic matching behavior. In S. J. Rogers & J. H. G. Williams (Eds.), *Imitation and the social mind: Autism and typical development* (pp. 71–95). New York: Guilford Press.

Morais, J., Cary, L., Alegria, J., & Bertelson, P. (1979). Does awareness of speech as a sequence of phones arise spontaneously? *Cognition, 7*(4), 323–331.

Morris, R. (1984). Multivariate methods for neuropsychology: Techniques for classification, identification, and prediction research, *International Neuropsychological Society Meeting*. Houston, TX.

Morton, J. (2004). *Understanding developmental disorders: A causal modeling approach*. UK: Blackwell Publishing.

Morton, J., & Frith, U. (1995). Causal modeling: A structural approach to developmental psychopathology. In D. Cicchetti & D. J. Cohen (Eds.), *Developmental psychopathology* (Vol. 1, pp. 357–390). New York: Wiley.

MTA. (1999). A 14-month randomized clinical trial of treatment strategies for attention-deficit/hyperactivity disorder. *Archives of General Psychiatry, 56*, 1073–1086.

Mundy, P., & Neal, R. (2000). Neural plasticity, joint attention, and a transactional social-orienting model of autism. *International Review of Research in Mental Retardation, 20*, 139–168.

Mundy, P., & Sigman, M. (1989). The theoretical implications of joint-attention deficits in autism. *Development and Psychopathology, 1*, 173–183.

Mundy, P., Sigman, M., Ungerer, J., & Sherman, T. (1986). Defining the social deficits of autism: The contribution of non-verbal communication measures. *Journal of Child Psychology and Psychiatry, 27*(5), 657–669.

Murphy, D. G., DeCarli, C., & Daly, E. M. (1993). X-chromosome effects on female brain: A magnetic resonance imaging study of Turner's syndrome. *Lancet, 342*(8881), 1197–1200.

Murray, C. J., & Lopez, A. D. (1996). Evidence-based health policy: Lessons from the Global Burden of Disease Study. *Science, 274*(5288), 740–743.

Nadel, L. (1986). Down syndrome in neurobiolgical perspective. In C. J. Epstein (Ed.), *The neurobiology of Down syndrome* (pp. 239–251). New York: Raven Press.

Nadel, L. (1999). Down syndrome in cognitive neuroscience perspective. In H. Tager-Flusberg (Ed.), *Neurodevelopmental disorders* (pp. 197–221). Cambridge, MA: MIT Press.

Nation, K. (2005). Children's reading comprehension difficulties. In M. J. Snowling & C. Hulme (Eds.), *The science of reading* (pp. 248–265). Oxford: Blackwell.

National Institute on Deafness and Other Communicative Disorders (NIDCD). (2004). *Auditory processing disorder in children.* Retrieved from *www.nidcd. gov/health/voice/auditory.asp.*

National Institutes of Health (NIH). (2000). *Phenylketonuria: Screening and management* (NIH Consensus Development Conference Statement). Retrieved from *consensus.nih.gov/2000/2000Phenylketonuria113.*

National Reading Panel. (2000). *Teaching children to read: An evidence-based assessment of the scientific research literature on reading and its implications for reading instruction.* Washington, DC: National Institute for Child Health and Human Development.

National Research Council. (2001). *Educating children with autism.* Washington, DC: National Academy Press.

Neuman, R. J., Lobos, E., Reich, W., Henderson, C. A., Sun, L. W., & Todd, R. D. (2007). Prenatal smoking exposure and dopaminergic genotypes interact to cause a severe ADHD subtype. *Biological Psychiatry, 61*(12), 1320–1328.

Newcomer, P. L., & Hammill, D. D. (2008). Test of Language Development— Primary (TOLD-P:4). Austin, TX: PRO-ED.

Newschaffer, C. J., & Curran, L. K. (2003). Autism: An emerging public health problem. *Public Health Report, 118*(5), 393–399.

Nichols, P. L. (1984). Twin studies of ability, personality, and interests. *Behavior Genetics, 14*, 161–170.

Nicolson, R. I., & Fawcett, A. J. (1990). Automaticity: A new framework for dyslexia research? *Cognition, 35*(2), 159–182.

Nigg, J. T., Willcutt, E. G., Doyle, A. E., & Sonuga-Barke, E. J. (2005). Causal heterogeneity in attention-deficit/hyperactivity disorder: Do we need neuropsychologically impaired subtypes? *Biological Psychiatry, 57*(11), 1224–1230.

Nittrouer, S. (1999). Do temporal processing deficits cause phonological processing problems? *Journal of Speech, Language, and Hearing Research, 42*(4), 925–942.

Nye, C., Foster, S. H., & Seaman, D. (1987). Effectiveness of language intervention with the language/learning disabled. *Journal of Speech and Hearing Disorders, 52*(4), 348–357.

Oliver, A., Johnson, M. H., Karmiloff-Smith, A., & Pennington, B. F. (2000). Deviations in the emergence of representations: A neuroconstructivist framework for analyzing developmental disorders. *Developmental Science, 3*, 1–40.

Olson, R. K., & Wise, B. (2006). Computer-based remediation for reading and related phonological disabilities. In M. C. McKenna, L. D. Labbo, R. D. Kieffer, & D. Reinking (Eds.), *International handbook of literacy and technology* (Vol. 2, pp. 57–74). Mahwah, NJ: Erlbaum.

O'Reilly, R. C. (2003). *Making working memory work: A computational model of learning in the prefrontal cortex and basal ganglia.* Boulder: Technical report, Institute of Cognitive Science, University of Colorado.

O'Reilly, R. C., Braver, T. S., & Cohen, J. D. (1999). A biologically based computational model of working memory. In A. Miyake & P. Shah (Eds.), *Mechanisms of active maintenance and executive control* (pp. 375–411). New York: Cambridge University Press.

O'Reilly, R. C., & Munakata, Y. (2000). *Computational explorations in cognitive neuroscience.* Cambridge, MA: MIT Press.

Orton, S. T. (1925). "Word-blindness" in school children. *Archives of Neurology and Psychiatry, 14,* 582–615.

Orton, S. T. (1937). *Reading, writing, and speech problems in children.* New York: Norton.

Osterling, J., & Dawson, G. (1994). Early recognition of children with autism: A study of first birthday home videotapes. *Journal of Autism and Developmental Disorders, 24*(3), 247–257.

Osterling, J. A., Dawson, G., & Munson, J. A. (2002). Early recognition of 1-year-old infants with autism spectrum disorder versus mental retardation. *Development and Psychopathology, 14*(2), 239–251.

Osterrieth, P. A. (1944). Le test d'une figure complexe. *Archives de Psychologie, 3,* 206–356.

Ozonoff, S., & Cathcart, K. (1998). Effectiveness of a home program intervention for young children with autism. *Journal of Autism and Developmental Disorders, 28*(1), 25–32.

Ozonoff, S., Goodlin-Jones, B. L., & Solomon, M. (2005). Evidence-based assessment of autism spectrum disorders in children and adolescents. *Journal of Clinical Child and Adolescent Psychology, 34*(3), 523–540.

Ozonoff, S., Pennington, B. F., & Rogers, S. J. (1990). Are there emotion perception deficits in young autistic children? *Journal of Child Psychology and Psychiatry, 31*(3), 343–361.

Ozonoff, S., Pennington, B. F., & Rogers, S. J. (1991). Executive function deficits in high-functioning autistic individuals: Relationship to theory of mind. *Journal of Child Psychology and Psychiatry, 32*(7), 1081–1105.

Palfrey, J. S., Levine, M. D., Walker, D. K., & Sullivan, M. (1985). The emergence of attention deficits in early childhood: A prospective study. *Journal of Developmental and Behavioral Pediatrics, 6*(6), 339–348.

Paracchini, S., Thomas, A., Castro, S., Lai, C., Paramasivam, M., Wang, Y., et al. (2006). The chromosome 6p22 haplotype associated with dyslexia reduces the expression of KIAA0319, a novel gene involved in neuronal migration. *Human Molecular Genetics, 15*(10), 1659–1666.

Patzer, D. K., & Volkmar, R. R. (1999). The neurobiology of autism and the pervasive developmental disorders. In D. S. Charney, E. J. Nestler, & B. S. Bunney (Eds.), *Neurobiology of mental illness* (pp. 761–778). New York: Oxford University Press.

Paulesu, E., Demonet, J. F., Fazio, F., McCrory, E., Chanoine, V., Brunswick, N., et al. (2001). Dyslexia: Cultural diversity and biological unity. *Science, 291*(5511), 2165–2167.

Peiffer, A. M., Rosen, G. D., & Fitch, R. H. (2002). Rapid auditory processing and MGN morphology in microgyric rats reared in varied acoustic environments. *Developmental Brain Research, 138*(2), 187–193.

Pelham, W. E., Jr., Wheeler, T., & Chronis, A. (1998). Empirically supported psychosocial treatments for attention deficit hyperactivity disorder. *Journal of Clinical Child Psychology, 27*(2), 190–205.

Pennington, B. F. (1991). *Diagnosing learning disorders: A neuropsychological framework*. New York: Guilford Press.

Pennington, B. F. (1994). The working memory function of the prefrontal cortices: Implications for developmental and individual differences in cognition. In M. M. Haith, J. Benson, R. Roberts, & B. F. Pennington (Eds.), *The development of future oriented processes* (pp. 243–289). Chicago: University of Chicago Press.

Pennington, B. F. (2002). *The development of psychopathology: Nature and nurture*. New York: Guilford Press.

Pennington, B. F. (2006). From single to multiple deficit models of developmental disorders. *Cognition, 101*, 385–413.

Pennington, B. F., Bender, B., Puck, M., Salbenblatt, J., & Robinson, A. (1982). Learning disabilities in children with sex chromosome anomalies. *Child Development, 53*(5), 1182–1192.

Pennington, B. F., & Bennetto, L. (1998). Toward a neuropsychology of mental retardation. In J. A. Burack, R. M. Hodapp, & E. Zigler (Eds.), *Handbook of mental retardation and development* (pp. 210–248). Cambridge, UK: Cambridge University Press.

Pennington, B. F., Filipek, P. A., Lefly, D., Churchwell, J., Kennedy, D. N., Simon, J. H., et al. (1999). Brain morphometry in reading-disabled twins. *Neurology, 53*(4), 723–729.

Pennington, B. F., Gilger, J. W., Pauls, D., Smith, S. A., Smith, S. D., & DeFries, J. C. (1991). Evidence for major gene transmission of developmental dyslexia. *Journal of the American Medical Association, 266*(11), 1527–1534.

Pennington, B. F., Heaton, R. K., Karzmark, P., Pendleton, M. G., Lehman, R., & Shucard, D. W. (1985). The neuropsychological phenotype in Turner syndrome. *Cortex, 21*(3), 391–404.

Pennington, B. F., & Lefly, D. L. (2001). Early reading development in children at family risk for dyslexia. *Child Development, 72*(3), 816–833.

Pennington, B. F., Lefly, D. L., Van Orden, G. C., Bookman, M. O., & Smith, S. D. (1987). Is phonology bypassed in normal or dyslexic development? *Annals of Dyslexia, 37*, 62–89.

Pennington, B. F., Moon, J., Edgin, J., Stedron, J., & Nadel, L. (2003). The neuropsychology of Down syndrome: Evidence for hippocampal dysfunction. *Child Development, 74*(1), 75–93.

Pennington, B. F., & Olson, R. K. (2005). Genetics of dyslexia. In M. Snowling & C. Hulme (Eds.), *The science of reading: A handbook* (pp. 453–472). Oxford: Blackwell.

Pennington, B. F., & Ozonoff, S. (1996). Executive functions and developmental psychopathology. *Journal of Child Psychology and Psychiatry, 37*(1), 51–87.

Pennington, B. F., Smith, S. D., Kimberling, W. J., Green, P. A., & Haith, M. M. (1987). Left-handedness and immune disorders in familial dyslexics. *Archives of Neurology, 44*(6), 634–639.

Pennington, B. F., & Welsh, M. C. (1995). Neuropsychology and developmental psychopathology. In D. Cicchetti & D. Cohen (Eds.), *Developmental Psychopathology* (Vol. 1, pp. 254–290). New York: Wiley.

Pennington, B. F., Willcutt, E. G., & Rhee, S. H. (2005). Analyzing comorbidity. *Advances in Child Development and Behavior, 33*, 263.

Perfetti, C. A., Beck, I., Bell, L. C., & Hughes, C. (1987). Phonemic knowledge and learning to read are reciprocal: A longitudinal study of first grade children. *Merrill–Palmer Quarterly, 33*(3), 283–219.

Petryshen, T. L., Kaplan, B. J., Fu Liu, M., de French, N. S., Tobias, R., Hughes, M. L., et al. (2001). Evidence for a susceptibility locus on chromosome 6q influencing phonological coding dyslexia. *American Journal of Medical Genetics, 105*(6), 507–517.

Pfeiffer, B., Kinnealey, M., Reed, C., & Herzberg, G. (2005). Sensory modulation and affective disorders in children and adolescents with Asperger's disorder. *American Journal of Occupational Therapy, 59*(3), 335–345.

Phinney, E., Pennington, B. F., Olson, R., Filley, C. M., & Filipek, P. A. (2007). Brain structure correlates of component reading processes: Implications for reading disability. *Cortex, 43*(6), 777–791.

Piaget, J. (1952). *The child's conception of number*. London: Routledge & Kegan Paul.

Pitcher, T. M., Piek, J. P., & Hay, D. A. (2003). Fine and gross motor ability in males with ADHD. *Developmental Medicine and Child Neurology, 45*(8), 525–535.

Piven, J. (1999). Genetic liability for autism: The behavioural expression in relatives. *International Review of Psychiatry, 11*(4), 299–308.

Piven, J., Arndt, S., Bailey, J., Havercamp, S., Andreasen, N. C., & Palmer, P. (1995). An MRI study of brain size in autism. *American Journal of Psychiatry, 152*(8), 1145–1149.

Plaisted, K., Saksida, L., Alcántara, J., & Weisblatt, E. (2003). Towards an understanding of the mechanisms of weak central coherence effects: Experiments in visual configural learning and auditory perception. *Philosophical Transactions of the Royal Society of London, Series B, 358*, 375–386.

Pless, M., & Carlsson, M. (2000). Effects of motor skill intervention on developmental coordination disorder: A meta-analysis. *Adapted Physical Activity Quarterly, 17*, 381–401.

Plomin, R., DeFries, J. C., McClearn, G. E., & Rutter, M. (1997). *Behavioral genetics*. New York: Freeman.

Pokorni, J. L., Worthington, C. K., & Maison, P. J. (2004). Phonological awareness intervention: Comparison of Fast ForWord, Earobics, and LiPS. *Journal of Educational Research, 97*, 147–157.

Polatajko, H. J. (1985). A critical look at vestibular dysfunction in learning-disabled children. *Developmental Medicine and Child Neurology, 27*, 283–292.

Polatajko, H. J., Rodger, S., Dhillon, A., & Hirji, F. (2004). Approaches to the management of children with motor problems. In D. Dewey & D. E. Tupper (Eds.), *Developmental motor disorders: A neuropsychological perspective* (pp. 461–486). New York: Guilford Press.

Pontius, A. A. (1973). Dysfunction patterns analogous to frontal lobe system and caudate nucleus syndromes in some groups of minimal brain dysfunction. *Journal of the American Women's Association, 28*(6), 285–292.

Popper, K. R. (1959). *The logic of scientific discovery.* London: Routledge.

Posthuma, D., & de Geus, E. J. C. (2006). Progress in the molecular-genetic study of intelligence. *Current Directions in Psychological Science, 15*(4), 151–155.

Price, C. J., & McCrory, E. (2005). Functional brain imaging studies of skilled reading and developmental dyslexia. In M. J. Snowling & C. Hulme (Eds.), *The science of reading* (pp. 473–496). Oxford: Blackwell.

Pringle-Morgan, W. P. (1896). A case of congenital word-blindness (inability to learn to read). *British Medical Journal, ii,* 1543–1544.

Proctor, R. A. (1873). Growth and decay of mind. *Cornhill Magazine, 28,* 541–555.

Pueschel, S. M., Gallagher, P. L., Zartler, A. S., & Pezzullo, J. C. (1987). Cognitive and learning processes in children with Down syndrome. *Research in Developmental Disabilities, 8*(1), 21–37.

Rae, C., Harasty, J. A., Dzendrowskyj, T. E., Talcott, J. B., Simpson, J. M., Blamire, A. M., et al. (2002). Cerebellar morphology in developmental dyslexia. *Neuropsychologia, 40*(8), 1285–1292.

Raitano, N. A., Pennington, B. F., Tunick, R. A., Boada, R., & Shriberg, L. D. (2004). Pre-literacy skills of subgroups of children with speech sound disorders. *Journal of Child Psychology and Psychiatry, 45*(4), 821–835.

Raitano-Lee, N. (2006). *An examination of the semantic and phonological contributions to the verbal short-term memory deficit in Down syndrome.* Unpublished manuscript, University of Denver.

Ramachandran, V. S., & Oberman, L. M. (2006). Broken mirrors: A theory of autism. *Scientific American, 295*(5), 62–69.

Ramey, S. L., Ramey, C. T., & Lanzi, R. G. (2007). Early intervention: Background, research findings, and future directions. In J. W. Jacobson, J. A. Mulick, & J. Rojahn (Eds.), *Handbook of intellectual and developmental disabilities* (pp. 445–463). New York: Springer.

Ramus, F. (2003). Developmental dyslexia: Specific phonological deficit or general sensorimotor dysfunction? *Current Opinion in Neurobiology, 13*(2), 212–218.

Ramus, F. (2004). Neurobiology of dyslexia: A reinterpretation of the data. *Trends in Neurosciences, 27*(12), 720–726.

Ramus, F. (2006). Genes, brain, and cognition: A roadmap for the cognitive scientist. *Cognition, 101*(2), 247–269.

Ramus, F., Rosen, S., Dakin, S. C., Day, B. L., Castellote, J. M., White, S., et al. (2003). Theories of developmental dyslexia: Insights from a multiple case study of dyslexic adults. *Brain, 126*(4), 841–865.

Rapin, I. (1987). Searching for the cause of autism: A neurological perspective. In

D. J. Cohen & A. M. Donnellan (Eds.), *Handbook of autism and pervasive developmental disorders* (pp. 710–717). New York: Wiley.

Rapin, I., & Allen, C. T. (1982). Developmental language disorders: Nosologic considerations. In U. Kirk (Ed.), *Neuropsychology of language, reading and spelling* (pp. 155–184). New York: Academic Press.

Raven, J. C. (1948). The comparative assessment of intellectual ability. *British Journal of Psychology, 28,* 12–19.

Raz, N., Torres, I. J., Briggs, S. D., Spencer, W. D., Thornton, A. E., Loken, W. J., et al. (1995). Selective neuroanatomic abnormalities in Down's syndrome and their cognitive correlates: Evidence from MRI morphometry. *Neurology, 45*(2), 356–366.

Redcay, E., & Courchesne, E. (2005). When is the brain enlarged in autism?: A meta-analysis of all brain size reports. *Biological Psychiatry, 58*(1), 1–9.

Reed, E. W., & Reed, S. C. (1965). *Mental retardation: A family study.* Philadelphia: Saunders.

Reeves, R. H., Baxter, L. L., & Richtsmeier, J. T. (2001). Too much of a good thing: Mechanisms of gene action in Down syndrome. *Trends in Genetics, 17*(2), 83–88.

Reiss, A. L., Aylward, E., Freund, L. S., Joshi, P. K., & Bryan, R. N. (1991). Neuroanatomy of fragile X syndrome: The posterior fossa. *Annals of Neurology, 29*(1), 26–32.

Reiss, A. L., & Freund, L. (1992). Behavioral phenotype of fragile X syndrome: DSM-III-R autistic behavior in male children. *American Journal of Medical Genetics, 43*(1–2), 35–46.

Reiss, A. L., Freund, L., Plotnick, L., Baumgardner, T., Green, K., Sozer, A. C., et al. (1993). The effects of X monosomy on brain development: Monozygotic twins discordant for Turner's syndrome. *Annals of Neurology, 34*(1), 95–107.

Reiss, A. L., Mazzocco, M. M., Greenlaw, R., Freund, L. S., & Ross, J. L. (1995). Neurodevelopmental effects of X monosomy: A volumetric imaging study. *Annals of Neurology, 38*(5), 731–738.

Reynolds, D., & Nicolson, R. I. (2007). Follow-up of an exercise-based treatment for children with reading difficulties. *Dyslexia, 13*(2), 78–96.

Reynolds, D., Nicolson, R. I., & Hambly, H. (2003). Evaluation of an exercise-based treatment for children with reading difficulties. *Dyslexia, 9*(1), 48–71. (Discussion, 46–47.)

Rice, M. L., Wexler, K., & Cleave, P. L. (1995). Specific language impairment as a period of extended optional infinitive. *Journal of Speech and Hearing Research, 38*(4), 850–863.

Richards, T. L., Aylward, E. H., Berninger, V. W., Field, K. M., Grimme, A. C., & Richards, A. L. (2006). Individual fMRI activation in orthographic mapping and morpheme mapping after orthographic or morphological spelling treatment in child dyslexics. *Journal of Neurolinguistics, 19*(1), 56–86.

Rimland, B. (1964). *Infantile autism.* New York: Meredith.

Rinehart, N. J., Bradshaw, J. L., Brereton, A. V., & Tonge, B. J. (2002). A clinical and neurobehavioural review of high-functioning autism and Asperger's disorder. *Australian and New Zealand Journal of Psychiatry, 36*(6), 762–770.

Rizzolatti, G., Fogassi, L., & Gallese, V. (2006). Mirrors in the mind. *Scientific American, 295*, 54–61.

Robichon, F., Levrier, O., Farnarier, P., & Habib, M. (2000). Developmental dyslexia: Atypical cortical asymmetries and functional significance. *European Journal of Neurology, 7*(1), 35–46.

Robinson, A., Lubs, H. A., & Bergson, D. (1979). *Sex chromosome aneuploidy: Prospective studies on children.* New York: Alan R. Liss.

Robison, J. E. (2007). *Look me in the eye: My life with Asperger's.* New York: Crown.

Rodier, P. M. (2000). The early origins of autism. *Scientific American, 282*(2), 56–63.

Rogers, S. J. (1998). Empirically supported comprehensive treatments for young children with autism. *Journal of Clinical Child Psychology, 27*(2), 168–179.

Rogers, S. J., & Pennington, B. F. (1991). A theoretical approach to the deficits in infantile autism. *Development and Psychopathology, 27*, 137–163.

Rogers, S. J., & Williams, H. G. (Eds.). (2006). *Imitation and the social mind: Autism and typical development.* New York: Guilford Press.

Rondal, J. A. (1993). Exceptional cases of language development in mental retardation: The relative autonomy of language as a cognitive system. In H. Tager-Flusberg (Ed.), *Constraints on language acquisition* (pp. 155–174). Hillsdale, NJ: Erlbaum.

Rosen, G. D., Bai, J., Wang, Y., Fiondella, C. G., Threlkeld, S. W., LoTurco, J. J., et al. (2007). Disruption of neuronal migration by RNAi of Dyx1c1 results in neocortical and hippocampal malformations. *Cerebral Cortex, 17*(11), 2562–2572.

Rosen, G. D., Herman, A. E., & Galaburda, A. M. (1999). Sex differences in the effects of early neocortical injury on neuronal size distribution of the medial geniculate nucleus in the rat are mediated by perinatal gonadal steroids. *Cerebral Cortex, 9*(1), 27–34.

Rosen, G. D., Press, D. M., Sherman, G. F., & Galaburda, A. M. (1992). The development of induced cerebrocortical microgyria in the rat. *Journal of Neuropathology and Experimental Neurology, 51*(6), 601–611.

Rosen, G. D., Waters, N. S., Galaburda, A. M., & Denenberg, V. H. (1995). Behavioral consequences of neonatal injury of the neocortex. *Brain Research, 681*(1), 177–189.

Rosen, S. (2003). Auditory processing in dyslexia and specific language impairment: Is there a deficit? What is its nature? Does it explain anything? *Journal of Phonetics, 31*, 509–527.

Rosenthal, R. H., & Allen, T. W. (1978). An examination of attention, arousal, and learning dysfunctions of hyperkinetic children. *Psychological Bulletin, 85*(4), 689–715.

Rourke, B. P. (1989). *Nonverbal learning disabilities.* New York: Guilford Press.

Rourke, B. P., & Finlayson, M. A. (1978). Neuropsychological significance of variations in patterns of academic performance: Verbal and visual–spatial abilities. *Journal of Abnormal Child Psychology, 6*(1), 121–133.

Rourke, B. P., & Strang, J. D. (1978). Neuropsychological significance of variations in patterns of academic performance: Motor, psychomotor, and tactile-perceptual abilities. *Journal of Pediatric Psychology, 2*, 62–66.

Rourke, B. P., Young, G. C., Strang, J. D., & Russell, D. L. (1986). Adult outcomes of central processing deficiencies in childhood. In I. Grant & K. M. Adams (Eds.), *Neuropsychological assessment in neuropsychiatric disorders: Clinical methods and empirical findings* (pp. 245–267). New York: Oxford University Press.

Rouse, C. E., & Krueger, A. B. (2004). Putting computerized instruction to the test: A randomized evaluation of a "scientifically-based" reading program. *Economics of Education Review, 23*(4), 323–338.

Rowe, D. C., Jacobson, K. C., & Van den Oord, E. J. (1999). Genetic and environmental influences on vocabulary IQ: Parental education level as moderator. *Child Development, 70*(5), 1151–1162.

Rumsey, J. M., Donohue, B. C., Brady, D. R., Nace, K., Giedd, J. N., & Andreason, P. (1997a). A magnetic resonance imaging study of planum temporale asymmetry in men with developmental dyslexia. *Archives of Neurology, 54*(12), 1481–1489.

Rumsey, J. M., Nace, K., Donohue, B., Wise, D., Maisog, J. M., & Andreason, P. (1997b). A positron emission tomographic study of impaired word recognition and phonological processing in dyslexic men. *Archives of Neurology, 54*(5), 562–573.

Russell, J. (1996). *Agency.* London: Taylor & Francis.

Russell, J. (1997). *Autism as an executive disorder.* New York: Oxford University Press.

Russell, J., & Hill, E. L. (2001). Action-monitoring and intention reporting in children with autism. *Journal of Child Psychology and Psychiatry, 42*(3), 317–328.

Russell, J., Jarrold, C., & Henry, L. (1996). Working memory in children with autism and with moderate learning difficulties. *Journal of Child Psychology and Psychiatry, 37*(6), 673–686.

Rutherford, M. D., Pennington, B. F., & Rogers, S. J. (2006). The perception of animacy in young children with autism. *Journal of Autism and Developmental Disorders, 36*(8), 983–992.

Rutter, M. (2000). Genetic studies of autism: From the 1970s into the millennium. *Journal of Abnormal Child Psychiatry, 28*(1), 3–14.

Rutter, M., Andersen-Wood, L., Beckett, C., Bredenkamp, D., Castle, J., Groothues, C., et al. (1999). Quasi-autistic patterns following severe early global privation: English and Romanian Adoptees (ERA) Study Team. *Journal of Child Psychology and Psychiatry, 40*(4), 537–549.

Rutter, M., Bailey, A., Berument, S. K., Lord, C., & Pickles, A. (2003). *Social Communication Questionnaire (SCQ).* Los Angeles: Western Psychological Services.

Rutter, M., & Mahwood, L. (1991). The long-term psychosocial sequelae of specific developmental disorders of speech and language. In M. Rutter & P. Casaer (Eds.), *Biological risk factors for psychosocial disorders* (pp. 233–259). Cambridge, UK: Cambridge University Press.

Rutter, M., & Quinton, D. (1977). Psychiatric disorders: Ecological factors and concepts of causation. In H. McGurk (Ed.), *Ecological factors in human development* (pp. 173–187). Amsterdam: North-Holland.

Sackett, D. L., Rosenberg, W. M. C., Gray, J. A. M., Haynes, R. B., & Richardson, W. S. (1996). Evidence-based medicine: What it is and what it isn't. *British Medical Journal, 312,* 71–72.

Sagan, C. (1995). *The demon-haunted world.* New York: Random House.

Sagvolden, T., Russell, V. A., Aase, H., Johansen, E. B., & Farshbaf, M. (2005). Rodent models of attention-deficit/hyperactivity disorder. *Biological Psychiatry, 57*(11), 1239–1247.

Salthouse, T. A. (1988). Initiating the formalization of theories of cognitive aging. *Psychology and Aging, 3*(1), 3–16.

Salthouse, T. A. (1991). Age and experience effects on the interpretation of orthographic drawings of three-dimensional objects. *Psychology of Aging, 6*(3), 426–433.

Samuel, V. J., Curtis, S., Thornell, A., George, P., Taylor, A., Brome, D., et al. (1997). The unexplored void of ADHD and African-American research: A review of the literature. *Journal of Attention Disorders, 1*(4), 197–207.

Sandak, R., Mencl, W. E., Frost, S. J., Rueckl, J. G., Katz, L., Moore, D. L., et al. (2004). The neurobiology of adaptive learning in reading: A contrast of different training conditions. *Cognitive, Affective, and Behavioral Neuroscience, 4*(1), 67–88.

Sattler, J. M., & Dumont, R. (2004). *Assessment of children: WISC-IV and WPPSI-III supplement.* San Diego, CA: Jerome M. Sattler.

Scarborough, H. S. (1990). Very early language deficits in dyslexic children. *Child Development, 61*(6), 1728–1743.

Scarborough, H. S. (1998). Early identification of children at risk for reading disabilities: Phonological awareness and some other promising predictors. In B. K. Shapiro, P. J. Accardo, & A. J. Capute (Eds.), *Specific reading disability: A view of the spectrum* (pp. 75–119). Timonium, MD: York Press.

Scarborough, H. S., & Parker, J. D. (2003). Children's learning and teachers' expectations: Matthew effects in children with learning disabilities: Development of reading, IQ, and psychosocial problems from grade 2 to grade 8. *Annals of Dyslexia, 53,* 47–71.

Scerri, T. S., Fisher, S. E., Francks, C., MacPhie, I. L., Paracchini, S., Richardson, A. J., et al. (2004). Putative functional alleles of DYX1C1 are not associated with dyslexia susceptibility in a large sample of sibling pairs from the UK. *Journal of Medical Genetics, 41*(11), 853–857.

Schaaf, R. C., & Miller, L. J. (2005). Occupational therapy using a sensory integrative approach for children with developmental disabilities. *Mental Retardation and Developmental Disabilities Research Reviews, 11*(2), 143–148.

Schain, R. J., & Yannet, H. (1960). Infantile autism: An analysis of 50 cases and a consideration of certain relevant neurophysiologic concepts. *Journal of Pediatrics, 57,* 560–567.

Schmahmann, J. D., & Caplan, D. (2006). Cognition, emotion and the cerebellum. *Brain, 129*(2), 290–292.

Schmidt-Sidor, B., Wisniewski, K. E., Shepard, T. H., & Serson, E. A. (1990). Brain growth in Down syndrome subjects 15–22 weeks of gestational age and birth to 60 months. *Clinical Neuropathology, 9*(4), 181–190.

Schultz, R. T. (2005). Developmental deficits in social perception in autism: The role of the amygdala and fusiform face area. *International Journal of Developmental Neuroscience, 23*(2), 125.

Schultz, R. T., Cho, N. K., Staib, L. H., Kier, L. E., Fletcher, J. M., Shaywitz, S. E., et al. (1994). Brain morphology in normal and dyslexic children: The influence of sex and age. *Annals of Neurology, 35*(6), 732–742.

Schultz, R. T., Gauthier, I., Klin, A., Fulbright, R. K., Anderson, A. W., Volkmar, F., et al. (2000). Abnormal ventral temporal cortical activity during face discrimination among individuals with autism and Asperger syndrome. *Archives of General Psychiatry, 57*(4), 331–340.

Schumacher, J., Anthoni, H., Dahdouh, F., Konig, I. R., Hillmer, A. M., Kluck, N., et al. (2006). Strong genetic evidence of DCDC2 as a susceptibility gene for dyslexia. *American Journal of Human Genetics, 78*(1), 52–62.

Sebat, J., Lakshmi, B., Malhotra, D., Troge, J., Lese-Martin, C., Walsh, T., et al. (2007). Strong association of *de novo* copy number mutations with autism. *Science, 316*, 445–449.

Seeger, G., Schloss, P., Schmidt, M. H., Ruter-Jungfleisch, A., & Henn, F. A. (2004). Gene–environment interaction in hyperkinetic conduct disorder (HD + CD) as indicated by season of birth variations in dopamine receptor (DRD4) gene polymorphism. *Neuroscience Letters, 366*(3), 282–286.

Semel, E., Wiig, E. H., & Secord, W. A. (2003). *Clinical Evaluation of Language Fundamentals, Fourth Edition*. San Antonio, TX: Psychological Corporation.

Semrud-Clikeman, M., Filipek, P. A., Biederman, J., Steingard, R., Kennedy, D., Renshaw, P., et al. (1994). Attention-deficit hyperactivity disorder: Magnetic resonance imaging morphometric analysis of the corpus callosum. *Journal of the American Academy of Child and Adolescent Psychiatry, 33*(6), 875–881.

Semrud-Clikeman, M., & Hynd, G. W. (1990). Right hemispheric dysfunction in nonverbal learning disabilities: Social, academic, and adaptive functioning in adults and children. *Psychological Bulletin, 107*(2), 196–209.

Sergeant, J. A. (2005). Modeling attention deficit/hyperactivity disorder: A critical appraisal of the cognitive–energetic model. *Biological Psychiatry, 57*, 1248–1255.

Shaffer, J. W. (1962). A specific cognitive deficit observed in gonadal aplasia (Turner's syndrome). *Journal of Clinical Psychiatry, 18*, 403–406.

Shalev, R. S., & Gross-Tsur, V. (2001). Developmental dyscalculia. *Pediatric Neurology, 24*(5), 337–342.

Shalev, R. S., Manor, O., & Kerem, B. (2001). Developmental dyscalculia is a familial learning disability. *Journal of Learning Disabilities, 34*, 59–65.

Shallice, T. (1988). *From neuropsychology to mental structure*. New York: Cambridge University Press.

Shanahan, M., McGrath, L., Santerre-Lemmon, L., Barnard, H., Willcutt, E. G., Olson, R. K., et al. (2007). *Shared cognitive deficits in reading disability and attention-deficit/hyperactivity disorder.* Paper presented at the biennial meeting of the Society for Research in Child Development. Boston.

Shanahan, M. A., Pennington, B. F., Yerys, B. E., Scott, A., Boada, R., Willcutt, E. G., et al. (2006). Processing speed deficits in attention deficit/hyperactivity disorder and reading disability. *Journal of Abnormal Child Psychology, 34*(5), 585–602.

Shankweiler, D. P., Liberman, I. Y., Mark, L. S., Fowler, C. A., & Fischer, F. W. (1979). The speech code and learning to read. *Journal of Experimental Psychology: Human Learning and Memory, 5,* 531–545.

Share, D. L., Jorm, A. F., Maclean, R., & Matthews, R. (2002). Temporal processing and reading disability. *Reading and Writing, 15*(1), 151–178.

Shaywitz, B. A., Shaywitz, S. E., Blachman, B. A., Pugh, K. R., Fulbright, R. K., Skudlarski, P., et al. (2004). Development of left occipitotemporal systems for skilled reading in children after a phonologically-based intervention. *Biological Psychiatry, 55*(9), 926–933.

Shaywitz, B. A., Shaywitz, S. E., Pugh, K. R., Mencl, W. E., Fulbright, R. K., Skudlarksi, P., et al. (2002). Disruption of posterior brain systems for reading in children with developmental dyslexia. *Biological Psychiatry, 52*(2), 101–110.

Shaywitz, S. E. (2003). *Overcoming dyslexia: A new and complete science-based program for reading problems at any level.* New York: Knopf.

Shaywitz, S. E., Shaywitz, B. A., Fletcher, J. M., & Escobar, M. D. (1990). Prevalence of reading disability in boys and girls: Results of the Connecticut Longitudinal Study. *Journal of the American Medical Association, 264*(8), 998–1002.

Shaywitz, S. E., Shaywitz, B. A., Fulbright, R. K., Skudlarski, P., Mencl, W. E., Constable, R. T., et al. (2003). Neural systems for compensation and persistence: Young adult outcome of childhood reading disability. *Biological Psychiatry, 54*(1), 25–33.

Shaywitz, S. E., Shaywitz, B. A., Pugh, K. R., Fulbright, R. K., Constable, R. T., Mencl, W. E., et al. (1998). Functional disruption in the organization of the brain for reading in dyslexia. *Proceedings of the National Academy of Sciences USA, 95*(5), 2636–2641.

Shaywitz, S. E., & Shaywitz, B. E. (1988). Attention deficit disorder: Current perspectives. In J. F. Kavanaugh & T. J. Truss (Eds.), *Learning disabilities: Proceedings of the national conference* (pp. 369–523). Parkton, MD: York Press.

Sherman, S. (1996). Epidemiology. In R. J. Hagerman & A. Cronister (Eds.), *Fragile X syndrome: Diagnosis, treatment, and research* (2nd ed., pp. 165–192). Baltimore: John Hopkins University Press.

Shermer, M. (1997). *Why people believe weird things: Pseudoscience, superstition, and other confusions of our time.* New York: Freeman.

Sheslow, D., & Adams, W. (1990). *Wide Range Assessment of Memory and Learning.* Wilmington, DE: Jastak Associates.

Shotwell, A. M., & Shipe, D. (1964). Effect of out-of-home care on the intellectual and social development of mongoloid children. *American Journal of Mental Deficiency, 90,* 693–699.

Shriberg, L. D., Tomblin, J. B., & McSweeny, J. L. (1999). Prevalence of speech delay in 6-year-old children and comorbidity with language impairment. *Journal of Speech, Language, and Hearing Research, 42*(6), 1461–1481.

Silbert, A., Wolff, P. H., & Lilienthal, J. (1977). Spatial and temporal processing in patients with Turner's syndrome. *Behavior Genetics, 7*(1), 11–21.

Silver, L. B. (1995). Controversial therapies. *Journal of Child Neurology, 10*(1), S96–S100.

Silverstein, A. B., Legutki, G., Friedman, S. L., & Takayama, D. L. (1982). Performance of Down syndrome individuals on the Stanford–Binet Intelligence Scale. *American Journal of Mental Deficiency, 86*(5), 548–551.

Simon, J. A., Keenan, J. M., Pennington, B. F., Taylor, A. K., & Hagerman, R. J. (2001). Discourse processing in women with fragile X syndrome: Evidence for a deficit establishing coherence. *Cognitive Neuropsychology, 18*, 1–18.

Simonoff, E., Bolton, P., & Rutter, M. (1998). Genetic perspectives on mental retardation. In J. A. Burack, R. M. Hodapp, & E. Zigler (Eds.), *Handbook of mental retardation and development* (pp. 41–79). Cambridge, UK: Cambridge University Press.

Sing, C. F., & Reilly, S. L. (1993). Genetics of common diseases that aggregate, but do not segregate in families. In C. F. Sing & C. L. Hanis (Eds.), *Genetics of cellular, individual, family and population variability* (pp. 140–161). New York: Oxford University Press.

Singer, H. S., Reiss, A. L., Brown, J. E., Aylward, E. H., Shih, B., Chee, E., et al. (1993). Volumetric MRI changes in basal ganglia of children with Tourette's syndrome. *Neurology, 43*(5), 950–956.

SLI Consortium. (2002). A genomewide scan identifies two novel loci involved in specific language impairment. *American Journal of Human Genetics, 70*(2), 384–398.

SLI Consortium. (2004). Highly significant linkage to the SLI1 locus in an expanded sample of individuals affected by specific language impairment. *American Journal of Human Genetics, 74*(6), 1225–1238.

Smith, S. D., Gilger, J. W., & Pennington, B. F. (2001). Dyslexia and other specific learning disorders. In D. L. Rimoin, J. M. Conner, & R. E. Pyeritz (Eds.), *Emery and Rimoin's principles and practice of medical genetics* (pp. 2827–2865). New York: Churchill Livingstone.

Smith, S. D., Pennington, B. F., Boada, R., & Shriberg, L. D. (2005). Linkage of speech sound disorder to reading disability loci. *Journal of Child Psychology and Psychiatry, 46*(10), 1045–1056.

Smith, T. (2005). The appeal of unvalidated treatments. In J. W. Jacobson, R. M. Foxx, & J. A. Mulick (Eds.), *Controversial therapies for developmental disorders* (pp. 45–57). Mahwah, NJ: Erlbaum.

Smith, T., Mruzek, D. W., & Mozingo, D. (2005). Sensory integrative therapy. In J. W. Jacobson, R. M. Foxx, & J. A. Mulick (Eds.), *Controversial therapies for developmental disabilities* (pp. 331–350). Mahwah, NJ: Erlbaum.

Snowling, M., Bishop, D. V., & Stothard, S. E. (2000). Is preschool language impairment a risk factor for dyslexia in adolescence? *Journal of Child Psychology and Psychiatry, 41*(5), 587–600.

Snowling, M. J., Gallagher, A., & Frith, U. (2003). Family risk of dyslexia is continuous: Individual differences in the precursors of reading skill. *Child Development, 74*(2), 358–373.

Sobcsky, W. E., Hull, C. E., & Hagerman, R. J. (1994). Symptoms of schizotypal personality disorder in fragile X women. *Journal of the American Academy of Child and Adolescent Psychiatry, 33*(2), 247–255.

Solan, H. A. (1990). An appraisal of the Irlen technique of correcting reading disorders using tinted overlays and tinted lenses. *Journal of Learning Disabilities, 23*, 621–623.

Sonuga-Barke, E. J. (2005). Causal models of attention-deficit/hyperactivity disorder: From common simple deficits to multiple developmental pathways. *Biological Psychiatry, 57*(11), 1231–1238.

Sparrow, S. S., Balla, D. A., & Cicchetti, D. (1984). *Vineland Adaptive Behavior Scales.* Circle Pines, MN: American Guidance Service.

Sparrow, S. S., Cicchetti, D., & Balla, D. A. (2005). *Vineland Adaptive Behavior Scales, Second Edition.* Circle Pines, MN: American Guidance Service.

Spreen, O., Tupper, D., Risser, A., Tuckko, H., & Edgell, D. (1984). *Human developmental neuropsychology.* New York: Oxford University Press.

Spring, B. (2007). Evidence-based practice in clinical psychology: What it is, why it matters; what you need to know. *Journal of Clinical Psychology, 63*(7), 611–631.

Staley, L. W., Hull, C. E., Mazzocco, M. M., Thibodeau, S. N., Snow, K., Wilson, V. L., et al. (1993). Molecular–clinical correlations in children and adults with fragile X syndrome. *American Journal of Diseases of Children, 147*(7), 723–726.

Stamm, J. S., & Kreder, S. V. (1979). Minimal brain dysfunction: Psychological and neuropsychological disorders in hyperkinetic children. In M. S. Gazzaniga (Ed.), *Handbook of behavioral neurology: Vol. 2. Neuropsychology* (pp. 237–307). New York: Plenum Press.

Stancliffe, R. J., & Keane, S. (2000). Outcomes and costs of community living: A matched comparison of group homes and semi-independent living. *Journal of Intellectual and Developmental Disability, 25*(4), 281–305.

Stanovich, K. E. (1986). Matthew effects in reading: Some consequences of individual differences in the acquisition of literacy. *Reading Research Quarterly, 21*, 360–406.

Steffenburg, S., Gillberg, C., Hellgren, L., Andersson, L., Gillberg, I. C., Jakobsson, G., et al. (1989). A twin study of autism in Denmark, Finland, Iceland, Norway and Sweden. *Journal of Child Psychology and Psychiatry, 30*(3), 405–416.

Stein, C. M., Millard, C., Kluge, A., Miscimarra, L. E., Cartier, K. C., Freebairn, L. A., et al. (2006). Speech sound disorder influenced by a locus in 15q14 region. *Behavior Genetics, 36*(6), 858–868.

Stein, C. M., Schick, J. H., Taylor, H., Shriberg, L. D., Millard, C., Kundtz-Kluge, A., et al. (2004). Pleiotropic effects of a chromosome 3 locus on speech-sound disorder and reading. *American Journal of Human Genetics, 74*(2), 283–297.

Stein, J. (2001). The sensory basis of reading problems. *Developmental Neuropsychology, 20*(2), 509–534.

Stein, J., & Walsh, V. (1997). To see but not to read: The magnocellular theory of dyslexia. *Trends in Neurosciences, 20*(4), 147–152.

Stein, M. T., Klin, A., & Miller, K. (2004). When Asperger's syndrome and a nonverbal learning disability look alike. *Journal of Developmental and Behavioral Pediatrics, 25*(5, Suppl.), S59–S64.

Stern, D. N. (1985). *The interpersonal world of the infant: A view from psycho-analysis and developmental psychology.* New York: Basic Books.

Sternberg, R. J. (1985). *Beyond IQ: A triarchic theory of human intelligence.* Cambridge, UK: Cambridge University Press.

Still, G. F. (1902). Some abnormal psychical conditions in children. *Lancet, i,* 1008–1012, 1077–1082, 1163–1168.

Stoodley, C. J., Talcott, J. B., Carter, E. L., Witton, C., & Stein, J. F. (2000). Selective deficits of vibrotactile sensitivity in dyslexic readers. *Neuroscience Letters, 295*(1–2), 13–16.

Stothard, S. E., Snowling, M. J., Bishop, D. V., Chipchase, B. B., & Kaplan, C. A. (1998). Language-impaired preschoolers: A follow-up into adolescence. *Journal of Speech, Language, and Hearing Research, 41*(2), 407–418.

Strang, J. D., & Rourke, B. P. (1985a). Adaptive behavior of children with specific arithmetic disabilities and associated neuropsychological abilities and deficits. In B. P. Rourke (Ed.), *Neuropsychology of learning disabilities: Essentials of subtype analysis* (pp. 167–183). New York: Guilford Press.

Strang, J. D., & Rourke, B. P. (1985b). Arithmetic disability subtypes: The neuropsychological significance of specific arithmetic impairment in childhood. In B. P. Rourke (Ed.), *Neuropsychology of learning disabilities: Essentials of subtype analysis* (pp. 167–183). New York: Guilford Press.

Stratton, K., Gable, A., & McCormick, M. C. (2001). *Immunization safety review: Thimerosal-containing vaccines and neurodevelopmental disorders.* Washington, DC: National Academy Press.

Strauss, A., & Lehtinen, L. (1947). *Psychopathology and education of the brain-injured child.* New York: Grune & Stratton.

Stuss, D. T., & Benson, D. F. (1986). *The frontal lobes.* New York: Raven Press.

Sudhalter, V., Cohen, I. L., Silverman, W., & Wolf-Schein, E. G. (1990). Conversational analyses of males with fragile X, Down syndrome, and autism: Comparison of the emergence of deviant language. *American Journal of Mental Retardation, 94*(4), 431–441.

Sudhalter, V., Scarborough, H. S., & Cohen, I. L. (1991). Syntactic delay and pragmatic deviance in the language of fragile X males. *American Journal of Medical Genetics, 38*(2–3), 493–497.

Swan, D., & Goswami, U. (1997a). Phonological awareness deficits in developmental dyslexia and the phonological representations hypothesis. *Journal of Experimental Child Psychology, 66*(1), 18–41.

Swan, D., & Goswami, U. (1997b). Picture naming deficits in developmental dyslexia: The phonological representations hypothesis. *Brain and Language, 56*(3), 334–353.

Swanson, H. L. (1999). Reading research for students with LD: A meta-analysis of intervention outcomes. *Journal of Learning Disabilities, 32*(6), 504–532.

Swanson, H. L. (2008). RTI, neuroscience, and sense: Chaos in the diagnosis and treatment of learning disabilities. In E. Fletcher-Janzen & C. R. Reynolds (Eds.), *Neuropsychological perspectives on learning disabilities in the era of RTI* (pp. 28–53). Hoboken, NJ: Wiley.

Szatmari, P., Offord, D. R., & Boyle, M. H. (1989). Correlates, associated impairments and patterns of service utilization of children with attention deficit disorder: Findings from the Ontario Child Health Study. *Journal of Child Psychology and Psychiatry, 30*(2), 205–217.

Szatmari, P., Peterson, A. D., Zwaigenbaum, L., Roberts, W., Brian, J., Xiao-Qing, L., et al. (2007). Mapping autism risk loci using genetic linkage and chromosomal rearrangements. *Nature Genetics, 39*(3), 319–328.

Tabuchi, K., Blundell, J., Etherton, M. R., Hammer, R. E., Liu, X., Powell, C. M., et al. (2007). A neuroligin-3 mutation implicated in autism increases inhibitory synaptic transmission in mice. *Science, 318*, 71–76.

Tager-Flusberg, H. (2001). A re-examination of the theory of mind hypothesis of autism. In J. Burack, T. Charman, N. Yirmiya, & P. Zelazo (Eds.), *The development of autism: Perspectives from theory and research* (pp. 173–194). Mahwah, NJ: Erlbaum.

Tager-Flusberg, H., Boshart, J., & Baron-Cohen, S. (1998). Reading the windows to the soul: Evidence of domain-specific sparing in Williams syndrome. *Journal of Cognitive Neuroscience, 10*(5), 631–639.

Tager-Flusberg, H., & Sullivan, K. (2000). A componential view of theory of mind: Evidence from Williams syndrome. *Cognition, 76*(1), 59–90.

Tager-Flusberg, M., Sullivan, K., & Boshart, J. (1997). Executive functions and performance on false belief tasks. *Developmental Neuropsychology, 13*, 487–493.

Taipale, M., Kaminen, N., Nopola-Hemmi, J., Haltia, T., Myllyluoma, B., Lyytinen, H., et al. (2003). A candidate gene for developmental dyslexia encodes a nuclear tetratricopeptide repeat domain protein dynamically regulated in brain. *Proceedings of the National Academy of Sciences USA, 100*(20), 11553–11558.

Tallal, P. (1980). Auditory temporal perception, phonics, and reading disabilities in children. *Brain and Language, 9*(2), 182–198.

Tallal, P., Miller, S. L., Bedi, G., Byma, G., Wang, X., Nagarajan, S. S., et al. (1996). Language comprehension in language-learning impaired children improved with acoustically modified speech. *Science, 271*(5245), 81–84.

Tallal, P., Miller, S. L., Jenkins, W. M., & Merzenich, M. M. (1997). The role of temporal processing in developmental language-based learning disorders: Research and clinical implications. In B. A. Blachman (Ed.), *Foundations of reading acquisition and dyslexia: Implications for early intervention* (pp. 49–66). Mahwah, NJ: Erlbaum.

Tallal, P., & Percy, M. (1973a). Defects of non-verbal auditory perception in children with developmental aphasia. *Nature, 241*(5390), 468–469.

Tallal, P., & Percy, M. (1973b). Developmental aphasia: Impaired rate of nonverbal processing as a function of sensory modality. *Neuropsychologia, 11*, 389–398.

Tallal, P., & Percy, M. (1975). Developmental aphasia: The perception of brief vowels and extended stop consonants. *Neuropsychologia, 13*, 69–74.

Taylor, B., Miller, E., Farrington, C. P., Petropoulos, M. C., Favot-Mayaud, I., Li, J., et al. (1999). Autism and measles, mumps, and rubella vaccine: no epidemiological evidence for a causal association. *Lancet, 353*(9169), 2026–2029.

Taylor, B., Miller, E., Lingam, R., Andrews, N., Simmons, A., & Stowe, J. (2002). Measles, mumps, and rubella vaccination and bowel problems or developmental regression in children with autism: Population study. *British Medical Journal, 324*(7334), 393–396.

Teicher, M. H., Polcari, A., English, C. D., Anderson, C. M., Anderson, S. L., Glod, C. A., et al. (1996). Dose-dependent effects of methylphenidate on activity, attention, and magnetic resonance imaging measures in children with ADHD [Abstract]. *Society for Neuroscience Abstracts, 22*, 1191.

Temple, E., Deutsch, G. K., Poldrack, R. A., Miller, S. L., Tallal, P., Merzenich, M. M., et al. (2003). Neural deficits in children with dyslexia ameliorated by behavioral remediation: Evidence from functional MRI. *Proceedings of the National Academy of Sciences USA, 100*(5), 2860–2865.

Temple, E., Poldrack, R. A., Salidis, J., Deutsch, G. K., Tallal, P., Merzenich, M. M., et al. (2001). Disrupted neural responses to phonological and orthographic processing in dyslexic children: An fMRI study. *NeuroReport, 12*(2), 299–307.

Thapar, A., Fowler, T., Rice, F., Scourfield, J., van den Bree, M., Thomas, H., et al. (2003). Maternal smoking during pregnancy and attention deficit hyperactivity disorder symptoms in offspring. *American Journal of Psychiatry, 160*(11), 1985–1989.

Thede, L. L., & Coolidge, F. L. (2007). Psychological and neurobehavioral comparisons of children with Asperger's disorder versus high-functioning autism. *Journal of Autism and Developmental Disorders, 37*(5), 847–854.

Theobold, T., Hay, D., & Judge, C. (1987). Individual variation and specific cognitive deficits in the fra(X) syndrome. *American Journal of Medical Genetics, 28*, 1–11.

Thomas, L. (1974). *Lives of a cell: Notes of a biology watcher.* New York: Viking Press.

Thompson, L. A., Detterman, D. K., & Plomin, R. (1991). Associations between cognitive abilities and scholastic achievement: Genetic overlap but environmental differences. *Psychological Science, 2*, 158–165.

Threlkeld, S. W., McClure, M. M., Bai, J., Wang, Y., LoTurco, J. J., Rosen, G. D., et al. (2007). Developmental disruptions and behavioral impairments in rats following in utero RNAi of Dyx1c1. *Brain Research Bulletin, 71*(5), 508–514.

Toal, F., Murphy, D. G., & Murphy, K. C. (2005). Autistic-spectrum disorders: Lessons from neuroimaging. *British Journal of Psychiatry, 187*, 395–397.

Torgesen, J. K. (2005). Recent discoveries on remedial interventions for children with dyslexia. In M. J. Snowling & C. Hulme (Eds.), *The science of reading: A handbook* (pp. 521–537). Oxford: Blackwell.

Torgesen, J. K., Alexander, A. W., Wagner, R. K., Rashotte, C. A., Voeller, K. K. S., & Conway, T. (2001). Intensive remedial instruction for children with severe reading disabilities: Immediate and long-term outcomes from two instructional approaches. *Journal of Learning Disabilities, 34*(1), 33–58.

Torgesen, J. K., Wagner, R. K., & Rashotte, C. A. (1999). *Test of Word Reading Efficiency (TOWRE).* Austin, TX: PRO-ED.

Torgesen, J. K., Wagner, R. K., Rashotte, C. A., & Herron, J. (2003). *Summary of outcomes from first grade study with Read, Write, Type and Auditory Discrimination in Depth instruction and software with at-risk children.* Tallahassee: Florida Center for Reading Research.

Tranel, D., Hall, L. E., Olson, S., & Tranel, N. N. (1987). Evidence for a right-hemisphere developmental learning disability. *Developmental Neuropsychology, 3,* 113–127.

Trauner, D., Wulfeck, B., Tallal, P., & Hesselink, J. (2000). Neurological and MRI profiles of children with developmental language impairment. *Developmental Medicine and Child Neurology, 42*(7), 470–475.

Treiman, R., & Breaux, A. M. (1982). Common phoneme and overall similarity relations among spoken syllables: Their use by children and adults. *Journal of Psycholinguistics Research, 11*(6), 569–598.

Trevarthen, C. (1979). Communication and cooperation in early infancy: A description of primary intersubjectivity. In M. Bullowa (Ed.), *Before speech: The beginning of human communication* (pp. 321–347). Cambridge, UK: Cambridge University Press.

Tupper, D. E., & Sondell, S. K. (2004). Motor disorders and neuropsychological development: A historical appreciation. In D. Dewey & D. E. Tupper (Eds.), *Developmental motor disorders: A neuropsychological perspective* (pp. 3–25). New York: Guilford Press.

Turkheimer, E., Haley, A., Waldron, M., D'Onofrio, B., & Gottesman, I. I. (2003). Socioeconomic status modifies heritability of IQ in young children. *Psychological Science, 14*(6), 623–628.

Unis, A. S., Munson, J. A., Rogers, S. J., Goldson, E., Osterling, J., Gabriels, R., et al. (2002). A randomized, double-blind, placebo-controlled trial of porcine versus synthetic secretin for reducing symptoms of autism. *Journal of the American Academy of Child and Adolescent Psychiatry, 41*(11), 1315–1321.

U.S. Department of Health and Human Services. (1999). *Mental health: A report of the Surgeon General.* Rockville, MD: Author.

Van Orden, G. C., Pennington, B. F., & Stone, G. O. (2001). What do double dissociations prove? *Cognitive Science, 25,* 111–172.

Vargha-Khadem, F., Gadian, D. G., Watkins, K. E., Connelly, A., Van Paesschen, W., & Mishkin, M. (1997). Differential effects of early hippocampal pathology on episodic and semantic memory. *Science, 277*(5324), 376–380.

Vargha-Khadem, F., Watkins, K. E., Price, C. J., Ashburner, J., Alcock, K. J., Connelly, A., et al. (1998). Neural basis of an inherited speech and language disorder. *Proceedings of the National Academy of Sciences USA, 95*(21), 12695–12700.

Veenstra-Vander Weele, J., & Cook, E. H. (2004). Molecular genetics of autism spectrum disorder. *Molecular Psychiatry, 9,* 819–832.

Vellutino, F. R. (1979). *Dyslexia: Theory and research.* Cambridge, MA: MIT Press.

Vellutino, F. R. (1987). Dyslexia. *Scientific American, 256*(3), 34–41.

Vellutino, F. R., Fletcher, J. M., Snowling, M. J., & Scanlon, D. M. (2004). Specific reading disability (dyslexia): What have we learned in the past four decades? *Journal of Child Psychology and Psychiatry, 45*(1), 2–40.

Vellutino, F. R., & Scanlon, D. M. (1989). Auditory information processing in poor and normal readers. In J. J. Dumont & H. Nakken (Eds.), *Learning disabilities* (Vol. 2, pp. 19–46). Amsterdam: Swets & Zeitlinger.

Veneri, M., Zalfa, F., & Bagni, C. (2004). FMRP and its target RNAs: fishing for the specificity. *NeuroReport, 15*(16), 2447–2450.

Verkerk, A. J., Pieretti, M., Sutcliffe, J. S., Fu, Y. H., Kuhl, D. P., Pizzuti, A., et al. (1991). Identification of a gene (FMR-1) containing a CGG repeat coincident with a breakpoint cluster region exhibiting length variation in fragile X syndrome. *Cell, 65*(5), 905–914.

Vig, S., & Jedrysek, E. (1999). Autistic features in young children with significant cognitive impairment: Autism or mental retardation? *Journal of Autism and Developmental Disorders, 29*(3), 235–248.

Vinckenbosch, E., Robichon, F., & Eliez, S. (2005). Gray matter alteration in dyslexia: Converging evidence from volumetric and voxel-by-voxel MRI analyses. *Neuropsychologia, 43*(3), 324–331.

Voeller, K. K. (1986). Right-hemisphere deficit syndrome in children. *American Journal of Psychiatry, 143*(8), 1004–1009.

Vyse, S. (2005). Where do fads come from? In J. W. Jacobson, R. M. Foxx, & J. A. Mulick (Eds.), *Controversial therapies for developmental disabilities* (pp. 3–17). Mahwah, NJ: Erlbaum.

Waber, D. P. (1979). Neuropsychological aspects of Turner's syndrome. *Developmental Medicine and Child Neurology, 21*(1), 58–70.

Wadsworth, S. J., DeFries, J. C., Fulker, D. W., & Plomin, R. (1995). Cognitive ability and academic achievement in the Colorado Adoption Project: A multivariate genetic analysis of parent–offspring and sibling data. *Behavior Genetics, 25*(1), 1–15.

Wadsworth, S. J., DeFries, J. C., Stevenson, J., Gilger, J. W., & Pennington, B. F. (1992). Gender ratios among reading-disabled children and their siblings as a function of parental impairment. *Journal of Child Psychology and Psychiatry, 33*(7), 1229–1239.

Wagner, R. K., Torgesen, J. K., & Rashotte, C. A. (1994). Development of reading-related phonological processing abilities: New evidence of bidirectional causality from a latent variable longitudinal study. *Developmental Psychology, 30*(1), 73–87.

Wagner, R. K., Torgesen, J. K., & Rashotte, C. A. (1999). *Comprehensive Test of Phonological Processing.* Austin, TX: PRO-ED.

Wahl, M., Robinson, C., & Torgesen, J. K. (2003). *Florida Center for Reading Research: Fast ForWord Language.* Retrieved from *www.fcrr.org/FCRReports/PDF/Fast_ForWord_Language_Report.pdf.*

Walley, A. C. (1993). The role of vocabulary development in children's spoken word recognition and segmentation ability. *Developmental Review, 13,* 286–350.

Wang, P. P., & Bellugi, U. (1994). Evidence from two genetic syndromes for a dissociation between verbal and visual–spatial short-term memory. *Journal of Clinical and Experimental Neuropsychology, 16,* 317–322.

Wang, P. P., Doherty, S., Rourke, S. B., & Bellugi, U. (1995). Unique profile of visuoperceptual skills in a genetic syndrome. *Brain and Cognition, 29*(1), 54–65.

Wang, Y., Paramasivam, M., Thomas, A., Bai, J., Kaminen-Ahola, N., Kere, J., et al. (2006). DYX1C1 functions in neuronal migration in developing neocortex. *Neuroscience, 143*(2), 515–522.

Watkins, K. E., Vargha-Khadem, F., Ashburner, J., Passingham, R. E., Connelly, A., Friston, K. J., et al. (2002). MRI analysis of an inherited speech and language disorder: Structural brain abnormalities. *Brain, 125*(Pt. 3), 465–478.

Wechsler, D. (1955). *Manual for the Wechsler scale*. New York: Psychological Corporation.

Wechsler, D. (1992). *Wechsler Individual Achievement Test*. San Antonio, TX: The Psychological Corporation.

Wechsler, D. (1997). *Wechsler Adult Intelligence Scale—Third Edition: Administration and scoring manual*. San Antonio, TX: Psychological Corporation.

Wechsler, D. (2001). *Wechsler individual achievement test 2nd Ed*. San Antonio, TX: Pearson.

Wechsler, D. (2002). *Wechsler Preschool and Primary Scale of Intelligence, Third Edition*. San Antonio, TX: Pearson.

Wechsler, D. (2003). *Wechsler Intelligence Scale for Children—Fourth Edition: Administration and scoring manual*. San Antonio, TX: Psychological Corporation.

Wegner, D. M. (2002). *The illusion of conscious will*. Cambridge, MA: MIT Press.

Weintraub, S., & Mesulam, M. M. (1983). Developmental learning disabilities of the right hemisphere: Emotional, interpersonal, and cognitive components. *Archives of Neurology, 40*(8), 463–468.

Weisberg, D. S., Keil, F. C., Goodstein, J., Rawson, E., & Gray, J. R. (2008). The seductive allure of neuroscience explanations. *Journal of Cognitive Neuroscience, 20*(3), 470–477.

Weismer, S. E., Plante, E., Jones, M., & Tomblin, J. B. (2005). A functional magnetic resonance imaging investigation of verbal working memory in adolescents with specific language impairment. *Journal of Speech, Language, and Hearing Research, 48*(2), 405–425.

Weiss, S. (1991). Morphometry and magnetic resonance imaging of the human brain in normal controls and Down's syndrome. *Anatomical Record, 231*(4), 593–598.

Welford, A. (1962). On changes of performance with age. *Lancet, ii*, 335–339.

Wender, E. H., & Lipton, M. A. (1980). *The National Advisory Committee report on hyperkinesis and food additives: Final report to the Nutrition Foundation*. Washington, DC: Nutrition Foundation.

Wertheimer, M. (1945). *Productive thinking*. New York: Harper.

West, S., King, V., Carey, T. S., Lohr, K. N., McKoy, N., Sutton, S. F., et al. (2002). *Systems to rate the strength of scientific evidence* (Agency for Healthcare Research and Quality Publication No. 02-E016). Rockville, MD: Agency for Healthcare Research and Quality.

Wiederholt, J., & Bryant, B. (2001). *Gray Oral Reading Test—Fourth Edition*. Austin, TX: PRO-ED.

Wigg, K. G., Couto, J. M., Feng, Y., Anderson, B., Cate-Carter, T. D., Macciardi, F., et al. (2004). Support for EKN1 as the susceptibility locus for dyslexia on 15q21. *Molecular Psychiatry, 9*(12), 1111–1121.

Willcutt, E. G., Brodsky, K., Chhabildas, N., Shanahan, M., Yerys, B., Scott, A., et al. (in press). The neuropsychology of ADHD: Validity of the executive function hypothesis. In D. Gozal & D. L. Molfese (Eds.), *Attention deficit hyperactivity disorder: From genes to animal models to patients*. Totowa, NJ: Humana Press.

Willcutt, E. G., & Pennington, B. F. (2000). Comorbidity of reading disability and attention-deficit/hyperactivity disorder: Differences by gender and subtype. *Journal of Learning Disabilities, 33*(2), 179–191.

Willcutt, E. G., Pennington, B. F., & DeFries, J. C. (2000). Etiology of inattention and hyperactivity/impulsivity in a community sample of twins with learning difficulties. *Journal of Abnormal Child Psychology, 28*(2), 149–159.

Willeford, J. A. (1977). *Assessing central auditory behavior in children: A test battery approach.* New York: Grune & Stratton.

Willey, L. H. (1999). *Pretending to be normal: Living with Asperger's syndrome.* London: Jessica Kingsley.

Williams, J. H. G., & Waiter, G. D. (2006). Neuroimaging self–other mapping in autism. In S. J. Rogers & J. H. G. Williams (Eds.), *Imitation and the social mind: Autism and typical development* (pp. 352–376). New York: Guilford Press.

Williams, J. H. G., Waiter, G. D., Gilchrist, A., Perrett, D. I., Murray, A. D., & Whiten, A. (2006). Neural mechanisms of imitation and 'mirror neuron' functioning in autistic spectrum disorder. *Neuropsychologia, 44*(4), 610–621.

Wilson, P. H., Maruff, P., Ives, S., & Currie, J. (2001). Abnormalities of motor and praxis imagery in children with DCD. *Human Movement Science, 17,* 491–513.

Wilson, P. H., Maruff, P., & Lum, J. (2003). Procedural learning in children with developmental coordination disorder. *Human Movement Science, 22*(4–5), 515–526.

Wing, L. (1991). The relationship between Asperger's syndrome and Kanner's autism. In U. Frith (Ed.), *Autism and Asperger syndrome* (pp. 93–121). Cambridge, UK: Cambridge University Press.

Wise, B. W., Ring, J., & Olson, R. K. (1999). Training phonological awareness with and without explicit attention to articulation. *Journal of Experimental Child Psychology, 72*(4), 271–304.

Wise, B. W., Ring, J., & Olson, R. K. (2000). Individual differences in gains from computer-assisted remedial reading. *Journal of Experimental Child Psychology, 77*(3), 197–235.

Wisniewski, K. E., Segan, S. M., Miezejeski, C. M., Sersen, E. A., & Rudelli, R. D. (1991). The Fra(X) syndrome: Neurological, electrophysiological, and neuropathological abnormalities. *American Journal of Medical Genetics, 38*(2–3), 476–480.

Witt, R. M., Kaspar, B. K., Brazelton, A. D., Comery, T. A., Craig, A. M., Weiler, I. J., et al. (1995). Developmental localization of fragile X mRNA in rat brain [Abstract]. *Society for Neuroscience Abstracts, 21,* 734.

Wolraich, M. L., Wilson, D. B., & White, J. W. (1995). The effect of sugar on behavior or cognition in children: A meta-analysis. *Journal of the American Medical Association, 274*(20), 1617–1621.

Woodcock, R. W., McGrew, K. S., & Mather, N. (2001). *Woodcock–Johnson III Tests of Achievement.* Itasca, IL: Riverside.

World Health Organization. (1992). *The ICD-10 classification of mental and behavioural disorders: Clinical descriptions and diagnostic guidelines.* Geneva: Author.

Wynn, K. (1998). Psychological foundations of number: Numerical competence in human infants. *Trends in Cognitive Sciences, 2,* 296–303.

Yerys, B. E., Hepburn, S. L., Pennington, B. F., & Rogers, S. J. (2007). Executive function in preschoolers with autism: Evidence consistent with a secondary deficit. *Journal of Autism and Developmental Disorders, 37*(6), 1068–1079.

Yochman, A., Parush, S., & Ornoy, A. (2004). Responses of preschool children with and without ADHD to sensory events in daily life. *American Journal of Occupational Therapy, 58*(3), 294–302.

Zametkin, A. J., Liebenauer, L. L., Fitzgerald, G. A., King, A. C., Minkunas, D. V., Herscovitch, P., et al. (1993). Brain metabolism in teenagers with attention-deficit hyperactivity disorder. *Archives of General Psychiatry, 50*(5), 333–340.

Zametkin, A. J., Nordahl, T. E., Gross, M., King, A. C., Semple, W. E., Rumsey, J., et al. (1990). Cerebral glucose metabolism in adults with hyperactivity of childhood onset. *New England Journal of Medicine, 323*(20), 1361–1366.

Zametkin, A. J., & Rapoport, J. L. (1986). The pathophysiology of attention deficit disorders. In B. B. Lahey & A. E. Kadzin (Eds.), *Advances in clinical child psychology* (pp. 177–216). New York: Plenum Press.

Zeaman, D., & House, B. (1963). The role of attention in retardate discriminant learning. In N. R. Ellis (Ed.), *Handbook of mental deficiency: Psychological theory and research* (pp. 159–223). New York: McGraw-Hill.

Zigler, E. (1969). Developmental versus difference theories of mental retardation and the problem of motivation. *American Journal of Mental Deficiency, 73*(4), 536–556.

Zimmer, C. (2004). *Soul made flesh: The discovery of the brain and how it changed the world.* New York: Free Press.

Zoia, S., Barnett, A., Wilson, P., & Hill, E. (2006). Developmental coordination disorder: Current issues. *Child: Care, Health, and Development, 32*(6), 613–618.

Index

Page numbers followed by an *f* or a *t* indicate figures or tables